Lippincott Certification Review:
Adult-Gerontology Acute Care Nurse Practitioner

Lippincott Certification Review:
Adult-Gerontology Acute Care Nurse Practitioner

Editor

Elizabeth Wirth-Tomaszewski, DNP, CRNP, CCRN, ACNP-BC, ACNPC

Track Director, Adult Gerontology Acute Care Nurse Practitioner Program
Assistant Clinical Professor
Drexel University
Philadelphia, Pennsylvania
Nurse Practitioner, Division of Critical Care Medicine
St. Luke's Health Network
Bethlehem, Pennsylvania

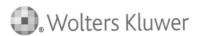

Philadelphia • Baltimore • New York • London
Buenos Aires • Hong Kong • Sydney • Tokyo

Acquisitions Editor: Nicole Dernoski/Jamie Blum
Development Editor: Maria M. McAvey
Senior Editorial Coordinator: Lindsay Ries
Production Project Manager: Kirstin Johnson
Design Coordinator: Elaine Kasmer
Manufacturing Coordinator: Kathleen Brown
Marketing Manager: Linda Wetmore
Prepress Vendor: SPi Global

Cataloging-in-Publication Data available on request from the Publisher

ISBN: 978-1975-1-4338-1

Dedication

This book is dedicated to all of the nurses, doctors, and advanced practitioners with whom I have had the honor of sharing this noble profession over the years. This is also dedicated to all of my students of the past, present, and future who will continue to push the art and science of nursing well beyond my own personal reach.

Contributors

Latesha Colbert-Mack, DNP, CRNP, AGACNP
Clinical Adjunct Faculty
Adult Gerontology Acute Care Nurse Practitioner
  Program
College of Nursing and Healthy Professions
Drexel University
Nurse Practitioner and Doctor of Nursing Practice
Department of Advanced Practice Nursing
Philadelphia, Pennsylvania

Kristy I. Dawe, MSN, AGACNP-BC, NP-C
Lead Critical Care Advanced Practitioner, Monroe
  Campus
St. Luke's University Health Network
Bethlehem, Pennsylvania

Patricia M. Dupak, MSN, AG-ACNP
Adjunct Professor
Acute Care Nurse Practitioner Program
Drexel University
Philadelphia, Pennsylvania
Critical Care Nurse Practitioner
Intensive Care Unit
Geisinger Wyoming Valley Hospital
Geisinger Hospital
Wilkes-Barre, Pennsylvania

Brenda Engler, MSN, CRNP, AGACNP-BC
Critical Care Nurse Practitioner
Department of Critical Care Medicine
Geisinger Health System
Danville, Pennsylvania

Kristen Scholz, MSN, CRNP, AGACNP
Acute Care Nurse Practitioner, Critical Care
St. Luke's University Health Network
Bethlehem, Pennsylvania

Rachel A. Schroy, DNP
Clinical Adjunct Facility for the Adult-Gerontology
  Acute Nurse Practitioner Program
College of Nursing and Healthy Professions
Drexel University
Philadelphia, Pennsylvania
Nurse Practitioner
Critical Care
St. Luke's University Hospital
Bethlehem, Pennsylvania

Binu Shajimon, DrNP
Adjunct Faculty
Department of Advanced Practice Nursing and
  Nurse Practitioner Program
Drexel University
Philadelphia, Pennsylvania

Traci Stahl, MSN, FNP-BC, AGACNP-BC
Clinical Adjunct Faculty
Adult Gero-Acute Care Nurse Practitioner Program
DeSales University
Center Valley, Pennsylvania
Critical Care Nurse Practitioner
Pulmonary Critical Care/Intensive Care Unit
Lehigh Valley University Health Network
East Stroudsburg, Pennsylvania

Elizabeth Wirth-Tomaszewski, DNP, CRNP,
  CCRN, ACNP-BC, ACNPC
Track Director, Adult Gerontology Acute Care Nurse
  Practitioner Program
Assistant Clinical Professor
Drexel University
Philadelphia, Pennsylvania
Nurse Practitioner, Division of Critical Care
  Medicine
St. Luke's Health Network
Bethlehem, Pennsylvania

Anne Dabrow Woods, DNP, RN, CRNP, ANP-BC,
  AGACNP-BC, FAAN
Critical Care Nurse Practitioner
Penn Medicine, Chester County Hospital
West Chester, Pennsylvania
Adjunct Faculty
College of Nursing & Health Professions
Drexel University
Philadelphia, Pennsylvania

Foreword

Graduate students are painfully aware of the dedication and sacrifices that are made to finish a degree that requires licensure. The anxiety created by the term "board examination" is common and often invokes more stress than the education required to sit for the examination. Over the years, my experience has been that acute care nurse practitioner students have a certain personality about them. They often appreciate a clear, concise, and cogent explanation of what they need to know and tend to prefer a quick way to evaluate their understanding of the concepts. These observations have led me to create a review book that allows the reader to determine where their personal needs are and return to their own educational references to enhance the learning in areas where needed. I have not included a comprehensive review of the material but instead test questions modeled after the two board examinations that adult gerontology acute care graduates are eligible to take. The goal is simple: promote conditioning to facilitate answering the complex questions found on the examinations.

Acknowledgments

First and foremost, I would like to thank my family for the encouragement and support to follow my path as a nurse practitioner and professor. I would also like to thank all of the contributors who have taken the time from their busy practices and lives to provide their specialty knowledge to those who are embarking on their own personal journeys as Adult Gerontology Acute Care Nurse Practitioners. It takes a village....

Elizabeth Wirth-Tomaszewski, DNP, CRNP, CCRN, ACNP-BC, ACNPC

Contents

CHAPTER 1

Introduction and Test-Taking Strategies

Elizabeth Wirth-Tomaszewski, DNP, CRNP, CCRN, ACNP-BC, ACNPC

Introduction

This book was conceived through discussion with many adult gerontology acute care nurse practitioner (NP) students and recent graduates. Most review books contain content that has already been taught in accredited programs. Students and graduates have indicated that they are looking for a simple question and answer format, with rationales for both correct and incorrect answers organized by systems. Graduates have also shown interest in a comprehensive, board-style examination that allows for diagnostic evaluation of their deficiencies. Both of these approaches provide information on the mastery of topics, while allowing the readers to return to their own materials to reinforce learning. The editor and expert contributors have responded with *Lippincott Certification Review: Adult Gerontology Acute Care Nurse Practitioner*.

This book is best utilized as a supplement to the content of an accredited adult-gerontology acute care nurse practitioner (AGACNP) program. Students and graduates may test their mastery of subjects as well as determine need for review of material through a systems-based approach. *Lippincott Certification Review: Adult Gerontology Acute Care Nurse*

Practitioner is not meant as a substitute for content review and textbook readings but rather a complement to enhance mastery of material presented.

Test-Taking Strategies

Most students and graduates are apprehensive of high-stakes examinations. Anxiety may originate from graduation potential, financial and social pressures, or meeting program expectations for high pass rates on the board examinations. In any case, test takers can be easily defeated if nerves are permitted to control their responses. Success is a matter of preparation, knowledge base, application of information, and techniques when handling difficult questions.

Preparation

Preparation should begin upon presentation of the information. Several factors have led to student difficulties when attempting to retain information. Note taking skills have declined in recent years, and test blueprints have provided specifics on which the students will be tested. The devil is in the details, however, in that the content is identified but often without explanation on how it will be tested.

Sadly, the art of note taking has declined in recent years due to the use of electronic devices to record lectures and many of those same lectures being available as files. Students have had less need to mentally participate in the absorption of knowledge, believing that review at a later date will suffice. Less effort is made to understand the concept and to commit the necessary information to memory. Imprinting the concepts and critical information is lost.

Handwriting notes requires a student to abbreviate what is understood, rather than what is said by the professor. This allows for processing the concept and imprinting of the information. Although seemingly redundant, recopying notes also reinforces the learning.

Knowing what topics will be presented on a test seems helpful; however, blueprints are often a misleading gift. The extent to which that knowledge is going to be evaluated is key. Will the examination test general knowledge of a concept, or will critical thinking be required to answer the question in a higher-level, multi-step function? Will multilogical thinking be required?

Studying versus cramming

Every person retains and utilizes information differently. In general, cramming should be avoided. Although information may be retained (and regurgitated) for the test, learning has likely not occurred. The ability to materialize answers comes from thorough understanding of the information presented. For instance, an algebraic equation can be memorized and numbers computed, but the purpose and utility of that equation may not be understood. Failure to comprehend basic concepts will affect later learning due to a weak foundation.

How can one study effectively? Studying is more than merely reading. Here are a few tips to maximize time when studying for a high-stakes examination:

1. *Scheduling.* Ensure multiple, short (1–2 hours) sessions that allow for breaks. This is known as "distributive practice." Attempt to avoid tight timetables, or where there is the possibility of interruptions. Pacing studying will improve retention of information.

2. *Environment.* For individual studying, a quiet area with minimal distractions may be best. Group studying is best in a library conference room or designated study area. Some find value in having more than one area, as not to associate any one particular location with "work." In either case, attempts should be made to reduce temptation to utilize technology for purposes other than studying (social media, etc.). Some feel that studying with quiet music helps with their retention, the choice of which is highly individualized (anything from Gregorian chants to heavy metal).

3. *Organization.* To be most effective, planning a study session is imperative. Specific goals for knowledge attainment should be established, and evaluated upon completion. Hardest material should be reviewed first, as this will require the most mental energy. Review the information, and note what should be revisited.

4. *Methods.* There are as many ways to study as there are test takers. Some have better success individually, whereas others excel in a group situation. Examples of study methods include pre- and posttests from notes, flashcards with questions/answers, rewriting notes and outlines with different colored inks, and mnemonics. Some study best from visual cues and others from verbal. Some students explain the concepts to classmates in their own words to better master the content. The test taker should take time to examine how he or she learns best and incorporate that into the study plan.

Know your examination

There are two different board examinations that adult gerontology acute care NP graduates can choose from, one from the American Nurses Credentialing Center (ANCC) and the other from the American Association of Critical Care Nurses (AACN). These examinations are similar but have some differences in their focus. Please refer to the appropriate Web site for the most updated information regarding the examination to be taken. The information presented is current as of this writing.

The ANCC offers a criterion-referenced examination, which scores a participant on his or her performance only and not in comparison to others.

The examination contains 200 questions, of which 25 questions are piloted and do not count toward the test taker's score. The scoring for the examination involves an initial raw score (how many questions answered correctly), which is then converted to a scaled score (based on the level of difficulty of the question). Candidates must score at least 350, with the highest score attainable being 500. The score reported to the participant is pass or fail.

The ANCC has provided extensive resources to allow graduates to prepare for their examination. This includes a blueprint with content information, as well as practice questions. The AGACNP examination is consensus based and focuses on the four domains of practice: Advanced Practice Registered Nurse (APRN) Core Competencies, Clinical Practice, Role-Professional Responsibility, and Health Care Systems. Each domain is outlined in the examination handbook.

The AACN also has a criterion-based examination that most states recognize for licensure. In addition to being a consensus-based certification, the Acute Care Nurse Practitioner Certification-Adult-Gerontology (ACNPC-AG) examination also incorporates the synergy model. The examination questions are designed to align with Bloom taxonomy at the application and analysis levels to ensure critical thinking abilities when caring for acutely and critically ill patients. The same process for scoring (modified Angoff) is used for the AACN examination as is used for the ANCC examination. Passing scores may change based on examination updates. Test takers have 3½ hours to answer 175 multiple choice items, of which 150 are scored. The remaining 25 questions are pilot questions and do not count positively or negatively toward the participant's score. The vast majority of the examination (approximately 73%–79%) tests clinical judgment, with the remaining questions testing nonclinical judgment.

The AACN web site also has a detailed handbook for the ACNPC-AG examination. The major content dimensions include patient care problems, skills and procedures, and validated competencies. Clinical and nonclinical judgments are further outlined into system-based categories to allow graduates a detailed blueprint of expectations. Sample questions are also provided.

Taking the examination

Scheduling. Avoid scheduling the board examination during times when increased stress could be reasonably expected. Some examples include after work, between other commitments, and even certain times of day (not everyone is a morning person). Although this would seem obvious, sometimes a reminder is helpful.

Time management. Be mindful of the timer. These examinations are a forced completion, meaning that there is not limitless time to be spent answering the questions. Budget time wisely, and avoid spending too much time on one perplexing item. Mark the item, and return to it if the examination allows.

Read the question. What is the question asking? The answer could be a diagnosis, treatment, assessment, or evaluation. There may be a long stem, with several distractors involved. Does all of the information pertain to the questions asked? Many times, this is not the case. Sometimes, the best course of action is to read the question at the end of the stem first. This allows for elimination of extraneous information that may cloud the answer. Another common error is adding more to the scenario or the question asked. Reading into the question goes further than critical thinking, adding details that are not presented in the item, which often yields an incorrect answer.

Read the answers. What choices are there? Always read all of the options. In general, an item asking about an intervention by the provider will include action such as "ordering" or "intubating" for example. Very rarely will an examination question be correctly answered by something passive, such as "continue to monitor" and "notifying the physician." If there is intervention the AGACNP should be performing, that is usually the answer. This includes "taking a detailed history" and prevention strategies. Carefully consider all the options.

What if none of the answers seem to make sense? Go back to the question! *The number one mistake made by test takers is misreading the question.*

Answer the question first. If an answer comes to mind quickly, search the answers to find a match. If it does not appear, re-read the question.

Eliminate wrong answers. If unsure about the answer, logically review the answers. Are there any that are simply wrong in any case? Eliminate those immediately. Be especially wary of absolutes (*always, never*) and negatives (*all except*).

Best guess. If that doesn't work, make the best guess possible. If possible, mark the question to return later. Sometimes answers are found in other questions on the examination.

Don't change answers. Repeat. Unless…. Only one case justifies changing an answer: another question on the examination solidified the answer to a previous item. This is the only case where a test taker should change his or her answer. Most times, first instinct is correct.

Example:

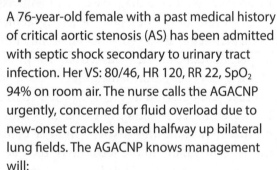

A 76-year-old female with a past medical history of critical aortic stenosis (AS) has been admitted with septic shock secondary to urinary tract infection. Her VS: 80/46, HR 120, RR 22, SpO$_2$ 94% on room air. The nurse calls the AGACNP urgently, concerned for fluid overload due to new-onset crackles heard halfway up bilateral lung fields. The AGACNP knows management will:

a. Require fluids to restore optimal filling pressures/preload

b. Require an immediate diuretic due to the nurse's assessment

c. Require pressors as her heart is unable to increase cardiac output to compensate

d. Require an inotrope to increase cardiac output

The above example requires the reader to examine several elements and apply knowledge to make a decision. Using the algorithm above:

Read the question. The question is asking how the AGACNP will manage the problem set forth in the stem. When reading the stem, choose the pertinent information to the situation. The patient has critical AS. She is hypotensive, tachycardic, and in septic shock. The nurse is reporting rales. This is objective, whereas her statement of concern about fluid overload is quite subjective. How does this information relate to the question?

Read the answers. The first choice refers to hypovolemia, which could be a concern given the hypotension and tachycardia but is not the only process that can cause this presentation. If volume is given in the setting of left heart failure, this could cause harm thereby making this answer not the *best* answer. The second choice is acting on the assessment of another, which should be assessed by the responsible NP. Also, administering a diuretic in someone with critical AS, the shock could worsen as the heart attempts to further compensate for loss in BP due to diuresis. The third choice recognizes that critical AS prohibits the heart from increasing cardiac output due to outflow obstruction and intervenes appropriately with pressors to treat the hypotension. The fourth choice is excluded as incorrect, as inotropes cannot increase cardiac output when critical AS exists.

A word about test anxiety

Board examination candidates are in control, even if test anxiety is a problem for them. There are several methods to help control this crippling phenomenon. The hardest task for most is identifying/admitting that test anxiety is a problem. Once identified, behavioral modification and other complementary therapies can prove successful. These methods can also be used when experiencing anxiety during role transition.

Be prepared. Preparedness is the best way to combat test anxiety, as this ensures efficient and productive studying. Arrive early to prevent rushing. Have all of the required identification and paperwork organized. Be mindful of time, but read each question thoroughly.

Focus point. If anxiety begins to build, pick a point on the screen to focus on (rather than elsewhere in the room, which could cause suspicion with a proctor). Allow the mind to rest a moment without analyzing, and return to the question when calm is restored.

Biofeedback. Similar to a focus point, the attention is taken away from the anxiety and placed on the body. Eyes should be closed and concentration placed on slowing one's breathing. The attention should be diverted for a moment to restore calm.

Aromatherapy. Often overlooked in the testing arena, aromatherapy can be the answer for some. Many essential oils are soothing and can help calm frayed nerves. Aromatherapy is also something that can be employed stealthily in a testing situation. One can apply some oil to pulse points such as behind the ear or on the wrist, and there are also lockets that hold a felt pad that can be impregnated with a choice of oils. Chamomile, sweet orange, peppermint, lavender, bergamot, and cardamom are some examples of relaxing and grounding oils that may help with test anxiety.

Results

What if I fail? Don't panic. Both examinations will provide a detailed report of deficiencies to assist in studying for the next attempt. Don't become discouraged. Use the information provided to brush up on material that wasn't the strongest suit. Continue to schedule study sessions or even take a review course. Not all graduates pass on the first attempt. The only interpretation that can be made is that there is some material yet to be mastered.

What if I pass? Congratulations! And please pay it forward. Once comfortable in the new role, consider being a preceptor or a mentor. Help others pass the examination. Teach the next generation. Be proactive and help push our profession forward.

References

AACN Certification Corporation. (2019). *ACNPC-AG exam handbook*. Aliso Viejo, CA: AACN.

ANCC Certification. (2017). Certification *general testing and renewal handbook*. Silver Spring, MD: ANCC.

Kang, E. (2019). *5 Research backed studying techniques*. George Lucas Educational Foundation. Retrieved November 10, 2019, from https://www.edutopia.org/article/5-research-backed-studying-techniques

Loveless, B. (2019). *10 Habits of highly effective students*. Education Corner. Retrieved November 10, 2019, from https://www.educationcorner.com/habits-of-successful-students.html

University of North Carolina at Chapel Hill. (2019). *Studying 101: Study smarter, not harder*. Retrieved November 10, 2019, from https://learningcenter.enc.edu/tips-and-tools/studying-101-study-smarter-not-harder/

CHAPTER 2

Professionalism, Roles, and Ethics

Kristy I. Dawe, MSN, AGACNP-BC, NP-C

Disease Questions

1 What is the definition of beneficence?

a. Acts that are performed by health care providers to help individuals stay well or help them regain their health

b. To do no harm

c. The capability of a person to make his or her own decisions without external influences

d. To keep medical information private

2 When prescribing morphine with the intent to reduce pain, the nurse practitioner also realizes that it can suppress a patient's respirations. The respiratory suppression is a secondary effect of the morphine but not the intended result of the medical treatment. This

scenario is an example of which principle of health care ethics?

a. Autonomy

b. Justice

c. Nonmaleficence

d. Confidentiality

3 A nurse practitioner working in a busy medical office is seeing a patient named Betty who has been recently diagnosed with terminal cancer. The nurse practitioner also cares for some of Betty's close friends. When Betty's close friend Tammy comes in for an appointment, she tries to discuss Betty's health issues with the nurse practitioner. The nurse practitioner refuses to even admit that Betty is a patient in the practice. What principle of health care ethics does the nurse practitioner exhibit here?

a. Justice

b. Confidentiality

c. Veracity

d. Role fidelity

4 A nurse practitioner is taking care of a critically ill patient in the hospital. The patient has given permission for the nurse practitioner to share his health information with his family. When the nurse practitioner tells the family that the patient's diagnosis is terminal, the patient's son requests that the patient not be given that information and should only be told that he will get better. The nurse practitioner obliges the son's request. What ethical principle is the nurse practitioner violating in this scenario?

a. Veracity

b. Role fidelity

c. Autonomy

d. Beneficence

5 A nurse practitioner is seeing a patient in her clinic today for complaints of heartburn. The medical assistant has taken the patient to the examination room as is the normal procedure. When the nurse practitioner enters the patient's room, the patient informs her that she feels much better now because she told the medical assistant that she was here for heartburn, and the medical assistant said it was likely just gastroesophageal reflux disease and nothing to worry about. What ethical principle was violated by the medical assistant?

a. Beneficence

b. Nonmaleficence

c. Veracity

d. Role fidelity

6 A nurse practitioner fails to meet her state's continuing education requirements. The nurse practitioner is guilty of:

a. Fraud

b. Deception

c. Unprofessional conduct

d. Health Insurance Portability and Accountability Act (HIPAA) violation

7 Which of the following is NOT one of the "four Ds of negligence"?

a. Duty

b. Deception

c. Direct cause

d. Damages

8 The failure of the nurse practitioner to act when he or she should is known as:

a. Misfeasance

b. Malfeasance

c. Nonfeasance

d. Incompetency

9 A new nurse practitioner is working the night shift in a small community hospital. Parts of her responsibilities are to be the team leader for codes and rapid responses throughout the hospital. Two hours into her shift, a code blue is called on a medical floor. The nurse practitioner is nervous and responds to the call but does not give any orders or lead the code team. The patient subsequently dies. This is an example of:

a. Nonfeasance

b. Misfeasance

c. Tortfeasor

d. Malfeasance

10 In which scenario did the nurse practitioner violate a patient's privacy?

a. A female patient is rushed into a trauma bay with multiple injuries and a male nurse practitioner performs the primary survey.

b. The nurse practitioner knocks on the examination room door and then enters once given the affirmation by the patient that it is ok to enter.

c. The nurse practitioner performs a physical examination on a 5-year-old patient with the patient's mother present.

d. The nurse practitioner leaves a message for a patient on her office voicemail that is accessible by her coworkers that her pregnancy test was positive.

11 It is expected that the nurse practitioner will keep up with the standard of care for his or her profession. How is the nurse practitioner expected to do this?

a. By reading professional articles

b. By attending continuing education presentations

c. By referring patients to specialists when appropriate

d. All of the above

12 What is the definition of malpractice?

a. A known side effect of aggressive treatment that causes the patient's condition to worsen

b. A failure by a health care provider or system that causes injury, damages, or loss to the patient

c. The death of a patient who has been admitted to a hospice agency

d. The determination that a nurse practitioner was legally responsible for a patient

13 Which of the following practice issues for nurse practitioners is NOT state regulated?

a. Scope of practice

b. Prescriptive authority

c. Reimbursement under private insurance

d. Requirement for collaboration or supervision

14 What is the purpose of HIPAA?

a. Protect the privacy and other health care rights of patients

b. A national health care fraud and abuse data collection system

c. A federal statute passed to improve the quality of health in the United States

d. A law enacted to expand health insurance coverage

15 Proper documentation in the medical record requires all of the following EXCEPT:

a. Identification of appropriate health risks

b. Reason for encounter and relevant history

c. Assessment, clinical impression, or diagnosis

d. Rationale for all diagnostics that are ordered

Disease Answers/Rationales

① The correct answer is A.

Rationales:

a. Beneficence is defined as acts performed by health care providers to help individuals stay well or help them regain health.

b. Nonmaleficence is the duty to do no harm.

c. Autonomy is an individual's capability to make his or her own decisions without external influences.

d. Confidentiality is the principle of keeping medical information private.

(Judson & Harrison, 2013, Chapter 2).

② The correct answer is C.

Rationales:

a. Autonomy is an individual's capability to make his or her own decisions without external influences.

b. Justice is what is due to an individual.

c. Nonmaleficence is the duty to do no harm. In this case, the intended effect of the morphine is to decrease pain, not suppress respirations. The benefit to the patient must always outweigh the potential harm.

d. Confidentiality is the principle of keeping medical information private.

(Judson & Harrison, 2013, Chapter 2).

③ The correct answer is B.

Rationales:

a. Justice is what is due to an individual.

b. Confidentiality is the principle of keeping medical information private, which the nurse practitioner did in this scenario.

c. Veracity is telling the truth.

d. Role fidelity is being true to the role in which you are licensed or certified.

(Judson & Harrison, 2013, Chapter 2).

④ The correct answer is A.

Rationales:

a. Veracity is the ethical principle that guides health care providers to tell patients the truth about their health.

b. Role fidelity is being true to the role in which you are licensed or certified.

c. Autonomy is an individual's capability to make his or her own decisions without external influences.

d. Beneficence is defined as acts performed by health care providers to help individuals stay well or help them regain health.

(Judson & Harrison, 2013, Chapter 2).

⑤ The correct answer is D.

Rationales:

a. Beneficence is defined as acts performed by health care providers to help individuals stay well or help them regain health.

b. Nonmaleficence is the duty to do no harm.

c. Veracity is the ethical principle that guides health care providers to tell patients the truth about their health.

d. Role fidelity is being true to the role in which you are licensed or certified. In this case, the medical assistant should not have given the patient a diagnosis.

(Judson & Harrison, 2013, Chapter 2).

6 **The correct answer is C.**

Rationales:

a. Fraud is the intent of a practitioner to deceive.

b. Deception is the act of deceiving.

c. The nurse practitioner is guilty of unprofessional conduct by not maintaining the minimum number of continuing education requirements.

d. The nurse practitioner did not violate any part of the HIPAA.

(Judson & Harrison, 2013, Chapter 3).

7 **The correct answer is B.**

Rationales:

a. Duty means the person charged with negligence owed a duty of care to the accuser.

b. Deception is not one of the four Ds of negligence. Dereliction is the fourth D and means that the health care provider in question breached his or her duty of care to the patient.

c. Direct cause means the breach in duty to care for the patient was the direct cause of the patient's injury.

d. Damages means there is a legally recognizable injury to the patient in question.

(Judson & Harrison, 2013, Chapter 5).

8 **The correct answer is C.**

Rationales:

a. Misfeasance is when a health care practitioner performs a completely wrongful or unlawful act.

b. Malfeasance is when a health care practitioner performs a lawful act in an improper or unlawful way.

c. Nonfeasance is the failure of a health care practitioner to act when he or she should.

d. Incompetency is the lack of ability or qualifications to perform an assigned task.

(Judson & Harrison, 2013, Chapter 5).

9 **The correct answer is A.**

Rationales:

a. Nonfeasance is the failure of a health care practitioner to act when he or she should. In this case, it was the nurse practitioner's duty to lead the code team.

b. Misfeasance is when a health care practitioner performs a completely wrongful or unlawful act.

c. Tortfeasor is a person who commits a tort.

d. Malfeasance is when a health care practitioner performs a lawful act in an improper or unlawful way.

(Judson & Harrison, 2013, Chapter 5).

Clinical Pearl

Nurse practitioners must practice in accordance with federal, state, and employer-based restrictions, in that order. For instance, a hospital practice may not allow a nurse practitioner to perform a procedure that is prohibited by the state in which he/she practices. It is the responsibility of the nurse practitioner to ensure that he/she is practicing within the scope of his/her board certification.

10 **The correct answer is D.**

Rationales:

a. This is not a violation of a patient's privacy.

b. There is no violation of the patient's privacy in this scenario.

c. Because the child is a minor, there is no violation of privacy.

d. Leaving a message with confidential health information is a violation of a patient's privacy.

(Judson & Harrison, 2013, Chapter 5).

11 **The correct answer is D.**

Rationales:

a. Reading professional articles is an example of the nurse practitioner keeping up the standards of care of his or her profession

b. Attending continuing education presentations is an example of the nurse practitioner keeping up the standards of care for his or her profession

c. Appropriately referring patients to specialists is an example of the nurse practitioner keeping up the standards of his or her practice.

d. All of the above are correct.

(Buppert, 2015, Chapter 8).

12 **The correct answer is B.**

Rationales:

a. The occurrence of a known side effect of a treatment, even if it causes the patient to worsen, is not the definition of malpractice.

b. Malpractice is the failure of a health care provider or system that causes injury, damages, or loss to a patient.

c. The death of a patient is not malpractice.

d. The determination that a nurse practitioner was legally responsible for a patient is the definition of liability.

(Buppert, 2015, Chapter 8).

13 **The correct answer is C.**

Rationales:

a. Individual states regulate a nurse practitioner's scope of practice.

b. Prescriptive authority is regulated by individual states.

c. Reimbursement under Medicaid is regulated by individual states, as opposed to private insurers.

d. Requirements for collaboration or supervision are regulated by each state.

(Buppert, 2015, Chapter 8).

14 **The correct answer is A.**

Rationales:

a. HIPAA is the federal law intended to protect the privacy and other health care right of patients.

b. The Healthcare Integrity and Protection Data Bank (HIPDB) is a national health care fraud and abuse data collection system established by HIPAA.

c. The Health Care Quality Improvement Act (HCQIA) of 1986 is a federal statute passed to improve the quality of health care in the United States.

d. The Patient Protection and Affordable Care Act (PPACA) is a federal law enacted in 2010 to expand health insurance coverage in the United States.

(Judson & Harrison, 2013, Chapter 3).

15 **The correct answer is D.**

Rationales:

a. Identification of appropriate health risks should be documented in the medical record.

b. The reason for the medical encounter and relevant history should be documented.

c. The nurse practitioner's assessment, clinical impression, or diagnosis should be documented in the medical record.

d. The rationale for ordering diagnostics does not need to be specified if the rationale can be easily inferred. For example, if the nurse practitioner is seeing a patient in an emergency room who presents with history of recent prolonged air travel and sudden onset of shortness of breath, tachycardia, and hypoxia, the rationale for ordering a chest computed tomography (CT) angiogram with contrast does not need to be explicitly documented. It is inferred that the CT scan is being ordered to evaluate the patient for a pulmonary embolus, as it is the first-choice diagnostic imaging to evaluate for this diagnosis.

(Buppert, 2015, Chapter 8).

References

Buppert, C. (2015). *Nurse practitioner's business practice and legal guide*. Burlington, MA: Jones & Bartlett Learning.

Judson, K., & Harrison, C. (2013). *Law & ethics for the health professions*. New York, NY: McGraw-Hill.

CHAPTER 3

Neurology

Patricia M. Dupak, MSN, AG-ACNP

Disease Questions

1 A 50-year-old male presents to the emergency department (ED) complaining of severe unilateral periorbital pain, nasal congestion, and lacrimation of eyes. The patient, noted to have ptosis and pupillary miosis, is restless and agitated with staff. The nurse practitioner determines the patient has which of the following?

a. Tension headaches

b. Cluster headaches

c. Subarachnoid hemorrhage (SAH)

d. Meningitis

2 A 67-year-old female presents with complaints of sudden stabbing facial pain near the right side of the mouth, radiating toward the ipsilateral ear, eye, and nostril. The pain is worsened by touch, movement, eating, and drafts. The patient's symptoms indicate which of the following?

a. Multiple sclerosis (MS)

b. Brain stem neoplasm

c. Cerebrovascular accident (CVA)

d. Trigeminal neuralgia

3 A throbbing headache that occurs episodically following onset of aura-type symptoms of visual disturbances, stars, sparks, light flashes, or zigzags of light, followed by nausea/vomiting, is common in which of the following?

a. Tension headache

b. Cluster headache

c. Migraine

d. Giant cell arteritis

4 A 79-year-old male presents to the ED for examination of headache with scalp tenderness, visual disturbances of loss of vision in one eye, and neck and jaw pain with eating. This patient is exhibiting signs of:

a. Giant cell arteritis

b. Rheumatoid arthritis

c. Plasma cell myeloma

d. Bacterial endocarditis

5 The urgency in diagnosing the patient with complaints of amaurosis fugax or diplopia with giant cell arteritis is to prevent permanent:

a. Double vision

b. Blindness

c. Blurred vision

d. Vascular occlusion

6 A patient is diagnosed with amaurosis fugax. The adult-gerontology acute care nurse practitioner (AGACNP) knows:

a. The patient can be admitted for observation.

b. The patient can be discharged once seen by ophthalmology.

c. The patient needs admission.

d. The patient can be discharged from emergency room/clinic and does not require admission.

7 Treatment of giant cell arteritis should begin immediately with:

a. Prednisone and temporal artery biopsy

b. Intravenous (IV) methylprednisolone and biopsy

c. Acetylsalicylic acid (ASA), IV methylprednisolone, and biopsy

d. Magnetic resonance imaging (MRI) or computed tomography (CT) angiography

8 An 85-year-old female is brought in for evaluation of confusion. Her family is at bedside and states that the patient has had progressive worsening of memory, difficulty finding words, inability to perform activities of daily living, and difficulty recognizing objects. The AGACNP recognizes these symptoms as:

a. Depression

b. Delirium

c. Polypharmacy

d. Dementia

9 Delirium can be distinguished from dementia by:

a. Acute onset, fluctuating course, attention deficit

b. Memory deficits, fluctuating course, onset

c. Rate of progression of deficits, behavioral changes

d. Persistent, progression, memory compromise

10 The AGACNP is called to the bedside of a 70-year-old male patient admitted for observation status post fall. His family states that he was fine during the day, but at night, he is confused, agitated, and has difficulty paying attention. The AGACNP knows this is likely caused by:

a. Dementia

b. Delirium

c. Polypharmacy

d. Depression

11 A patient presents to the ED after a witnessed loss of consciousness. The patient fell to the ground, had twitching to bilateral arms/legs, and turned blue. Emergency medical services (EMS) noted that the patient does not respond to stimuli and may have bitten his tongue. The patient is at risk for:

a. Status epilepticus

b. Serial seizures

c. Absence seizure

d. Syncope

12 A seizure with consciousness preserved, convulsive jerking, sensory flashing lights, and nausea are symptoms of:

a. Simple partial seizure

b. Complex partial seizure

c. Generalized seizure

d. Tonic–clonic seizure

13 This seizure is generally preceded by an aura, loss of consciousness, falling, and respiratory compromise:

a. Simple partial seizure

b. Complex partial seizure

c. Generalized seizure

d. Tonic–clonic seizure

14 Prolonged seizure and recurring convulsions lasting longer than 5 minutes should be considered to be:

a. Complex partial seizure

b. Generalized seizure

c. Tonic–clonic seizure

d. Status epilepticus

15 In patients with new onset of seizures without identifiable cause, who do not return to normal level of consciousness, which testing is necessary to identify nonconvulsive status epilepticus?

a. CT of brain

b. Chest x-ray

c. Lumbar puncture (LP)

d. Electroencephalography (EEG)

16 A seizure that starts in one part of the brain and affects the part of body controlled by that part of the brain describes which of the following?

a. Focal seizure

b. Generalized seizure

c. Tonic–clonic seizure

d. Status epilepticus

17 A loss of awareness and fall with observed clonic jerking motions describe which of the following?

a. Syncope

b. Myocardial infarction (MI)

c. Cerebrovascular accident

d. Seizure

18 Status epilepticus is a medical emergency with initial management to ensure that airway, breathing, and hemodynamics are addressed. These patients are immediately medicated with:

a. Benzodiazepines

b. Antiepileptic drugs (AEDs)

c. Glucose

d. Normal saline

19 Which of the following is required for patients with refractory status epilepticus not terminated by benzodiazepines and AEDs during emergent treatment?

a. Intubation, ventilation, and drug-induced coma with midazolam or propofol

b. Midazolam or propofol infusions

c. Additional AEDs

d. Additional benzodiazepines

20 Under which of the following conditions must a patient be admitted?

a. Status epilepticus

b. Frequent seizures requiring medication titration and electroencephalographic monitoring

c. Inpatient monitor when psychogenic nonepileptic seizures suspected

d. All of the above

21 A 45-year-old female is admitted to the hospital for complaints of weakness, paresthesia, unsteady gait, urinary urgency, and diplopia. MRI of the brain and cervical cord was completed with the presence of multiple lesions. This likely indicates which of the following?

a. Vitamin E deficiency

b. Wernicke encephalopathy

c. Multiple sclerosis

d. Vitamin B12 deficiency

22 Treatment for multiple sclerosis begins with:

a. Corticosteroids

b. Benzodiazepines

c. Ocrelizumab

d. Dalfampridine

23 Patients with multiple sclerosis who do not respond to glucocorticoid therapy and have acute central nervous system inflammatory demyelinating disease should be treated with:

a. Benzodiazepines

b. Plasma exchange

c. Methylprednisolone

d. Dalfampridine

24 When do patients with multiple sclerosis require admission?

a. When plasma exchange is required for severe relapses

b. During severe relapses

c. When patients are unable to manage at home

d. All of the above

25 A patient is admitted to the hospital for progressive, symmetrical muscle weakness with absent deep tendon reflexes. The patient states that symptoms started a few days ago, and now includes difficulty walking. The concern is for:

a. Multiple sclerosis

b. Peripheral neuropathy

c. Tick paralysis

d. Guillain–Barré syndrome

26 Treatment for Guillain–Barré syndrome begins with:

a. Corticosteroids

b. Gabapentin

c. Plasmapheresis and intravenous immunoglobulin (IVIG)

d. Mechanical ventilation

27 When does a patient with Guillain–Barré syndrome require admission?

a. Never—this is not an immediate emergency.

b. If the patient needs mechanical ventilation.

c. All patients should be hospitalized.

d. Hospitalization may be needed for initial treatment.

28 A 35-year-old female presents to hospital with complaints of ptosis, diplopia, difficulty swallowing, dyspnea, and weakness to arms/legs. The AGACNP suspects which of the following?

a. Myasthenia gravis

b. Multiple sclerosis

c. Guillain–Barré syndrome

d. Acute cervical disk protrusion

29 Which of the following is a life-threatening complication of myasthenia gravis that may lead to respiratory weakness requiring intensive care unit (ICU) monitoring?

a. Myasthenic syndrome

b. Myasthenic crisis

c. Acetylcholine receptor antibody

d. Thymoma

30 Patients with myasthenia gravis require admission:

a. When there is acute exacerbation or respiratory involvement

b. When plasmapheresis is necessary

c. When thymectomy is medically necessary

d. All of the above

31 Symptomatic treatment for myasthenia gravis includes which of the following?

a. Acetylcholinesterase, IVIG, glucocorticoid and nonsteroidal immunomodulating treatments, thymectomy

b. Thymectomy

c. Acetylcholinesterase, glucocorticoids

d. IVIG

32 A 78-year-old female presents to the ED after suffering sudden onset of dysarthria and paresthesia/weakness of contralateral arm, leg, and face lasting several minutes and resolves quickly. This patient's symptoms are classic findings in:

a. Subclavian steal syndrome

b. Transient ischemic attack (TIA)

c. Focal seizure

d. Brain tumor

33 A 46-year-old female presents with TIA, which has now resolved. When would this patient require admission?

a. The patient is seen within 1 week of symptoms.

b. The patient is seen within 1 month.

c. The patient has a history of TIA.

d. The patient has a history of heart disease.

34 Anticoagulation is recommended in those with TIA:

a. Who also have atrial fibrillation

b. Who have mechanical heart valves

c. Who have a left ventricular thrombus

d. All of the above

35 Which of the following are antiplatelet recommendations in patients with TIA?

a. In those with contraindications to full anticoagulation

b. Dual platelet therapy with aspirin and clopidogrel

c. Short-term use of aspirin and clopidogrel

d. All of the above

36 A 67-year-old male with a past medical history for hypertension (HTN), diabetes mellitus (DM), tobacco abuse, atrial fibrillation, and atherosclerosis presents with complaints of acute left-sided paralysis, poor balance, poor coordination, and tiredness. The AGACNP suspects

a. TIA

b. CVA

c. Guillain–Barré syndrome

d. Myasthenia gravis

37 Small lesions usually less than 1.5 cm in diameter that occur in the distribution of short penetrating arteries of the basal ganglia, cerebellum, pons, internal capsule, thalamus, and less commonly the cerebral white matter describe which of the following conditions?

a. Lacunar infarction

b. Carotid circulation obstruction

c. TIA

d. Vertebrobasilar occlusion

38 Thrombotic or embolic occlusion of a major vessel leads to:

a. Lacunar infarction

b. Carotid circulation obstruction

c. Cerebral infarction

d. Intracerebral hemorrhage (ICH)

39 Which of the following vascular distributions is described by contralateral leg weakness and sensory loss, and an area least affected by strokes?

a. Middle cerebral artery

b. Anterior cerebral artery

c. Posterior cerebral artery

d. Vertebral basilar artery

40 Which of the following vascular distributions is described by facial asymmetry, arm weakness, and speech deficits?

a. Middle cerebral artery

b. Anterior cerebral artery

c. Posterior cerebral artery

d. Vertebral basilar artery

41 Which of the following vascular distributions is described by visual disturbance due to occipital lobe circulation?

a. Middle cerebral artery

b. Anterior cerebral artery

c. Posterior cerebral artery

d. Vertebral basilar artery

42 Intracerebral hemorrhage is defined as intraparenchymal bleeding due to which of the following causes?

a. Spontaneous, nontraumatic, no angiographic evidence of vascular anomaly

b. Traumatic injury

c. Aneurysm

d. Angioma

43 Most frequent cause of intracerebral (intraparenchymal) hemorrhage is:

a. DM

b. Infection

c. Trauma

d. HTN

44 Which of the following leads to sudden onset of nausea and vomiting, uncoordinated movements, unsteady gait, headache, and loss of consciousness that may result in coma or death?

a. Cerebellar hemorrhage

b. Intracerebral hemorrhage

c. Subarachnoid hemorrhage

d. Subdural hematoma (SDH)

45 A 35-year-old male complains of a sudden acute headache that radiates into the posterior aspect of the neck and is worsened by movement, described as a "thunderclap." He has not experienced headache of this severity before. This would be highly suspicious for:

a. ICH

b. Cerebellar hemorrhage

c. SAH

d. SDH

46 Lumbar puncture with the presence of xanthochromia indicates

a. ICH

b. Cerebellar hemorrhage

c. SAH

d. SDH

47 Lumbar puncture should not be performed in the initial evaluation of the unconscious patient due to the risk for:

a. Tonsillar herniation

b. Epidural hematoma

c. Intracranial hematoma

d. Subarachnoid hemorrhage

48 A rapid systematic neurologic examination of a patient is performed and repeated frequently to assess the three components of Glasgow Coma Scale (GCS). A patient presents opening eyes to voice, motor response to command, and verbal response being confused but comprehensible. What is the GCS score for this patient?

a. 10

b. 12

c. 13

d. 9

49 A 26-year-old female presents status post head injury. Neurologic examination reveals eye opening to painful stimuli, withdraws to pain, and has incomprehensible sounds. Her GCS would be calculated at:

a. 10

b. 12

c. 8

d. 6

50 A 75-year-old male presents to the ED after being found by the neighbor lying on the ground. He complains of headache and has a laceration to the right side of the forehead. The patient takes warfarin for Afib. His lab work reveals international normalized ratio (INR) of 3.5. His GCS is 15, and CT scan of the head determines small hematoma formation with no midline shift. The patient should be:

a. Admitted for observation, INR reversal, and follow-up CT scan

b. Discharged to his family with close observation

c. Discharged to home and told to stop warfarin

d. Admitted to unit bed for frequent neuro checks, INR reversal, and neurosurgery evaluation

51 A 50-year-old male presents to the ED after falling off ladder while fixing his roof. EMS reports that the patient is awake, alert, and moving all extremities while on scene but in the ambulance deteriorated to only opening eyes to stimulation. He does not look toward sound, extremities have abnormal flexion response to stimuli, and he produces incomprehensible sounds when questioned. Which of the following is the most appropriate care for this condition?

a. Transport the patient to the closest hospital.

b. Apply cervical collar prior to transport.

c. Apply oxygen to keep oxygen saturations greater than 90% en route.

d. Intubate the patient maintaining cervical spine precautions, and transport to the closest trauma center.

52 A 54-year-old male presents to the ED after skiing accident involving hitting a tree. He is awake and alert and has a GCS of 15. CT scan of the head reveals a skull fracture and biconvex collection of blood in the low to mid-temporal lobe not causing midline shift but with bruising on opposite side of the brain. Which of the following is the most appropriate care for this condition?

a. Stat neurosurgery consults for epidural hematoma.

b. Stat neurosurgery consults for SDH.

c. Admit to observation and monitor GCS; hold all anticoagulants.

d. Monitor the patient in the ED and discharge if repeat neurologic examination unchanged.

53 A 75-year-old female presents with acute mental status changes after a fall. The AGACNP needs to explain to the patient's family the results of the CT scan of the head on the family member

with the radiology impression for hyperdense "crescents" as the blood spreads around the surface of the brain. Which of the following is this condition most consistent with?

a. Epidural hematoma

b. Acute SDH

c. Chronic SDH

d. Intraparenchymal hemorrhage

54 A 45-year-old female status post traumatic brain injury has been admitted. The nurse calls with a concern of a BP 200/102, bradycardia, and irregular respiratory rate. This likely represents signs of:

a. Decreased intracranial pressure

b. Increased intracranial pressure

c. Emergent need to intubate

d. Hypertensive emergency

55 A 32-year-old male presents with intracranial hemorrhage. He takes novel oral anticoagulation for deep vein thrombosis (DVT). INR reversal should be instituted with a goal of:

a. INR $\leq$ 1.4, PTT $\leq$ 40, platelets >100,000

b. INR $\leq$ 2, PTT $\leq$ 45, platelets >50,000

c. INR $\leq$ 2, PTT $\leq$ 45, platelets >100,000

d. INR $\leq$ 1.8, PTT $\leq$ 40, platelets >50,000

56 Patients with severe head injury are:

a. Not at risk of developing DVT/PE

b. At risk of developing DVT only if on prolonged bed rest

c. At risk of developing DVT only if INR reversed

d. At high risk of developing DVT/PE

57 A 30-year-old female presented to the ED, whose family stated that she complained of headache, stiff neck, nausea, and vomiting earlier in the day with fever. The patient is now lethargic. The AGACNP's first priority is to order:

a. Lumbar puncture

b. CT scan of the head

c. Blood work

d. Arterial blood gas (ABG)

58 A 30-year-old female presented to the ED, whose family stated that she complained of headache, stiff neck, nausea, and vomiting earlier in the day with fever. The patient is now lethargic. The AGACNP suspects:

a. Encephalitis

b. Viral meningitis

c. Bacterial meningitis

d. CVA

59 The AGACNP suspects a patient has viral meningitis. The treatment includes which of the following?

a. No specific treatment; resolves in 7–10 days

b. Early use of antibiotics and herpes coverage

c. Early coverage with antibiotics and steroids

d. Antibiotics, steroids, and phenytoin generic

60 When should emergency transfer of a patient suspected of spinal cord compression occur?

a. When the acute care facility treating the patient cannot provide advanced imaging and neurosurgical specialists.

b. Before the facility has stabilized the patient.

c. After all imaging and specialists have assessed the patient.

d. The patient does not need to be transferred.

Disease Answers/Rationales

1 The correct answer is B.

Rationales:

a. Tension headaches: most common type of headache and generally chronic in nature; headaches can be triggered by stress, fatigue, noise, or glare. Pain is described as mild to moderate bilateral, nonthrobbing headache.

b. Cluster headaches: severe episodes of unilateral periorbital pain, nasal congestion, lacrimation of eyes, redness of the eye, Horner syndrome (ptosis, pupillary meiosis, and diminished ability to sweat).

c. Subarachnoid hemorrhage: "worst headache in my life," with sudden onset, no precipitating factors, no relief with medications (over the counter or opioids).

d. Meningitis: classic triad of bacterial meningitis: fever, nuchal rigidity, and change in mental status.

(Rabow, McPhee, & Papadakis, 2018, p. 992).

2 The correct answer is D.

Rationales:

a. Multiple sclerosis: symptoms are optic neuritis (pain and temporary vision loss); long tract symptoms of the spinal cord numbness, paresthesia, or weakness; internuclear ophthalmoplegia (impairment of eye of adduction); and/or transverse myelitis.

b. Brain stem neoplasm: symptoms include double vision, movement of eyelids, drooping eye, facial muscle weakness (swallowing, controlling secretions); depends on the area of brain affected by tumor.

c. CVA: classic symptoms are facial droop, speech difficulties, muscle weakness, paresthesia of one side of the body.

d. Trigeminal neuralgia: pain described as unilateral stabbing, intense, excruciating, on one side of the mouth traveling to ipsilateral ear, eye, nostril, or side of the face, facial flushing, salivation, and headache; worsened by touch, movement, eating, and drafts.

(Rabow et al., 2018, pp. 994–997).

3 **The correct answer is C.**

Rationales:

a. Tension headache: most common type of headache and generally chronic in nature; headaches can be triggered by stress, fatigue, noise, or glare. Pain is described as mild to moderate bilateral, nonthrobbing headache.

b. Cluster headaches: severe, episodes of unilateral periorbital pain, nasal congestion, lacrimation of eyes, redness of the eye, Horner syndrome (ptosis, pupillary meiosis, and diminished ability to sweat).

c. Migraine: typically has aura-type symptoms of visual disturbance, photophobia, phonophobia, nausea, vomiting; typically, but not always unilateral; lasts 4–72 hours; aggravated by physical activity.

d. Giant cell arteritis: central and branch retinal artery occlusion: sudden blockage of central or branches of artery causing sudden loss of vision or loss of visual fields; permanent partial visual loss or complete loss without intervention. Sudden, "painless," amaurosis fugax (ipsilateral intermittent monocular blindness), central retinal artery occlusion; branch retinal artery occlusion, sudden loss of vision with loss of visual field, fundal signs of retinal swelling, sometimes "cotton wool spots" are identified in the area of retina supplied by the occluded artery.

(Rabow et al., 2018, pp. 990–992).

4 **The correct answer is A.**

Rationales:

a. Giant cell arteritis: also known as Horton disease, cranial arteritis and temporal arteritis, central and branch retinal artery occlusion: "classic" systemic rheumatic disease of older adults greater than 50 years of age, mean onset at 79 years with complaints of "scalp tenderness, visual disturbance (amaurosis fugax or diplopia), jaw pain (claudication), or throat pain." Suspicion should be with symptoms of new headaches, abrupt onset of visual disturbances, monocular loss of vision, jaw claudication, fever, anemia, high sedimentation rate (ESR), and/or C-reactive protein (CRP).

b. Rheumatoid arteritis: inflammatory polyarthritis, symptoms have been present for a short time (weeks), joint pain and swelling (especially hand, wrist, forefoot) along with "morning stiffness," decreased strength to areas with grip.

c. Plasma cell myeloma: fever, bone pain, fatigue, weakness, weight loss, anemia, hepatomegaly, splenomegaly, lymphadenopathy.

d. Bacterial endocarditis: acute rapidly progressive infection, low-grade fever with nonspecific symptoms (chills, anorexia, weight loss, headache, myalgias, arthralgias, night sweats, abdominal pain, and dyspnea).

(Rabow et al., 2018, p. 868).

5 **The correct answer is B.**

Rationales:

a. Double vision is not a permanent sequela of giant cell arteritis.

b. Amaurosis fugax (painless, temporary loss of vision in one eye or diplopia) is considered a medical emergency and requires STAT ophthalmologist consultation.

Blindness occurs if treatment is not started within a few hours of onset of symptoms. This is considered an emergency, and there is risk of loss of vision to other eye without prompt treatment.

c. Blurred vision is not a sequela of giant cell arteritis

d. Vascular occlusion is not a permanent sequela of giant cell arteritis.

(Rabow et al., 2018, p. 196).

6 **The correct answer is C.**

Rationales:

a. The patient requires admission, not observation.

b. The patient must be admitted.

c. Patients with visual loss or blindness due to giant cell arteritis require admission and stat consultation by ophthalmology, high-dose corticosteroid therapy, and close monitoring to ensure adequate treatment and monitoring of another eye.

d. The patient requires admission.

(Rabow et al., 2018, p. 196).

7 **The correct answer is C.**

Rationales:

a. Intravenous steroids and aspirin are preferred over oral steroids; biopsy is required.

b. Aspirin must be given with IV steroids and biopsy.

c. Treatment is considered a medical emergency, and the patient is at risk for blindness if not promptly treated. All patients should receive initial IV methylprednisolone, ASA, monitoring to ensure that symptoms don't worsen, and temporal artery biopsy. Imaging with ultrasonography, MRI, or CT angiography is useful and can sometimes avoid biopsy but should not precede medication treatment.

d. Imaging does not treat the urgent medical condition. IV steroids and aspirin are necessary to prevent blindness.

(Rabow et al., 2018, p. 869).

8 **The correct answer is D.**

Rationales:

a. Depression: in elderly persistent sadness, anxious or worrying, weight changes/loss, difficulty sleeping.

b. Delirium: hyperactive: acute onset of confusion, excitement, incoherent speech/conversation, agitation; hypoactive delirium: somnolence, lethargy, confusion, inactivity.

c. Polypharmacy: symptoms due to types of medications involved, but symptoms resolve once absence of medications typically antipsychotics, benzodiazepines, opioids.

d. Dementia: is progressive, gradual, weeks/months/years; memory loss, decreased intellectual functioning, loss of short-term memory.

(Marino, 2014, pp. 800–805; Rabow et al., 2018, p. 57).

9 **The correct answer is A.**

Rationales:

a. Delirium is acute in nature with hyperactive and hypoactive symptoms of confusion, attention, rapid onset, and fluctuating course; primary deficit in attention and memory.

b. An essential component of delirium is inattention.

c. Dementia is progressive weeks/months/years of memory loss, decreased intellectual functioning, and decreased ability to perform activities of daily living.

Patients with dementia can develop delirium while hospitalized due to change in habit, normal surroundings, and change in medications.

d. An essential component of delirium is inattention with abrupt onset.

(Marino, 2014, pp. 801–805; Rabow et al., 2018, p. 61).

10 **The correct answer is D.**

Rationales:

a. Dementia: symptoms are progressive with gradual onset.

b. Delirium: acute confusion, rapid onset of symptoms, inability to concentrate.

c. Polypharmacy: depending on medications involved, elderly: histamines, cardiac medications (digoxin, beta-blockers), steroids nonsteroidal anti-inflammatory drugs (NSAIDs) and antibiotics.

d. Depression: elderly less likely to report symptoms, sadness, anxious or worrying, weight changes/loss, difficulty sleeping.

(Marino, 2014, pp. 801–805; Rabow et al., 2018, pp. 61–62).

Clinical Pearl

Status epilepticus: aggressive requires rapid treatment, most life threatening and least common.

11 **The correct answer is A.**

Rationales:

a. Status epilepticus: tonic–clonic, (grand mal) seizures, loss of consciousness and falling, respiratory arrest, muscle rigidity-tonic, muscle twitching/jerking clonic, urinary incontinence, lasts a few minutes; some patients may have aura, and proceeds with postictal state (sleep, headache, muscle soreness, nausea, confusion of event).

b. Serial seizures: partial seizure: conscious, convulsive jerking, paresthesia to limbs or body, flashing lights, nausea; complex seizure: patient may complain of aura type: fear, anxiety, dyspnea, alteration of consciousness.

c. Absence seizure: "petit mal" seizure, fluttering of eyelids, but body tone is maintained and no falling. One minute or longer, patient abruptly regains contact and will continue conversation or activity.

d. Syncope: transient loss of consciousness with inability to maintain postural tone with spontaneous recovery.

(Claassen & Goldstein, 2017, pp. 152–158; Marino, 2014, pp. 817–822; Rabow et al., 2018, pp. 998–1002).

12 **The correct answer is A.**

Rationales:

a. Simple partial seizure is characterized by preserved consciousness, convulsive jerking movements, sensory complaints of flashing lights, buzzing noises, hallucinations, and nausea.

b. Complex partial seizure is characterized by focal seizure with alteration of consciousness, and the patient complains of feeling emotional, fear, breathless, and abdominal sensations, followed by involuntary lip smacking, chewing, sucking, or picking at things/clothes.

c. Generalized seizures is characterized by simple or complex seizure progressing to generalized seizures with loss of consciousness and motor activity (convulsions), classified as nonmotor (absence seizures) and motor seizures (tonic–clonic, clonic, tonic, myoclonic, epileptic spasms).

d. Tonic–clonic seizure is characterized by grand mal, usually preceded by an aura, yelling, loss of consciousness, falling, and respiratory arrest.

(Claassen & Goldstein, 2017, pp. 152–158; Marino, 2014, pp. 817–822; Rabow et al., 2018, pp. 997–1002).

13 **The correct answer is D.**

Rationales:

a. Simple partial seizure is characterized by preserved consciousness, convulsive jerking movements, sensory complaints of flashing lights, buzzing noises, hallucinations, and nausea.

b. Complex partial seizure is characterized by focal seizure with alteration of consciousness, and the patient complains of feeling emotional, fear, breathless, and abdominal sensations, followed by involuntary lip smacking, chewing, sucking, or picking at things/clothes.

c. Generalized seizures is characterized by simple or complex seizure progressing to generalized seizures with loss of consciousness and motor activity (convulsions), classified as nonmotor (absence seizures) and motor seizures (tonic–clonic, clonic, tonic, myoclonic, epileptic spasms).

d. Tonic–clonic seizure is characterized by grand mal, usually preceded by an aura, yelling, loss of consciousness, falling, and respiratory arrest.

(Claassen, & Goldstein, 2017, pp. 152–158; Marino, 2014, pp. 817–822; Rabow et al., 2018, pp. 997–1002).

14 **The correct answer is D.**

Rationales:

a. Complex partial seizure is characterized by focal seizure with alteration of consciousness, and the patient complains of feeling emotional, fear, breathless, and abdominal sensations, followed by involuntary lip smacking, chewing, sucking, or picking at things/clothes.

b. Generalized seizures is characterized by simple or complex seizure progressing to generalized seizures with loss of consciousness and motor activity (convulsions), classified as nonmotor (absence seizures) and motor seizures (tonic–clonic, clonic, tonic, myoclonic, epileptic spasms).

c. Tonic–clonic seizure is characterized by grand mal, usually preceded by an aura, yelling, loss of consciousness, falling, and respiratory arrest.

d. Status epilepticus is characterized by tonic–clonic (grand mal) seizures, loss of consciousness, falling, respiratory arrest, muscle rigidity-tonic, muscle twitching/jerking clonic, urinary incontinence, lasts a few minutes; some patients may have aura and proceeds with postictal state.

(Claassen & Goldstein, 2017, pp. 152–158; Marino, 2014, pp. 817–822; Rabow et al., 2018, pp. 997–1002).

15 **The correct answer is D.**

Rationales:

a. CT of the brain can provide information regarding brain tissue and structures to identify injuries and disease but not active seizure.

b. Chest x-ray will not be able to identify active seizure.

c. LP provides information about cerebrospinal fluid, with the purpose of ruling out

life-threatening conditions such as bacterial meningitis or SAH.

d. EEG: EEG is an essential component in identifying and diagnosing seizures; EEGs can detect the presence and location of seizure.

(Claassen & Goldstein, 2017, pp. 152–158; Marino, 2014, pp. 817–822; Rabow et al., 2018, pp. 997–1002).

16 **The correct answer is A.**

Rationales:

a. Focal seizure: symptoms and EEG manifestations indicate only a restricted part of one cerebral hemisphere has been activated.

b. Generalized seizure: rapidly spread activity to bilateral hemispheres.

c. Tonic–clonic: grand mal seizure; paroxysmal neuronal discharge spreads throughout the cerebral cortex.

d. Status epilepticus: acute prolonged, life-threatening neurologic disorder, which if left untreated will have permanent neuronal injury in the hippocampus, cerebellum, and neocortex.

(Claassen & Goldstein, 2017, pp. 152–158; Marino, 2014, pp. 817–822; Rabow et al., 2018, pp. 997–1002).

17 **The correct answer is D.**

Rationales:

a. Syncope is characterized by transient loss of consciousness with inability to maintain postural tone with spontaneous recovery.

b. An MI may cause cerebral hypoperfusion due to cardiac arrhythmia can cause loss of consciousness and fall, not normally clonic type jerking motions.

c. CVA is characterized by classic symptoms: facial droop, speech difficulties, hemiplegia/paresthesia; loss of consciousness when suspecting brainstem ischemia.

d. Seizure is characterized by loss of awareness, fall, and clonic jerking motions.

(Claassen & Goldstein, 2017, pp. 152–158; Marino, 2014, pp. 817–822; Rabow et al., 2018, pp. 997–1002).

18 **The correct answer is A.**

Rationales:

a. Benzodiazepines are recommended as initial therapy followed by antiepileptics and glucose. Benzodiazepines result in higher rate of cessation of status.

b. Antiepileptic patient can be on multiple medications in order to control seizures.

c. Empiric administration of glucose is not warranted unless hypoglycemia is suspected, due to easy access to point of care glucose testing devices.

d. Normal saline is not proven to prevent seizures.

(Brophy & Human, 2017, pp. 51–73; Claassen & Goldstein, 2017, pp. 152–158; Rabow et al., 2018, pp. 997–1002).

19 **The correct answer is A.**

Rationales:

a. Status epilepticus lasting several minutes with ongoing use of respiratory sedating medications puts the patient at risk for respiratory depression and cardiac arrest. Providers need vigilant monitoring of refractory convulsions with emergent treatment to protect the brain from further injury.

b. Propofol infusions should never be used in nonmechanically ventilated patients with protected airways.

c. Additional AEDs are not indicated in status epilepticus, as they are not used in acute seizures.

d. Additional benzodiazepines may suppress respiratory status, requiring airway protection.

(Rajajee, Riggs, & Seder, 2017, pp. 4–28).

20 **The correct answer is D.**

Rationales:

a. Patients with status epilepticus must be admitted for close monitoring.

b. Patients with frequent seizures requiring medication and long-term EEG must be hospitalized.

c. Inpatient monitoring requires admission.

d. In hospital mortality rates: generalized status epilepticus 21%, nonconvulsive status epilepticus 52%, and refractory status epilepticus 61%.

(Claassen & Goldstein, 2017, pp. 152–158; Marino, 2014, pp. 817–822; Rabow et al., 2018, p. 997–1002).

Clinical Pearl

Jacksonian march movements: simple partial seizure of convulsive jerking or paresthesia, which spread to different parts of the limb, body, or face.

21 **The correct answer is C.**

Rationales:

a. Vitamin E deficiency: progresses from hyporeflexia, ataxia, limitation in upward gaze, visual field deficits.

b. Wernicke encephalopathy: confusion, ataxia, nystagmus, peripheral neuropathy.

c. Multiple sclerosis: common initial complaints of weakness, numbness, tinkling or unsteadiness in limbs, spastic paraparesis; optic neuritis, diplopia urinary urgency.

d. Vitamin B12 deficiency: fatigue, weakness, numbness, poor balance, memory loss.

(Rabow et al., 2018, pp. 1036–1040).

22 **The correct answer is A.**

Rationales:

a. Corticosteroids are given for partial recovery from acute exacerbations; preventing relapses are treated by corticosteroids.

b. Benzodiazepines show no support in management of multiple sclerosis.

c. Ocrelizumab is the only medication effective in slowing progression in primary progressive multiple sclerosis and approved by FDA.

d. Dalfampridine improves walking by improving speed of walking.

(Rabow et al., 2018, pp. 1036–1040).

23 **The correct answer is B.**

Rationales:

a. Benzodiazepines do not improve multiple sclerosis.

b. Plasma exchange is used to treat relapses not responding to steroids.

c. Methylprednisolone is used for initial treatment.

d. Dalfampridine has been shown to offer improvement with walking, but not immediate therapy.

(Rabow et al., 2018, pp. 1036–1040).

24 **The correct answer is D.**

Rationales:

Patients with multiple sclerosis require admission to the hospital when there is a need for plasma exchange for severe relapse, during a severe relapse, and when patients are unable to manage the condition at home.

(Rabow et al., 2018, pp. 1036–1040).

25 **The correct answer is D.**

Rationales:

a. Multiple sclerosis: common initial complaints of weakness, numbness, tinkling or unsteadiness in limbs, spastic paraparesis; optic neuritis, diplopia urinary urgency.

b. Peripheral neuropathy: symmetric distal sensory loss, sensation of burning or weakness of limbs.

c. Tick paralysis: paresthesia, fatigue and weakness, muscular pain.

d. Guillain–Barré syndrome: (acute idiopathic polyneuropathy) "progressive" symmetric muscle weakness with absent deep tendon reflexes.

(Marino, 2014, p. 823; Rabow et al. 2018, p. 1051).

26 **The correct answer is C.**

Rationales:

a. Corticosteroids are not beneficial.

b. Gabapentin is not beneficial.

c. Plasmapheresis and IVIG are best performed within the first few days of illness, useful during severe/rapidly progressive cases or those requiring ventilatory support.

d. Mechanical ventilation is required only if the patient is having difficult time clearing secretions, aspirating, diminished vital capacity, or dyspnea.

(Marino, 2014, p. 823; Rabow et al., 2018, p. 1051).

27 **The correct answer is C.**

Rationales:

a. Guillain-Barre syndrome can cause emergent airway/ventilation issues.

b. The patient may deteriorate quickly and should be monitored closely.

c. Patients diagnosed with GBS should be admitted to the hospital for close monitoring and until it has been determined that the course of the disease has plateaued or has shown sign of reversal.

d. Subsequent hospitalization may be required.

(Marino, 2014, p. 823; Rabow et al., 2018, p. 1051).

28 **The correct answer is A.**

Rationales:

a. Myasthenia gravis: fluctuating weakness of commonly used voluntary muscles producing symptoms of ptosis, diplopia, difficulty swallowing, dyspnea, and arm/leg weakness.

b. Multiple sclerosis: common initial complaints of weakness, numbness, tinkling or unsteadiness in limbs, spastic paraparesis; optic neuritis, diplopia urinary urgency.

c. Guillain–Barré syndrome: (acute idiopathic polyneuropathy) "progressive" symmetric muscle weakness with absent deep tendon reflexes.

d. Acute cervical disk protrusion: herniated disc: common complaint neck pain, numbness or tingling in unilateral limb, weakness to limb, loss of balance, problems with fine motor skills.

(Marino, 2014, pp. 822–823; Rabow et al., 2018, pp. 1058–1059).

29 **The correct answer is B.**

Rationales:

a. Myasthenic syndrome variable weakness, typically improves with activity.

b. Myasthenic crisis: typically, patients experience respiratory distress out of proportion to limb/bulbar weakness; weak respiratory muscles may fatigue suddenly producing respiratory collapse.

c. Acetylcholine receptor antibody: laboratory test found in myasthenia gravis patients, normally negative.

d. Thymoma: frequently associated tumor of the thymus in patients with MG requiring a thymectomy.

(Marino, 2014, pp. 822–823; Rabow et al., 2018, pp. 1058–1059).

30 **The correct answer is D.**

Rationales:

a. Those with acute exacerbation require admission.

b. Those requiring plasmapheresis should be admitted.

c. Those requiring thymectomy must be admitted.

d. Myasthenia gravis occurs at all ages, is associated with thymic tumor or thyrotoxicosis, and is most common in young women while thymoma is associated in older men. Admission and prevention of exacerbation of respiratory depression should be considered for all patients presenting with symptoms of myasthenia gravis.

(Marino, 2014, pp. 822–823; Rabow et al., 2018, pp. 1058–1059).

Clinical Pearl

Therapeutic plasma exchange is the removal of the patient's plasma and replacement with another fluid (donor plasma, colloid, crystalloid); the removal of plasma and certain harmful substances will reduce further damage and may improve or reverse the pathologic process of certain immunomodulated neurologic and hematologic disorders.

31 **The correct answer is A.**

Rationales:

a. Acetylcholinesterase, IVIG, glucocorticoid and nonsteroidal immunomodulating treatments, and thymectomy are the four basic therapies for MG to render the patient's symptoms better while minimizing side effects.

b. Thymectomy is performed only when a thymoma is present.

c. Acetylcholinesterase and glucocorticoids are partial treatment, along with IVIG and thymectomy for treatment of MG.

d. IVIG is only partial treatment.

(Marino, 2014, pp. 822–823; Rabow et al., 2018, pp. 1058–1059).

32 **The correct answer is B.**

Rationales:

a. Subclavian steal syndrome: flow reversal in a branch of the subclavian artery that is the result of an ipsilateral lesion of the proximal subclavian artery. Syndrome may occur when a significant stenosis in the subclavian artery compromises distal perfusion to the inferior mesenteric artery (IMA), vertebral artery, or axillary artery.

b. TIA is the correct answer. Classic signs and symptoms of TIA include sudden or rapid onset of neurologic deficit caused by ischemia lasting a few minutes to 24 hours with reversal of symptoms.

c. Focal seizure: lateralizing features can occur during or after a focal seizure; unilateral automatisms are ipsilateral to the seizure focus; contralateral clonic activity is unusual, and postictal confusion usually resolves within minutes.

d. Brain tumor: clinical manifestations with headache, seizures, focal deficits, sensory loss, aphasia, and visual spatial dysfunction.

(Gross & Grose, 2017, pp. 102–115; Marino, 2014, p. 832; Rabow et al., 2018, pp. 1004–1006).

33 **The correct answer is A.**

Rationales:

a. Patients seen within 1 week of attack and when they are at increased risk of recurrence require admission.

b. TIA is subacute after 1 week, less than 1 month and does not require admission.

c. Patients with history of TIA are likely to have recurrence but do not require hospitalization.

d. Heart disease does not make admission imperative.

(Gross & Grose, 2017, pp. 102–115; Marino, 2014, p. 832; Rabow et al., 2018, pp. 1004–1006).

34 **The correct answer is D.**

Rationales:

a. Patients with TIA in the setting of atrial fibrillation should be anticoagulated.

b. Patients with TIA who have had mechanical heart valves should be anticoagulated.

c. Patients with left ventricular thrombus should be anticoagulated.

d. All of the above are correct.

(Gross & Grose, 2017, pp. 102–115; Marino, 2014, p. 832; Rabow et al., 2018, pp. 1004–1006).

35 **The correct answer is D.**

Rationales:

a. All patients who are not a candidate for anticoagulation should be treated with antiplatelet therapy to reduce the frequency of TIAs/strokes.

b. Dual antiplatelet therapy is preferred.

c. Short-term use of dual antiplatelet therapy has been shown to reduce the frequency of TIA.

d. All of the above is correct.

(Gross & Grose, 2017, pp. 102–115; Marino, 2014, p. 832; Rabow et al., 2018, pp. 1004–1006).

36 **The correct answer is B.**

Rationales:

a. TIA: classic signs and symptoms of TIA include sudden or rapid onset of neurologic deficit caused by ischemia lasting a few minutes to 24 hours with reversal of symptoms.

b. CVA: classic signs and symptoms of CVA include sudden onset of neurologic deficit in patients often with history for HTN, DM, tobacco use, atrial fibrillation, or atherosclerosis.

c. Guillain–Barré syndrome: classic signs and symptoms include (acute idiopathic polyneuropathy) progressive symmetric muscle weakness with absent deep tendon reflexes.

d. Myasthenia gravis: classic signs and symptoms include fluctuating weakness of commonly used voluntary muscles producing symptoms of ptosis, diplopia, difficulty swallowing, dyspnea, and arm/leg weakness.

(Gross & Grose, 2017, pp. 102–115; Marino, 2014, p. 832; Rabow et al., 2018, pp. 1004–1006).

37 **The correct answer is A.**

Rationales:

a. Lacunar infarction consists of small lesions usually less than 1.5 cm and is commonly associated with uncontrolled HTN.

b. Carotid circulation obstruction: signs vary depending on occluded.

c. TIA: classic signs and symptoms of TIA include sudden or rapid onset of neurologic deficit caused by ischemia lasting a few minutes to 24 hours with reversal of symptoms.

d. Vertebrobasilar occlusion: symptoms based on location of occluded vessel.

(Gross & Grose, 2017, pp. 102–115; Marino, 2014, p. 832; Rabow et al., 2018, pp. 1004–1006).

38 **The correct answer is C.**

Rationales:

a. Lacunar infarction consists of small lesions usually less than 1.5 cm and is commonly associated with uncontrolled HTN.

b. Carotid circulation obstruction: signs vary depending on occluded vessel, similar to CVA symptoms.

c. Cerebral infarction: caused by disruption of blood flow to a major vessel, onset is usually abrupt, and there may be little progression except cerebral edema.

d. Intracerebral hemorrhage: loss of consciousness, vomiting at the onset of bleeding, headache, and focal symptoms.

(Gross & Grose, 2017, pp. 102–115; Marino, 2014, p. 832; Rabow et al., 2018, pp. 1004–1008).

39 **The correct answer is B.**

Rationales:

a. Middle cerebral artery: occlusion leads to contralateral hemiplegia, hemisensory loss, and bilateral symmetric loss of vision in half of visual field, with eyes deviated to the side affected by lesion.

b. Anterior cerebral artery: occlusion causes weakness and sensory loss in the contralateral leg, mild weakness of the arm, and urinary incontinence.

c. Posterior cerebral artery: contralateral homonymous hemianopsia, cortical blindness, dyslexia, memory deficit, visual agnosia.

d. Vertebral basilar artery: vertigo, nausea, vomiting, headache, nystagmus, lateral gaze, diplopia, pupillary changes.

(Gross & Grose, 2017, pp. 102–115; Marino, 2014, p. 832; Rabow et al., 2018, pp. 1004–1008).

40 **The correct answer is A.**

Rationales:

a. Middle cerebral artery: occlusion leads to contralateral hemiplegia, hemisensory loss, and bilateral symmetric loss of vision in half of visual field, with eyes deviated to the side affected by lesion.

b. Anterior cerebral artery: occlusion causes weakness and sensory loss in the contralateral leg, mild weakness of the arm, and urinary incontinence.

c. Posterior cerebral artery: contralateral homonymous hemianopsia, cortical blindness, dyslexia, memory deficit, visual agnosia.

d. Vertebral basilar artery: vertigo, nausea, vomiting, headache, nystagmus, lateral gaze, diplopia, pupillary changes.

(Rabow et al., 2018, p. 1008).

Clinical Pearl

Guillain–Barré syndrome/acute polyneuropathy: characterized by "symmetric" rapidly progressive muscular weakness, distal sensory loss, and autonomic dysfunction beginning after a recent infectious disorder, surgery, or immunization.

41 **The correct answer is C.**

Rationales:

a. Middle cerebral artery: occlusion leads to contralateral hemiplegia, hemisensory loss, and bilateral symmetric loss of vision in half of visual field, with eyes deviated to the side affected by lesion.

b. Anterior cerebral artery: occlusion causes weakness and sensory loss in the contralateral leg, mild weakness of the arm, and urinary incontinence.

c. Posterior cerebral artery: vision is primary affected due to occipital lobe circulation, contralateral homonymous hemianopsia, cortical blindness, dyslexia, memory deficit, visual agnosia.

d. Vertebral basilar artery: vertigo, nausea, vomiting, headache, nystagmus, lateral gaze, diplopia, pupillary changes.

(Rabow et al., 2018, p. 1008).

42 **The correct answer is A.**

Rationales:

a. ICH is spontaneous, nontraumatic parenchymal bleeding in patients with no angiographic evidence associated with a vascular anomaly such as an aneurysm or angioma, usually due to HTN.

b. Traumatic injury is not implicated in intraparenchymal bleeding.

c. Aneurysm is not implicated in intraparenchymal bleeding.

d. Angioma is not implicated in intraparenchymal bleeding.

(Garvin & Mangat, 2017, pp. 159–169; Hemphill & Lam, 2017; Rabow et al., 2018, p. 27).

43 **The correct answer is D.**

Rationales:

a. DM is not implicated in intraparenchymal bleeding.

b. Infection is not implicated in intraparenchymal bleeding.

c. Traumatic injury is not implicated in intraparenchymal bleeding. Aneurysm is not implicated in intraparenchymal bleeding.

d. Hypertension is the leading cause of intraparenchymal bleeding.

(Garvin & Mangat, 2017, pp. 159–169; Hemphill & Lam, 2017; Rabow et al., 2018, pp. 1010–1011).

44 **The correct answer is A.**

Rationales:

a. Cerebellar hemorrhage is characterized by sudden onset of vomiting, uncoordinated movements, unsteady gait, headache, and loss of consciousness that may lead to coma or death.

b. ICH is a spontaneous, nontraumatic hemorrhage in patients with no angiographic evidence associated with a vascular anomaly such as an aneurysm or angioma, usually due to HTN.

c. SAH: abrupt onset, "thunderclap" headache with exertion or Valsalva maneuver, neck stiffness, alterations in mental status.

d. SDH: usual mechanism of injury trauma to brain after high-speed impact to the skull, causes the brain to accelerate or decelerate relative to the fixed structures of the dura and tearing of blood vessels; falls, violence or motor vehicle accidents, blunt head trauma.

(Garvin & Mangat, 2017, pp. 159–169; Hemphill & Lam, 2017; Rabow et al., 2018, pp. 1010–1011).

45 **The correct answer is C.**

Rationales:

a. ICH is a spontaneous, nontraumatic hemorrhage in patients with no angiographic evidence associate with a vascular anomaly such as an aneurysm or angioma, usually due to HTN.

b. Cerebellar hemorrhage is characterized by sudden onset of vomiting, uncoordinated movements, unsteady gait, headache, and loss of consciousness that may lead to coma or death.

c. SAH: abrupt onset, "thunder clap" headache with exertion or Valsalva maneuver, neck stiffness, alterations in mental status.

d. SDH: usual mechanism of injury trauma to brain after high speed impact to the skull, causes the brain to accelerate or decelerate relative to the fixed structures of the dura and tearing of blood vessels; falls, violence or motor vehicle accidents, blunt head trauma.

(Edlow & Samuels, 2017, pp. 116–123; Garvin & Mangat, 2017, pp. 159–169; Rabow et al., 2018, pp. 1010–1011).

46 **The correct answer is C.**

Rationales:

a. ICH does not cause xanthrochromia.

b. Cerebellar hemorrhage does not cause xanthochromia.

c. LP with xanthochromia indicates the yellowish discoloration of CSF that results from the degradation of hemoglobin into bilirubin and is present 12 hours after onset of bleed. CT scan of head is preferred with angiography to diagnose SAH, but in the instance CT scan is negative, LP can demonstrate an elevated red blood cell count and the presence of xanthochromia.

d. SDH does not cause xanthochromia.

(Edlow & Samuels, 2017, pp. 116–123; Garvin & Mangat, 2017, pp. 159–169; Rabow et al., 2018, p. 1012).

47 **The correct answer is A.**

Rationales:

a. LP should not be performed as the initial evaluation due to risk of increased intracranial pressure, and CT scan is needed to identify cerebral edema that could increase chances of herniation upon LP.

b. Epidural hematoma is not a risk of lumbar puncture.

c. Intracranial hematoma is not a risk of lumbar puncture.

d. Subarachnoid hemorrhage is not a risk of lumbar puncture.

(Garvin & Mangat, 2017, pp. 159–169; Rabow et al., 2018, pp. 1010–1012).

48 **The correct answer is C.**

Rationales:

Glasgow Coma Scale:

Best eye response: open eyes spontaneously 4, open to verbal command 3, open to pain 2, no eye opening 1.

Best verbal response: oriented 5, confused 4, inappropriate words 3, incomprehensible sounds 2, no verbal response 1.

Best motor response: obeys commands 6, localizing pain 5, withdrawal from pain 4, flexion to pain 3, extension to pain 2, no motor response 1.

(Cadena & Sarwal, 2017, pp. 74–81).

49 **The correct answer is C.**

Rationales:

Glasgow Coma Scale:

Best eye response: open eyes spontaneously 4, open to verbal command 3, open to pain 2, no eye opening 1.

Best verbal response: oriented 5, confused 4, inappropriate words 3, incomprehensible sounds 2, no verbal response 1.

Best motor response: obeys commands 6, localizing pain 5, withdrawal from pain 4, flexion to pain 3, extension to pain 2, no motor response 1.

(Cadena & Sarwal, 2017, pp. 74–81).

50 **The correct answer is D.**

Rationales:

a. Patient should be admitted, rather than observation status.

b. Patient must be admitted for INR reversal and close monitoring.

c. Patient must be admitted for INR reversal and close monitoring.

d. Patient requires INR reversal, close monitoring in ICU, and repeat CT scan to reevaluate. Intracranial trauma and bleeding require frequent neurological evaluation and reversal of bleeding with blood products and other agents for a goal INR ≤ 1.4, prothrombin time PTT ≤ 40 seconds, and platelets ≥100,000.

(Aziz et al., 2012, pp. 767–784; Edlow & Samuels, 2017, pp. 116–123; Garvin & Mangat, 2017, pp. 159–169).

Clinical Pearl

Kernig and Brudzinski signs are indicative of meningeal irritation, heightening suspicion for meningitis.

51 **The correct answer is D.**

Rationales:

a. The patient should be immobilized and transported to the nearest trauma center with neurosurgery capacity.

b. Although the patient requires cervical spine immobilzation, his airway is a priority.

c. The patient's airway is at risk and must be protected.

d. The priority is to intubate to protect the patient's airway while maintaining cervical spine precautions. Severe head injury quickly leads to failure of oxygenation, ventilation, and airway protection, and intubation is essential. Cervical spine stabilization should be in place and transport to nearest trauma center with neurosurgery capability.

(Aziz et al., 2012, pp. 767–784; Garvin & Mangat, 2017, pp. 159–169).

52 **The correct answer is A.**

Rationales:

a. Stat neurosurgery consults for epidural hematoma: epidural hematomas can cause rapid neurologic deterioration and usually require surgical intervention/evacuation if they cause mass effect greater than 1 cm. Epidural hematomas classically present with a "lucid interval" after injury with rapid deterioration, results from laceration of the middle meningeal artery due to fracture of the squamosal portion of the temporal bone. CT scan demonstrates "biconvex hyperdensities" or collections of blood in the low to mid temporal lobe.

b. Biconvex densities describe epidural hematomas, as opposed to the crescent shape of subdural hematomas.

c. Epidural hematomas require immediate neurosurgical consultation

d. Epidural hematomas require immediate neurosurgical consultation

(Aziz et al., 2012, pp. 767–784; Garvin & Mangat, 2017, pp. 159–169; Stein & Knight, 2017, pp. 170–180).

53 **The correct answer is B.**

Rationales:

a. Epidural hematoma: biconvex hyperdensities of collection of blood from laceration of the middle meningeal artery due to fracture of the squamosal portion of the temporal bone.

b. Acute SDH: hyperdense crescents as the blood spreads around the surface of the brain. Symptoms appear suddenly, most times with an inciting event.

c. Chronic SDH: collection of blood below the layer of the dura but external to the brain and arachnoid membrane. Symptoms are gradual and usually insidious.

d. Intraparenchymal hemorrhage: focal areas of hyperdensity, typically with hypodense surroundings of edema.

(Aziz et al., 2012, pp. 767–784; Garvin & Mangat, 2017, pp. 159–169).

54 **The correct answer is B.**

Rationales:

a. Elevated BP, bradycardia, and irregular respiratory patterns are characteristic of Cushing triad, which is consistent with increased ICP.

b. Elevated intracranial pressure with signs of HTN, bradycardia, and irregular respiratory rate should alert the provider of worsening bleeding and neurological deterioration; HTN should be treated to control the risk of further association of rebleeding. Hypotension should be avoided and has been associated with increased risk of deterioration in head-injured patients; bradycardia and irregular respirations are hemodynamic signs of increased pressure within the skull causing decreased blood flow to the brain. Cushing reflex classically presents as an increase in systolic BP, bradycardia, and irregular respiration, caused by increased intracranial pressure inside the skull.

c. The patient does not exhibit impending respiratory failure or airway compromise.

d. Although the BP is severely elevated, the acceleration in BP is directly related to compensatory mechanisms attempting to overcome the high ICP.

(Aziz et al., 2012, pp. 767–784; Garvin & Mangat, 2017, pp. 159–169; Rabow et al., 2018, pp. 1010–1013).

55 **The correct answer is A.**

Rationales:

a. Intracranial trauma and bleeding require frequent neurological evaluation, reversal of bleeding with blood products, and other agents for a goal INR ≤ 1.4, prothrombin time PTT ≤ 40 seconds, and platelets ≥100,000.

b. The INR should be reversed to <1.4, PT <40, and platelets >100,000.

c. The INR should be reversed to <1.4, and PTT to <40

d. The INR should be reversed to <1.4, and platelets >100,000

(Aziz et al., 2012, pp. 767–784; Edlow & Samuels, 2017, pp. 116–123; Garvin & Mangat, 2017, pp. 159–169; Rabow et al., 2018, pp. 1010–1013).

56 **The correct answer is D.**

Rationales:

a. These patients are at high risk for developing DVT/PE.

b. These patients are at high risk for developing DVT/PE.

c. These patients are at high risk for DVT/PE regardless of INR reversal.

d. Patients with severe head injury are at high risk of developing deep venous thrombosis and pulmonary embolism, early use of mechanical compression devices is imperative.

(Aziz et al., 2012, pp. 767–784; Garvin & Mangat, 2017, pp. 159–169; Rabow et al., 2018, pp. 1010–1013).

57 **The correct answer is B.**

Rationales:

a. LP provides information about cerebrospinal fluid, with the purpose of ruling out life-threatening conditions such as bacterial endocarditis or SAH.

b. CT of the brain can provide information regarding brain tissue and structures to identify injuries.

c. Blood work is important to contribute to the patient's diagnosis, but a CT scan of the head should be first priority.

d. ABG is not of primary importance but can be included in workup.

(Aziz et al., 2012, pp. 767–784; Rabow et al., 2018, pp. 1010–1013).

58 **The correct answer is C.**

Rationales:

a. Encephalitis: acute inflammation of the brain caused by viral or other systemic infection, herpes virus, arboviruses, rabies virus, West Nile encephalitis, Japanese encephalitis; symptoms of anxiety, lethargy, fever, nystagmus, ocular paralysis, nausea, vomiting, nuchal rigidity, severe headache, ataxia, dysphagia, hemiparesis, progression to coma.

b. Viral meningitis: inflammation of the leptomeninges from central nervous system infection; causative agents are enteroviruses, coxsackievirus, echovirus.

c. Bacterial meningitis: most common *Streptococcus pneumoniae, Neisseria meningitides, Haemophilus influenzae, Escherichia coli, Enterobacter, Klebsiella,* and *Proteus*. Symptoms: fever, stiff neck, altered mental status, severe headache, photophobia, chills, + Kernig sign, + Brudzinski sign.

d. CVA: facial droop, altered speech, hemiplegia; symptoms alter depending on area affected.

(Gaieski, O'Brien, & Hernandez, 2017, pp. 124–133; Rabow et al., 2018, pp. 1304–1305).

59 The correct answer is A.

Rationales:

a. Treatment for viral meningitis (aseptic meningitis) is mostly supportive; rest, hydration, antipyretics, and pain or anti-inflammatory medications; caused by herpes simplex virus and the *Enterovirus* (coxsackieviruses and echoviruses).

b. Antibiotics do not treat viral meningitis.

c. Antibiotics do not treat viral meningitis.

d. There is no role for antibiotics or phenytoin in treating viral meningitis.

(Gaieski et al., 2017, pp. 124–133; Rabow et al., 2018, pp. 1304–1305).

60 The correct answer is A.

Rationales:

a. Spinal cord compression can be a complication of metastatic tumor, lymphoma, or plasma cell myeloma. Back pain is most common presenting symptom. Emergent treatment may prevent or possibly reverse paresis and urinary and bowel incontinence. The patient should be stabilized prior to transfer.

b. All patients should be stabilized prior to transport to a tertiary facility

c. Transfer should not be delayed for imaging or specialist assessments.

d. This patient requires tertiary care for neurosurgery if the facility lacks the services.

(O'Phelan, 2017, pp. 144–151; Rabow et al., 2018, pp. 1670–1671; Stein & Knight, 2017, pp. 170–180).

References

Aziz, A., Fox, A., Porembka, M., & Klingensmith, M. (2012). *The Washington manual of surgery* (6th ed.). Philadelphia, PA: Wolters Kluwer Health/Lippincott Williams & Wilkins.

Brophy, G. M., & Human, T. (2017). Pharmacotherapy pearls for emergency neurological life support. *Neurocritical Care, 27*(S1), 51–73. https://doi.org/10.1007/s12028-017-0456-x

Cadena, R. S., & Sarwal, A. (2017). Emergency neurological life support: Approach to the patient with coma. *Neurocritical Care, 27*(S1), 74–81. https://doi.org/10.1007/s12028-017-0452-1

Claassen, J., & Goldstein, J. N. (2017). Emergency neurological life support: Status epilepticus. *Neurocritical Care, 27*(S1), 152–158. https://doi.org/10.1007/s12028-017-0460-1

Edlow, B. L., & Samuels, O. (2017). Emergency neurological life support: Subarachnoid hemorrhage. *Neurocritical Care, 27*(S1), 116–123. https://doi.org/10.1007/s12028-017-0458-8

Gaieski, D. F., O'Brien, N. F., & Hernandez, R. (2017). Emergency neurologic life support: Meningitis and encephalitis. *Neurocritical Care, 27*(S1), 124–133. https://doi.org/10.1007/s12028-017-0455-y

Garvin, R., & Mangat, H. S. (2017). Emergency neurological life support: Severe traumatic brain injury. *Neurocritical Care, 27*(S1), 159–169. https://doi.org/10.1007/s12028-017-0461-0

Gross, H., & Grose, N. (2017). Emergency neurological life support: Acute ischemic stroke. *Neurocritical Care, 27*(S1), 102–115. https://doi.org/10.1007/s12028-017-0449-9

Hemphill, J. C., & Lam, A. (2017). Emergency neurological life support: Intracerebral hemorrhage. *Neurocritical Care, 27*(S89–S101). doi:10.1007/s12028*017-0453

Marino, P. L. (2014). *Marino's the ICU book.* Philadelphia, PA: Wolters Kluwer Health/Lippincott Williams & Wilkins.

O'Phelan, K. H. (2017). Emergency neurologic life support: Spinal cord compression. *Neurocritical Care, 27*(S1), 144–151. https://doi.org/10.1007/s12028-017-0459-7

Rabow, M. W., McPhee, S. J., & Papadakis, M. A. (2018). *Current medical diagnosis and treatment 2019* (58th ed.). New York, NY: McGraw-Hill Education.

Rajajee, V., Riggs, B., & Seder, D. B. (2017). Emergency neurological life support: Airway, ventilation, and sedation. *Neurocritical Care, 27*(S1), 4–28. https://doi.org/10.1007/s12028-017-0451-2.

Stein, D. M., & Knight, W. A. (2017). Emergency neurological life support: Traumatic spine injury. *Neurocritical Care, 27*(S1), 170–180. https://doi.org/10.1007/s12028-017-0462-z

CHAPTER 4

Cardiology

Anne Dabrow Woods, DNP, RN, CRNP, ANP-BC, AGACNP-BC, FAAN

Disease Questions

1 The adult-gerontology acute care nurse practitioner (AGACNP) is evaluating a 46-year-old man who has a history of type 2 diabetes, dyslipidemia, and hypertension. He has been taking metformin 1,000 mg by mouth twice daily, atorvastatin 40 mg by mouth daily, lisinopril 10 mg by mouth daily, and hydrochlorothiazide 12.5 mg daily. Last week, his primary care provider increased his lisinopril dose to 20 mg daily and the hydrochlorothiazide to 25 mg daily. He presents to the emergency department (ED) with swelling of his lips, tongue, and eyes. Which medication most likely caused these symptoms?

a. Metformin

b. Lisinopril

c. Hydrochlorothiazide

d. Atorvastatin

2 The AGACNP is evaluating a 42-year-old man who was admitted to telemetry for angina. He develops acute midsternal chest pain that radiates to his jaw and left arm. He also is diaphoretic and nauseated. A 12-lead electrocardiogram (ECG) is done and shows ST elevation in leads II, III, and aVF. What coronary vessel is being affected?

a. Left anterior descending

b. Left circumflex

c. Right coronary artery

d. Left main

3 The AGACNP is called to the bedside of a 40-year-old male who is having midsternal chest pain with radiation to his left arm and jaw and is nauseated. He has received three sublingual nitroglycerin, and he is still having chest pain. He has ST elevation on his 12-lead ECG in leads V2, V3, and V4. His blood pressure (BP) is 145/53, and his heart rate (HR) is 100 bpm. What intervention is most appropriate for this patient?

a. Make the patient nothing by mouth (NPO); draw stat coagulation studies, complete blood count (CBC), troponin, and a chemistry; start the patient on a heparin infusion and a nitroglycerin infusion; administer four 81-mg non–enteric-coated aspirin, give metoprolol 5 mg IV every 15 minutes for three doses; administer morphine 2 mg IV prn for chest pain; and call the cardiac catheterization lab team.

b. Draw stat coagulation studies, CBC, troponin, and a chemistry. Start the patient on a heparin infusion and a nitroglycerin infusion and send him for a stat computed tomography (CT) angiogram of the chest.

c. Make the patient NPO; draw stat coagulation studies, CBC, troponin, and a chemistry; start the patient on a heparin infusion; administer a crystalloid fluid bolus; give him morphine 2 mg IV as needed for the chest pain; give him aspirin 324 mg orally; and call the cardiac catheterization lab team.

d. Give the patient four 81-mg aspirin, order an additional three nitroglycerin sublingually as needed for the chest pain, and start the patient on heparin infusion if he still has chest discomfort after three additional sublingual nitroglycerin.

4 The AGACNP auscultates an S3 heart sound on a patient. This heart sound is often heard with which condition?

a. Uncontrolled hypertension

b. Aortic stenosis

c. Tricuspid regurgitation

d. Volume overload

5 The AGACNP auscultates an S4 heart sound on a patient. This heart sound is often heard with which condition?

a. Uncontrolled hypertension

b. Aortic stenosis

c. Tricuspid regurgitation

d. Volume overload

6 The AGACNP auscultates a harsh, noisy, systolic murmur at the right sternal border, 2nd intercostal space, that radiates to the carotids. This murmur is due to which valve disorder?

a. Tricuspid regurgitation

b. Mitral stenosis

c. Mitral regurgitation

d. Aortic stenosis

7 The AGACNP auscultates a holosystolic murmur at the left, 5th intercostal space at the apex. This murmur is due to which valve disorder?

a. Tricuspid regurgitation

b. Mitral stenosis

c. Mitral regurgitation

d. Aortic stenosis

8 The AGACNP is evaluating a 62-year-old man who was admitted for palpitations. He is found to be in atrial fibrillation with an HR of 130 bpm and has a BP of 110/68 mm Hg. Two days ago, the patient had a nonpharmacologic stress test and was in normal sinus rhythm. What is the best course of action for this patient?

a. Give diltiazem 0.25 mg/kg followed by an infusion at 5–15 mg/hr.

b. Give metoprolol 20 mg IV bolus.

c. Give adenosine 6 mg IV bolus.

d. Immediately cardiovert the patient.

9 The AGACNP is called to the bedside of a 46-year-old man who has a history of hypertension and myocardial infarction (MI) and who was admitted for a bowel resection due to acute diverticulitis and perforated bowel. On day 1 postop, the AGACNP is called to his bedside because his BP is 70/52, his HR is 150 bpm, and his rhythm is irregularly irregular. A 12-lead ECG shows he is now in uncontrolled atrial fibrillation. What is the best course of action for this patient?

a. Immediately give metoprolol 5 mg IV bolus.

b. Immediately give him diltiazem 10 mg IV bolus.

c. Prepare for stat synchronized cardioversion and sedate the patient if possible.

d. Prepare for stat defibrillation and sedate the patient if possible.

10 The AGACNP is evaluating a 52-year-old patient who had an ST elevation MI of the anterior wall and had a drug-eluting stent placed in his left anterior descending coronary artery. The AGACNP knows it is vital for the patient to receive which drug combination to keep his drug-eluting stent patent?

a. Warfarin and aspirin

b. Ticagrelor and aspirin

c. Metoprolol and aspirin

d. Diltiazem and aspirin

11 The AGACNP is admitting a 54-year-old man who has a history of cardiomyopathy and two MIs, and his admitting diagnosis is heart failure with reduced ejection fraction and left ventricle (LV) function. Based on his echocardiogram, his ejection fraction is 30%. The patient is prescribed carvedilol, furosemide, lisinopril, and losartan. Which medication treats the symptoms of heart failure and DOES NOT affect the pathophysiology?

a. Carvedilol

b. Furosemide

c. Lisinopril

d. Losartan

12 In patients who are in acute pulmonary edema, which medication should NOT be given?

a. Calcium channel blockers

b. Digoxin

c. Angiotensin converting enzyme (ACE) inhibitors

d. Nitrates

13 In black patients diagnosed with hypertension, which antihypertensive class is considered first-line therapy?

a. Beta-blockers

b. Central alpha agonists

c. Loop diuretics

d. Calcium channel blockers

14 In patients with diabetes and hypertension, which antihypertensive class is considered first-line therapy?

a. Beta-blockers

b. Central alpha agonists

c. ACE inhibitors

d. Thiazide diuretics

15 According to the latest BP guidelines, what is the systolic BP goal for patients with hypertension over the age of 65 years?

a. Less than 120 mm Hg

b. Less than 130 mm Hg

c. Less than 140 mm Hg

d. Less than 150 mm Hg

16 The AGACNP is evaluating a 48-year-old woman diagnosed with variant angina/Prinzmetal angina. What is the drug of choice for this patient to control variant angina?

a. Metoprolol

b. Diltiazem

c. Lisinopril

d. Losartan

17 In patients with chronic stable angina with normal left ventricular function, which drug class is recommended as first-line treatment?

a. Beta-blockers

b. Nitrates

c. Calcium channel blockers

d. Anticoagulants

18 The AGACNP is called to the bedside of a 72-year-old patient who complains his left foot turns white and he has pain when his leg is elevated and he has cramping in the leg with walking. The AGACNP notices that his left lower extremity develops rubor when it is put into a dependent position and he has minimal hair growth on his lower extremities. He has palpable but diminished pulses in both lower extremities. What is the next best course of action?

a. Measure his ankle–brachial index (ABI) in both legs.

b. Send him immediately for an angiogram of his lower extremities.

c. Order a Doppler ultrasound to assess for a deep vein thrombosis.

d. Order compression stockings.

19 A 24-year-old male who has a history of intravenous drug abuse is admitted with a fever of 3 weeks' duration, weight loss, and fatigue, and he states that he has dyspnea on exertion. On examination, the AGACNP notices that he has painful red nodules in the distal phalanges and small white retina infarcts. What diagnosis would be included in the differentials?

a. Pericarditis

b. Myocarditis

c. Endocarditis

d. Pneumonia

20 A patient is diagnosed with suspected methicillin-resistant *Staphylococcus aureus* (MRSA) endocarditis. Which antibiotic is recommended for empiric coverage until culture results are available?

a. Ceftriaxone

b. Nafcillin

c. Vancomycin

d. Aztreonam

21 The AGACNP is called to the bedside to evaluate a 30-year-old man who complains of precordial chest pain that increases with deep inspiration, coughing, and lying flat. The AGACNP orders a 12-lead ECG and notices that he has widespread ST-segment elevation. What is the most likely differential diagnosis for this patient?

a. ST-segment elevation myocardial infarction (STEMI)

b. Pericarditis

c. Endocarditis

d. Pleuritis

22 The AGACNP is called to the bedside to evaluate a 32-year-old woman who complains of acute onset of shortness of breath that came on about an hour ago. She is vice president of a global pharmaceutical company and states that she has never experienced anything like this before. She states that she just came off a 16-hour flight yesterday. What questions related to her history would be of particular importance?

a. Recent travel history, birth control use, pain and swelling in her calves

b. History of asthma or smoking

c. Family history of lung cancer and chronic obstructive pulmonary disease (COPD)

d. Recent upper respiratory or lower respiratory infection

23 The AGACNP is admitting a 50-year-old man who has a history of hypertension and dyslipidemia, and he complains of fatigue, myalgias, and leg pain and is being ruled out for a deep vein thrombosis. He takes atorvastatin 80 mg daily and lisinopril 20 mg daily. His alanine aminotransferase (ALT) is 350 units/L, aspartate aminotransferase (AST) is 325 units/L, creatine phosphokinase (CPK) is over 10 times the upper limit of normal, and creatinine is 3 mg/dL. What would be the first action?

a. Decrease the atorvastatin dose to 40 mg daily and recheck his liver function tests (LFTs) and CPK in 2 days.

b. Hold the atorvastatin for one day and recheck the LFTs and CPK levels.

c. Stop the atorvastatin, start a crystalloid IV and recheck LFTs, creatinine, blood urea nitrogen (BUN), and CPK levels every few hours to monitor for trending.

d. Stop the atorvastatin and initiate fibrates and niacin.

24 The AGACNP is called to evaluate a 65-year-old man admitted for a gastrointestinal (GI) bleed with a history of American Heart Association (AHA) stage B heart failure. He was given 2,000 mL of normal saline (NSS), 4 units of packed red blood cells, and 2 units of fresh frozen plasma and has been on a pantoprazole infusion at 8 mg/hr and NSS at 125 mL/hr for the past 24 hours. He now complains of shortness of breath, and he is acutely diaphoretic. His vital signs are BP 170/100, HR 86/minute, respiratory rate 38/minute, and SpO$_2$ 86%. He has crackles apices to bases bilaterally. What is the best course of action?

a. Stop the IV NSS and place him on 2 L nasal cannula.

b. Stop the IV NSS give him furosemide 40 mg IV, place him on bilevel positive airway pressure (BiPap), and start a nitroglycerin infusion at 10 μg/min.

c. Stop the IV NSS and give him metoprolol 5 mg IV.

d. Stop the IV NSS and start him on a nitroglycerin infusion at 50 μg/min.

25 What is the fastest way to decrease an elevated bradykinin level in a patient who develops angioedema from being on an ACE inhibitor?

a. Administer diphenhydramine

b. Administer methylprednisolone

c. Administer epinephrine

d. Administer fresh frozen plasma

26 What is considered the standard for dyslipidemia management based on the latest guidelines?

a. Therapy is based on the low–density lipoprotein (LDL) goal.

b. Therapy is based on the future risk of cardiovascular events.

c. Therapy is based on the LDL/high-density lipoprotein (HDL) ratio.

d. Therapy is based on the number of cardiovascular events the patient has already experienced.

27 Which cardiovascular drug class blocks the sympathetic output?

a. ACE inhibitors

b. Angiotensin receptor blockers

c. Calcium channel blockers

d. Beta-blockers

28 A patient with hypertension is on lisinopril, and his BP is not adequately controlled. What drug is NOT recommended to be combined with lisinopril in order to achieve BP control?

a. Losartan

b. Metoprolol

c. Amlodipine

d. Hydrochlorothiazide

29 The AGACNP is called to the bedside to evaluate a 32-year-old landscaper who has a history of syncope and is feeling light-headed and tired. He states that the symptoms started about 6 weeks ago, and he noticed on his wearable device that his resting HR has decreased from 60 bpm to 40 bpm. Which diagnostic study should be ordered immediately?

a. Stat CT of his head

b. Stat ECG and Lyme titer

c. Stat troponin

d. Stat orthostatic BP assessments

30 A 24-year-old man who was admitted to the telemetry unit after being involved in a head-on motor vehicle crash and had fractured his sternum. The AGACNP is called to his room because he is hypotensive and tachycardic. On physical examination, his neck veins are grossly distended and his heart sounds are distant. What is the most likely diagnosis?

a. Hypovolemic shock

b. Acute fat embolism

c. Acute cardiac tamponade

d. Acute pulmonary embolism

31 The AGACNP is called to the bedside of a 72-year-old man who is in complete heart block with an HR of 30/minute and a BP of 78/40 mm Hg. What would be the most appropriate immediate action?

a. Give the patient atropine 1 mg IV.

b. Immediately start transcutaneous pacing.

c. Give the patient 1,000 mL of NSS.

d. Give the patient digoxin immune fab.

32 A 24-year-old patient develops a narrow complex tachycardia with an HR of 170 bpm. The patient's BP is 130/82 mm Hg. Vagal maneuvers have been unsuccessful in breaking the rhythm. What would be the best intervention for this patient?

a. Administer digoxin 0.25 mg IV.

b. Administer diltiazem 10 mg IV.

c. Administer metoprolol 5 mg IV.

d. Administer adenosine 6 mg IV.

33 The AGACNP is called to evaluate a 54-year-old man who complains of a sudden onset of a severe ripping and tearing sensation in his back and substernally, and he states that he feels very faint. Which would be the most likely differential diagnosis?

a. Acute coronary syndrome

b. Acute pulmonary embolism

c. Acute aortic dissection

d. Acute tension pneumothorax

34 In a patient complaining of an acute tearing and ripping sensation in the back and substernally, which diagnostic test should be ordered as soon as the diagnosis is suspected?

a. Stat 12-lead ECG

b. Stat cardiac enzymes

c. Stat arterial blood gas

d. Stat CT angiography of the chest, abdomen, and pelvis

35 A patient experiences a cardiac arrest and is found to be in ventricular fibrillation. Which intervention should immediately be done after cardiopulmonary resuscitation (CPR) is initiated?

a. Defibrillation

b. Synchronized cardioversion

c. Administer 1 mg epinephrine intravenously

d. Intubate the patient to secure the airway

36 The AGACNP is seeing a patient who had an MI who had a drug-eluting stent placed in his left anterior descending coronary artery. Which medications should be ordered to ensure the patient's stent remains patent?

a. Aspirin 324 mg twice daily and ticagrelor 180 mg daily

b. Aspirin 81 mg daily and clopidogrel 300 mg daily

c. Aspirin 324 mg daily and ticagrelor 90 mg twice daily

d. Aspirin 81 mg daily and ticagrelor 90 mg twice daily

37 A patient develops an acute holosystolic blowing murmur at the apex that radiates to the axilla, an S3 heart sound, and shortness of breath 24 hours after having an acute STEMI. What is the most likely cause of the patient's symptoms?

a. Acute rupture of the papillary muscles and chordae tendineae

b. Acute aortic regurgitation

c. Acute mitral stenosis

d. Acute aortic stenosis

38 A 48-year-old patient experiences sinus bradycardia with an HR of 40/minute. The patient denies chest pain or shortness of breath, and his BP is 120/68 mm Hg. What would be the best course of action?

a. Administer atropine 0.5 mg IV stat and consult cardiology.

b. Administer atropine 1 mg IV stat and consult cardiology.

c. Start transcutaneous pacing and consult cardiology.

d. Watchful waiting and consult cardiology.

39 A patient is experiencing symptomatic bradycardia, and he has received 3 mg of atropine. What would be the best medication to order next for this patient?

a. Dopamine 2–10 µg/kg/min

b. Dobutamine 2–10 µg/kg/min

c. Norepinephrine 5 mg/min

d. Dopamine 20 µg/kg/min

40 In patients who have a systolic BP less than 85 mm Hg, have an ejection fraction of 20%, and need additional inotropic support, which agent is recommended?

a. Dobutamine

b. Milrinone

c. Diltiazem

d. Metoprolol

41 What arrhythmia is NOT commonly seen in patients with Wolff–Parkinson–White (WPW) syndrome?

a. AV reentrant tachycardia

b. Atrial flutter

c. Atrial fibrillation

d. AV block

42 In patients who have a coronary artery bypass and graft using the saphenous vein, which antiplatelet agent should be initiated within 6 hours postoperatively to reduce saphenous vein graft closure?

a. Aspirin

b. Unfractionated heparin

c. Low molecular weight heparin

d. Argatroban

43 Which class of antiarrhythmic agent is diltiazem?

   a. Class I

   b. Class II

   c. Class III

   d. Class IV

44 Which antiarrhythmic/rate control agent prolongs the action potential phase 3?

   a. Metoprolol

   b. Amiodarone

   c. Diltiazem

   d. Digoxin

45 According to the latest hypertension guidelines, which diuretic is preferred due to its long half-life and proven reduction of cardiovascular disease risk?

   a. Hydrochlorothiazide

   b. Chlorthalidone

   c. Furosemide

   d. Spironolactone

46 How many minutes per week should the average adult engage in moderate-intensity exercise?

   a. 200 minutes

   b. 150 minutes

   c. 100 minutes

   d. 75 minutes

47 How many months should patients be on dual antiplatelet therapy who have had a bare metal stent or a drug-eluting stent placed for acute coronary syndrome?

   a. 3 months

   b. 6 months

   c. 9 months

   d. 12 months

48 How many months should elective noncardiac surgery be delayed after a bare metal stent has been placed?

   a. 1 month

   b. 3 months

   c. 6 months

   d. 12 months

49 How many months should elective, noncardiac surgery be delayed after a drug-eluting stent has been placed?

   a. 1 month

   b. 3 months

   c. 6 months

   d. 12 months

50 A patient is diagnosed with atrial fibrillation, and her CHA2DS2-VASc score is 0. What is the most reasonable course of therapy?

   a. It is reasonable to omit antithrombotic therapy.

   b. Start the patient on a direct oral anticoagulant.

   c. Start the patient on a direct oral anticoagulant and 75 mg of aspirin.

   d. The patient should be scheduled for an ablation.

51 A patient has ST elevation in leads I, aVL, V5, and V6 on his 12-lead ECG. Which type of MI is the patient experiencing?

   a. Anterior

   b. Lateral

   c. Inferior

   d. Posterior

52 A patient is having a STEMI with a percutaneous intervention and requires P2Y12 inhibitor therapy. Which loading dose is correct?

a. Clopidogrel 75 mg

b. Prasugrel 180 mg

c. Ticagrelor 180 mg

d. Ticagrelor 90 mg

53 For patients who are having a STEMI who go to a PCI-capable hospital, what is the first medical contact to device time recommendation?

a. 90 minutes or less

b. 120 minutes or less

c. 180 minutes or less

d. 240 minutes or less

54 A patient is admitted with shortness of breath. A transcutaneous echocardiogram is done and reveals an ejection fraction of 42%. What is the heart failure classification?

a. Heart failure with reduced ejection fraction

b. Heart failure with preserved ejection fraction

c. Heart failure with borderline ejection fraction

d. Heart failure with acute decompensation

55 A 68-year-old man with a history of heart failure is admitted to the hospital with community-acquired pneumonia. The patient is currently receiving furosemide 80 mg orally daily, carvedilol 25 mg orally twice a day, and enalapril 20 mg orally twice a day. The patient develops pink frothy sputum and crackles from the apices to bases bilaterally and is acutely short of breath after receiving 2 L of crystalloids over the past 8 hours. Current vital signs are 140/90 mm Hg, 86 bpm, and 36 resp/min. Which is the correct dose of furosemide for this patient?

a. 20 mg IV stat

b. 40 mg IV stat

c. 60 mg IV stat

d. 80 mg IV stat

56 Which antihypertensive agent is associated with the adverse effect of lower extremity edema?

a. ACE inhibitors

b. Beta-blockers

c. Dihydropyridine calcium channel blockers

d. Nondihydropyridine calcium channel blockers

57 The AGACNP is called to evaluate a 52-year-old man who is having chest pain after having sexual intercourse. He states that he has erectile dysfunction and took sildenafil earlier today. Which medication should NOT be given to this patient?

a. Nitrates

b. Beta-blockers

c. Morphine

d. Heparin

58 A 28-year-old landscaper is admitted with chest pain. He complains of chest pain more prevalent on the right side, it is worse with movement, and he has tenderness across the costochondral joints and sternoclavicular joint and rib tenderness on the right side. What is the most likely diagnosis for this patient?

a. Acute pulmonary embolism

b. Acute coronary syndrome

c. Pneumothorax

d. Costochondritis

59 An 82-year-old with a history of dementia and atrial fibrillation is admitted with an HR of 30 bpm, hypotension with BP of 90/50 mm Hg, nausea, vomiting, diarrhea, lethargy, weakness, and increased confusion and states that he is seeing yellow halos around objects. The patient is afebrile, and his respiratory rate is 18 resp/min. These symptoms are most likely due to which condition?

a. Digoxin toxicity

b. ACE inhibitor toxicity

c. Beta-blocker toxicity

d. Calcium channel blocker toxicity

60 A 78-year-old with a history of heart failure and cognitive impairment is brought to the hospital because he felt light-headed and very lethargic. On arrival, his vital signs were 90/50 mm Hg, 30 bpm, and 18 resp/min. His family states that he had just refilled his medications and there was only 1 metoprolol tablet in the bottle. What would be the best course of action?

a. Administer atropine 1 mg IV stat; may repeat up to 5 mg in total.

b. Start an epinephrine infusion.

c. Administer glucagon 1–5 mg IV stat; may repeat up to 15 mg in total; consider a continuous infusion.

d. Start digoxin immune fab.

Disease Answers/Rationales

1 **The correct answer is B.**

Rationales:

a. Metformin is not associated with angioedema.

b. ACE inhibitors can cause angioedema due to the elevation of the bradykinin, which manifests as swelling of the mucous membranes including the lips, tongue, and eyes in less than 1% of the population.

c. Hydrochlorothiazide is not associated with angioedema.

d. Atorvastatin is not associated with angioedema.

(Arcangelo et al., 2017, p. 296).

2 **The correct answer is C.**

Rationales:

a. The left anterior descending coronary artery perfuses the anterior wall of the LV and is reflected in leads V2, V3, and V4 on the 12-lead ECG.

b. The left circumflex coronary artery perfuses the lateral wall of the LV and is reflected in leads I, aVL, V5, and V6.

c. The right coronary artery perfuses the inferior wall of the LV and is reflected in leads II, III, and aVF.

d. The left main coronary artery is the origination of the left anterior descending coronary artery and the left circumflex coronary artery and is reflected in V1, V2, V3, and V4 and potentially the lateral wall leads.

(Thaler, 2015, p. 241)

3 **The correct answer is A.**

Rationales:

a. In an acute STEMI, the goal is to reestablish perfusion to the myocardium as quickly as possible, within 90 minutes of recognition of the event to percutaneous intervention. The patient needs to be NPO, draw stat labs, place the patient on a heparin and nitroglycerin infusion, give four 81 mg non–enteric-coated aspirin, give metoprolol 5 mg IV every 5 minutes for 3 doses, administer morphine IV as needed, and call the cardiac catheterization team stat.

b. The CT angiography of the chest is not indicated because this patient is having a STEMI.

c. The patient's BP is sufficient, so there is no need to administer a crystalloid fluid bolus.

d. Continued medical therapy is not indicated; this patient needs percutaneous coronary intervention (PCI).

(Advanced Cardiac Life Support, 2015).

4 **The correct answer is D.**

Rationales:

a. An S4 heart sound is often associated with uncontrolled hypertension and is heard immediately before the S1 heart sound.

b. Aortic stenosis is associated with a systolic murmur heard best at the 2nd intercostal space, right sternal border, and often radiates to the carotids.

c. Tricuspid regurgitation causes a systolic murmur and is best heard at the lower left sternal border.

d. An S3 heart sound is often associated with volume overload due to the rush of blood into a dilated LV such as in systolic heart failure.

(Bickley, 2017, p. 348).

5 **The correct answer is A.**

Rationales:

a. An S4 heart sound is associated with uncontrolled hypertension and occurs immediately before S1.

b. A systolic ejection murmur heard at the right sternal border, 2nd intercostal space and radiating to the carotids is associated with aortic stenosis.

c. Tricuspid regurgitation is associated with a systolic ejection murmur heard best at the lower left sternal border.

d. Volume overload is associated with an S3 heart sound, which is heard immediately after the S2 heart sound.

(Bickley, 2017, p. 348).

Clinical Pearl

An S3 heart sound is most often associated with volume overload, whereas an S4 heart sound is most often associated with uncontrolled hypertension.

6 **The correct answer is D.**

Rationales:

a. Tricuspid regurgitation is a systolic murmur that is best heard at the lower left sternal border.

b. Mitral stenosis is a diastolic murmur that is low pitched and best heard with patient in the left lateral lean position with the bell of the stethoscope.

c. Mitral regurgitation is a holosystolic murmur best heard on the left side, 5th intercostal space at the apex of the heart.

d. Aortic stenosis is a systolic murmur that is best heard at the right sternal border, 2nd intercostal space, and often radiates to the carotid arteries.

(Bickley, 2017, p. 350).

7 **The correct answer is C.**

Rationales:

a. Tricuspid regurgitation is a systolic murmur that is best heard at the lower left sternal border.

b. Mitral stenosis is a diastolic murmur that is low pitched and best heard with the patient in the left lateral lean position with the bell of the stethoscope.

c. Mitral regurgitation is a holosystolic murmur best heard on the left side, 5th intercostal space at the apex of the heart.

d. Aortic stenosis is a systolic murmur that is best heard at the right sternal border, 2nd intercostal space, and often radiates to the carotid arteries.

(Bickley, 2017, p. 350).

> **Clinical Pearl**
>
> Murmurs occur due to turbulent blood flow. In systole, the right and LVs are contracting; thus any impingement to flow such as aortic stenosis, pulmonic stenosis, or backflow of blood such as in mitral regurgitation or tricuspid regurgitation will result in systolic murmurs. In diastole, the right and LVs are filling. If the aortic valve or pulmonic valve is incompetent or the mitral valve or tricuspid valve is stenosed, diastolic murmurs will occur.

8 The correct answer is A.

Rationales:

a. Diltiazem 0.25 mg/kg IV bolus followed by an infusion at 5–15 mg/hr is the correct drug and dosage to slow the HR in a patient with uncontrolled atrial fibrillation.

b. The metoprolol dose of 20 mg IV bolus is too high; the correct dose is 2.5–5 mg IV bolus to slow the HR in uncontrolled atrial fibrillation.

c. Adenosine is used to treat tachycardia with a narrow QRS complex that is regular. Atrial fibrillation is irregular; therefore, adenosine would not be advised.

d. The patient is hemodynamically stable and therefore would not require synchronized cardioversion.

(Advanced Cardiac Life Support, 2015).

9 The correct answer is C.

Rationales:

a. The patient is hemodynamically unstable; therefore, IV metoprolol would not be indicated.

b. The patient is hemodynamically unstable; therefore, IV diltiazem would not be indicated.

c. The patient is hemodynamically unstable and would require immediate synchronized cardioversion, and the patient should be sedated if possible.

d. The patient is hemodynamically unstable and requires immediate synchronized cardioversion and not unsynchronized defibrillation.

(Advanced Cardiac Life Support, 2015).

10 The correct answer is B.

Rationales:

a. Warfarin is best suited for blood clot prevention and anticoagulation; however, it is more effective in areas of slower blood flow such as in veins. Because the coronary arteries are considered high blood flow areas, warfarin is not recommended to keep bare metal and drug-eluting stents patent.

b. Ticagrelor and aspirin are recommended to keep bare metal and drug-eluting stents patent because they both decrease platelet aggregation and are most effective in high blood flow areas.

c. Metoprolol does not affect platelet function.

d. Diltiazem does not affect platelet function.

(Levine et al., 2016).

11 The correct answer is B.

Rationales:

a. Carvedilol directly impacts the pathophysiology of heart failure by decreasing the endothelial dysfunction.

b. Furosemide does not impact the pathophysiology of heart failure; it decreases the signs and symptoms of heart failure such as shortness of breath and volume overload by its action on the loop of Henle in the kidney.

c. Lisinopril is an ACE inhibitor, and it directly impacts the pathophysiology of heart failure by decreasing endothelial dysfunction.

d. Losartan is an angiotensin receptor blocker, and it directly impacts the pathophysiology of heart failure by decreasing endothelial dysfunction.

(Yancy et al., 2017).

12 The correct answer is A.

Rationales:

a. Calcium channel blockers decrease myocardial contractility and therefore should not be given in acute pulmonary edema.

b. Digoxin increases myocardial contraction and decreases the HR; it is not contraindicated in acute pulmonary edema.

c. ACE inhibitors do not affect myocardial contractility and are not contraindicated in acute pulmonary edema.

d. Nitrates vasodilate the blood vessels and exert the majority of their action on the veins and, as a result, decrease venous return to the heart. They are not contraindicated in acute pulmonary edema.

(Arcangelo et al., 2017, pp. 297–299).

13 **The correct answer is D.**

Rationales:

a. Beta-blockers are considered second-line therapy for hypertension in black people.

b. Central alpha agonists are not considered first-line therapy for black people with hypertension; they are considered adjuvant agents.

c. Loop diuretics are not recommended in the management of hypertension; they are used in heart failure to control symptoms.

d. Calcium channel blockers and thiazide-based diuretics are considered first-line agents for hypertension in black people.

(Whelton, 2018, p. e188).

14 **The correct answer is C.**

Rationales:

a. Beta-blockers are considered second-line therapy for hypertension in adults with diabetes and hypertension.

b. Central alpha agonists are considered adjuvant therapy for hypertension in adults with diabetes and hypertension.

c. ACE inhibitors are considered first-line therapy for patients with hypertension, diabetes, and albuminuria due to their renal protective properties.

d. Thiazide diuretics are considered second-line therapy for patients with hypertension and diabetes.

(Whelton, 2018, p. e183).

> **Clinical Pearl**
>
> Angiotensin converting enzyme inhibitors are first-line therapy for hypertension in patients with the comorbidities of diabetes and albuminuria due to their renal protective properties.

15 **The correct answer is B.**

Rationales:

a. The systolic BP goal for patients with hypertension over the age of 65 years is less than 130 mm Hg.

b. The systolic BP goal for patients with hypertension over the age of 65 years is less than 130 mm Hg.

c. The systolic BP goal for patients with hypertension over the age of 65 years is less than 130 mm Hg.

d. The systolic BP goal for patients with hypertension over the age of 65 years is less than 130 mm Hg.

(Whelton, 2018, p. e190).

16 **The correct answer is B.**

Rationales:

a. Beta-blockers such as metoprolol are the drug class of choice in stable angina that is not caused by vasospasm. If beta-blockers are used in variant angina, they may induce coronary vasospasm from unopposed alpha-receptor activity.

b. Diltiazem is the drug of choice for Prinzmetal angina because this type of angina is caused by vasospasm of the coronary artery, and calcium channel blockers decrease vasospasm.

c. ACE inhibitors such as lisinopril are used to treat heart failure and hypertension; they do not affect coronary vasospasm.

d. Angiotensin receptor blockers such as losartan are used to treat heart failure and hypertension, they do not decrease coronary vasospasm.

(Arcangelo et al., 2017, pp. 298–299).

17 **The correct answer is A.**

Rationales:

a. Beta-blockers are recommended as first-line treatment in patients with chronic stable angina who have normal left ventricular function.

b. Nitrates are considered second-line therapy for patients with chronic stable angina who have normal left ventricular function.

c. Calcium channel blockers are considered second-line therapy for patients with chronic stable angina who have normal left ventricular function.

d. Anticoagulants are not recommended for patients with chronic stable angina.

(Kannam & Gersh, 2019).

18 **The correct answer is A.**

Rationales:

a. When peripheral arterial disease (PAD) of the lower extremities is suspected, obtaining the ABI will identify patients at risk for PAD and those who need additional diagnostic studies. In this case, the patient still had palpable pulses so obtaining the ABI is the most prudent diagnostic.

b. If the patient did not have a pulse in his lower extremity, immediate angiogram of his lower extremities would be recommended.

c. The patient does not have signs or symptoms of peripheral venous disease such as edema, darkening of the skin when the leg is dependent, and pain when the leg is lower than the heart, so an ultrasound of the lower extremities to rule out deep vein thrombosis is not warranted.

d. Compression stockings are contraindicated in patients with PAD due to their compression.

(Bickley, 2017, pp. 519–520).

19 **The correct answer is C.**

Rationales:

a. Patients with pericarditis will have a pericardial friction rub and muffled heart tones if the effusion is large enough.

b. Myocarditis symptoms are often nonspecific but may include fever and myalgia. There are no associated skin lesions or retinal infarcts with myocarditis.

c. Endocarditis presents with fever, weight loss, fatigue, and dyspnea on exertion. The patient may also have red nodules in the distal phalanges on the pads of the fingers and toes (Osler nodes); Janeway lesions, which are nontender red macules on the palms and soles; and small white retina infarcts that are called Roth spots.

d. Pneumonia presents as a cough, shortness of breath, and fever, and the patient will have an infiltrate on chest x-ray.

(Bhat et al., 2014, p. 429).

Clinical Pearl

Always remember to look at the skin on the soles of the feet and the hands to help determine if a patient has endocarditis.

20 **The correct answer is C.**

Rationales:

a. Ceftriaxone does not cover MRSA infection.

b. Nafcillin does not cover MRSA infection.

c. The patient is suspected of having MRSA and needs to be on vancomycin until cultures come back definitively.

d. Aztreonam does cover MRSA; however, the patient is not allergic to vancomycin, so vancomycin would still be the first-line antimicrobial until cultures are finalized.

(Gilbert, Eliopoulos, Chambers, & Saag, 2019).

21 **The correct answer is B.**

Rationales:

a. STEMI usually manifests in midsternal chest pain that radiates to the neck and left arm and can be associated with nausea, shortness of breath, and diaphoresis.

b. Pericarditis is associated with precordial chest pain that increases with deep inspiration, coughing, and lying flat.

c. Endocarditis presents with fever, weight loss, fatigue, and dyspnea on exertion. The patient may also have red nodules in the distal phalanges on the pads of the fingers and toes (Osler nodes); Janeway lesions, which are nontender red macules on the palms and soles; and small white retina infarcts that are called Roth spots.

d. Pleuritis is associated with chest wall pain that is exacerbated with coughing and deep breaths.

(Bhat et al., 2014, p. 435).

22 **The correct answer is A.**

Rationales:

a. This 32-year-old patient is of childbearing age and works for a global pharmaceutical company and most likely travels. With her symptoms of acute shortness of breath, one must consider pulmonary embolism in the differential; therefore, travel history, birth control use, and asking about pain and swelling in her calves would be of most importance.

b. Although history of asthma and smoking is important, the patient stated that she has never experienced a symptom like this before and smoking would not cause acute onset shortness of breath.

c. Having a family history of lung cancer and COPD would be important to note in the history; however, they would not cause acute shortness of breath.

d. Having a recent upper or lower respiratory infection would not cause an acute onset of shortness of breath.

(Bhat et al., 2014, p. 636).

23 **The correct answer is C.**

Rationales:

a. The patient has a CPK level of greater than 10 times the normal limit, and his creatinine is elevated in addition to the elevated LFTs. This indicates the patient is in acute rhabdomyolysis and the statin needs to be discontinued, a crystalloid solution needs to be started to flush the myoglobin from the kidneys, and labs need to be trended. Decreasing the dose of statin is incorrect.

b. The patient has a CPK level of greater than 10 times the normal limit, and his creatinine is elevated in addition to the elevated LFTs. This indicates the patient is in acute rhabdomyolysis and the statin needs to be discontinued, a crystalloid solution needs to be started to flush the myoglobin from the kidneys, and labs need to be trended. Stopping the statin for one day is incorrect.

c. The patient has a CPK level of greater than 10 times the normal limit, and his creatinine is elevated in addition to the elevated LFTs. This indicates the patient is in acute rhabdomyolysis and the statin needs to be discontinued, a crystalloid solution needs to be started to flush the myoglobin from the kidneys, and labs need to be trended.

d. The patient has a CPK level of greater than 10 times the normal limit, and his creatinine is elevated in addition to the elevated LFTs. This indicates the patient is in acute rhabdomyolysis and the statin needs to be discontinued, a crystalloid solution needs to be started to flush the myoglobin from the kidneys, and labs need to be trended. Initiating fibrates and niacin would exacerbate the rhabdomyolysis.

(Grundy et al., 2019, p. e324).

24 **The correct answer is B.**

Rationales:

a. Placing him on 2 L nasal cannula is not adequate treatment. The patient is experiencing pulmonary edema secondary to volume overload and needs diuresis and more aggressive oxygenation.

b. Stopping the NSS, giving him a diuretic, and placing him on BiPap and starting nitroglycerin at a low dose will work to decrease the pulmonary edema in the patient.

c. Stopping the NSS is correct; however, giving a patient in acute pulmonary edema a beta-blocker is incorrect because it decreases the cardiac output.

d. Stopping the NSS is correct; however, the 50 μg/min of nitroglycerin is too high of a dose to start, and without a diuretic, the patient will not get out of pulmonary edema.

(Bhat et al., 2014, pp. 154–156).

25 **The correct answer is D.**
Rationales:

a. ACE inhibitors prevent the degradation of bradykinin, which results in angioedema in a small percentage of the population. Administering diphenhydramine does not decrease bradykinin levels.

b. Administering methylprednisolone does not decrease bradykinin levels.

c. Administering epinephrine does not decrease bradykinin levels.

d. Transfusing the patient with fresh frozen plasma will decrease the circulating bradykinin levels resulting in a decrease in angioedema.

(Vaeskar & Craig, 2012, pp. 72–78).

Clinical Pearl

ACE inhibitors prevent the degradation of bradykinin, which results in angioedema; the fastest way to decrease bradykinin levels is to transfuse fresh frozen plasma.

26 **The correct answer is B.**
Rationales:

a. Treating to a target LDL number is no longer recommended in managing dyslipidemia.

b. Treating patients based on their future risk of cardiovascular events is now the standard of dyslipidemia management.

c. The LDL/HDL ratio is not the standard way dyslipidemia is now managed.

d. The number of cardiovascular events is important; however, the goal of dyslipidemia therapy is based on decreasing the risk of future cardiovascular events.

(Grundy et al., 2019, p. e295).

27 **The correct answer is D.**
Rationales:

a. ACE inhibitors block the conversion of angiotensin to angiotensin II.

b. Angiotensin receptor antagonists block angiotensin from activating the angiotensin receptor.

c. Calcium channel antagonists block the slow-moving calcium channels.

d. Beta-blockers antagonize the beta receptors in the heart and the lungs so that epinephrine and norepinephrine cannot activate them.

(Arcangel et al., 2017, pp. 297–298).

28 **The correct answer is A.**
Rationales:

a. In managing hypertension, an ACE inhibitor such as lisinopril should not be combined with an angiotensin receptor blocker.

b. Metoprolol, which is a beta-blocker, can be given to a patient on an ACE inhibitor.

c. Amlodipine, which is a dihydropyridine calcium channel blocker, can be given to a patient on an ACE inhibitor.

d. Hydrochlorothiazide, which is a thiazide diuretic, can be given to a patient on an ACE inhibitor.

(Whelton, 2018, p. e164).

29 **The correct answer is B.**

Rationales:

a. The patient has no neurological symptoms that would require a CT of the head.

b. The patient needs a 12-lead ECG to verify the rhythm, and because this patient is a landscaper and at risk for Lyme disease, which can cause bradycardia, a Lyme titer should be drawn.

c. The patient is not having chest discomfort, so cardiac enzymes would not need to be drawn stat unless the 12-lead ECG revealed ST abnormalities.

d. Orthostatic BP assessment is important; however, it is more prudent to obtain the 12-lead ECG and Lyme titer first.

(Linden, 2019).

30 **The correct answer is C.**

Rationales:

a. This patient is hypotensive and tachycardic; however, his distended neck veins and distant heart sounds are indicative of acute cardiac tamponade due to blood accumulating in the pericardial sac. In hypovolemic shock, the neck veins would be flat.

b. Fat embolism occurs 24–72 hours after a traumatic fracture such as a femur fracture, and the symptoms include hypoxemia, neurologic abnormalities/confusion, and petechial rash.

c. Distended neck veins, distant heart sounds, tachycardia, and hypotension is the classic presentation for acute cardiac tamponade from blood accumulating very quickly in the pericardial sac.

d. Pulmonary embolism symptoms include acute shortness of breath, hypoxemia, and cardiac compromise; however, the patient would not have distant heart sounds.

(Bhat et al., 2014, pp. 168–169).

31 **The correct answer is B.**

Rationales:

a. The patient is experiencing complete heart block, and in this case atropine is often not effective because it affects the SA node and not the ventricles.

b. In complete heart block, transcutaneous pacing is the best intervention because there is no communication between the atria and ventricles.

c. A fluid bolus will not increase the patient's HR, which is causing the hypotension. Addressing the HR first is the best intervention.

d. Digoxin immune fab is not recommended unless the patient is suspected of having digoxin poisoning.

(Advanced Cardiac Life Support, 2015).

32 **The correct answer is D.**

Rationales:

a. Digoxin does not take effect quickly and is not recommended to break a supraventricular tachycardia (SVT).

b. Diltiazem is not recommended as first line to break an SVT.

c. Metoprolol is not recommended as first line to break an SVT.

d. Adenosine 6 mg IV given as a bolus followed by a NSS flush and elevating the extremity with the IV is recommended for stopping a narrow complex SVT. The dose may be followed by adenosine 12 mg IV bolus.

(Advanced Cardiac Life Support, 2015).

Clinical Pearl

Adenosine is the recommended drug of choice for narrow complex, supraventricular tachycardias.

33 **The correct answer is C.**

Rationales:

a. The symptoms of acute coronary syndrome are midsternal chest pain that radiates to the neck and left arm and is associated with nausea, diaphoresis, and shortness of breath.

b. The symptoms of acute pulmonary embolism are acute shortness of breath, tachycardia, and hypoxemia.

c. The symptoms of sudden onset of a severe ripping and tearing sensation in the back and substernal accompanied by feeling light-headed and dizzy is the classic presentation of aortic dissection.

d. Acute tension pneumothorax symptoms are shortness of breath, hypotension, and tracheal deviation to the contralateral side.

(Bhat et al., 2014, pp. 73, 121).

34 **The correct answer is D.**

Rationales:

a. A 12-lead ECG is important, but a stat CT angiography of the chest, abdomen, and pelvis is standard of care to identify the dissecting aortic aneurysm and its location.

b. Cardiac enzymes are important, but a stat CT angiography of the chest, abdomen, and pelvis is standard of care to identify the dissecting aortic aneurysm and its location.

c. Arterial blood gases are not needed at this point; a stat CT angiography of the chest, abdomen, and pelvis is standard of care to identify the dissecting aortic aneurysm and its location.

d. This patient requires immediate confirmation of the dissecting aortic aneurysm. A stat angiography of the chest, abdomen, and pelvis is standard of care to identify the dissecting aortic aneurysm and its location.

(Bhat et al., 2014, pp. 73, 121).

35 **The correct answer is A.**

Rationales:

a. A patient in cardiac arrest with ventricular fibrillation needs immediate defibrillation to stop the rhythm and allow the SA node to restore a normal sinus rhythm.

b. Synchronized cardioversion is not recommended in ventricular fibrillation due to the chaos of the rhythm.

c. Administering epinephrine is done after the patient is defibrillated and only if the patient does not convert into a normal sinus rhythm.

d. Securing the airway is not the first priority; early defibrillation has been shown to the most effective intervention in ventricular fibrillation cardiac arrest.

(Advanced Cardiac Life Support, 2015).

36 **The correct answer is A.**

Rationales:

a. Low-dose aspirin and ticagrelor 90 mg twice daily after the patient receives the loading dose of 180 mg of ticagrelor.

b. Although low-dose aspirin is correct, the clopidogrel dose is the loading dose and subsequent doses are 75 mg daily.

c. The dose of aspirin is too high; low-dose aspirin is recommended.

d. Low-dose aspirin is appropriate, but ticagrelor 90 mg should be given twice daily to ensure stent patency.

(Levine et al., 2016, pp. 1090–1094).

37 **The correct answer is A.**

Rationales:

a. Development of an acute holosystolic blowing murmur at the apex that radiates to the axilla, an S3 heart sound, and shortness of breath 24 hours of having an acute ST-segment elevation MI indicates there is acute mitral regurgitation due to rupture of the papillary muscles and chordae tendineae.

b. Acute aortic regurgitation would result in a diastolic murmur.

c. Acute mitral stenosis would result in a diastolic murmur.

d. Acute aortic stenosis would result in a systolic murmur and would be heard at the 2nd intercostal space, right sternal border, and radiate to the carotids.

(Bickley, 2017, p. 350).

38 **The correct answer is D.**

Rationales:

a. The patient is asymptomatic and does not require drug intervention.

b. The patient is asymptomatic and does not require drug intervention.

c. The patient is asymptomatic and does not require transcutaneous pacing.

d. The patient is asymptomatic, so no intervention is required at this time except for monitoring and consulting cardiology.

(Advanced Cardiac Life Support, 2015).

39 **The correct answer is A.**

Rationales:

a. Patients who are experiencing symptomatic bradycardia and have received atropine should be started on dopamine 2–10 µg/kg/min, and a transcutaneous pacemaker should be applied.

b. Dobutamine increases the strength of the myocardial contraction; it does not affect HR.

c. Norepinephrine affects the alpha and beta receptors but does not have as potent beta 1 receptor activation as dopamine.

d. Dopamine from 10–20 µg/kg/min affects the alpha receptors resulting in vasoconstriction as well as an increase in HR from beta receptor activation. However, the dose is too high to start.

(Advanced Cardiac Life Support, 2015).

40 **The correct answer is A.**

Rationales:

a. In patients who are hypotensive and require inotropic support, dobutamine is recommended as the first-line agent because milrinone causes more vasodilation than does dobutamine.

b. Milrinone causes more vasodilation than dobutamine, so using it in a hypotensive patient is not recommended until the BP is restored to a more optimum level.

c. Diltiazem is a calcium channel blocker and has negative inotropic and chronotropic activity and will not increase the cardiac output.

d. Metoprolol is a beta-blocker and has negative inotropic and chronotropic activity and will not increase the cardiac output.

(Bhat et al., 2014, pp. 154–156).

41 **The correct answer is D.**

Rationales:

a. AV reentrant tachycardia is often seen in WPW syndrome.

b. Atrial flutter is often seen in WPW syndrome.

c. Atrial fibrillation is often seen in WPW syndrome.

d. AV block is usually not seen in WPW syndrome.

(Bhat et al., 2014, p. 189).

Clinical Pearl

The arrhythmias most often associated with Wolff-Parkinson-White syndrome are AV reentrant tachycardia, atrial flutter, and atrial fibrillation.

42 **The correct answer is A.**

Rationales:

a. Aspirin is recommended as the antiplatelet agent of choice to reduce saphenous vein graft closure as per the most recent research studies and guidelines.

b. Unfractionated heparin effect occurs by the deactivation of thrombin and the activated factor X and as a result prevents fibrin formation and inhibits thrombin-induced activation of platelets and factors V and VIII. Research has found aspirin to be superior in preventing saphenous vein graft closure.

c. Low molecular weight heparin has a reduced ability to inactivate thrombin; however, it still inactivates factor Xa. Research has found aspirin to be superior in preventing saphenous vein graft closure.

d. Argatroban stops the activation of factors V, VIII, and XIII and protein C and inhibits platelet aggregation. Research has shown aspirin to be superior in preventing saphenous vein graft closure.

(Hillis, 2011, p. e149).

43 **The correct answer is D.**

Rationales:

a. Class I antiarrhythmics agents block the voltage gated sodium channels such as lidocaine, quinidine, and flecainide.

b. Class II antiarrhythmic agents are those that inhibit or activate the autonomic nervous system such as beta-blockers, muscarinic receptor inhibitors such as atropine and digoxin, and adenosine receptor activators such as adenosine.

c. Class III antiarrhythmics are drugs that affect the potassium channels such as amiodarone or sotalol.

d. Class IV antiarrhythmics are drugs that affect the calcium channels such as calcium channel blockers.

(Lei et al., 2018, p. 1879–1896).

44 **The correct answer is B.**

Rationales:

a. Class II antiarrhythmic agents are those that inhibit or activate the autonomic nervous system such as beta-blockers, muscarinic receptor inhibitors such as atropine and digoxin, and adenosine receptor activators such as adenosine.

b. Class III antiarrhythmics are drugs that affect the potassium channels such as amiodarone or sotalol.

c. Class IV antiarrhythmics are drugs that affect the calcium channels such as calcium channel blockers.

d. Class II antiarrhythmic agents are those that inhibit or activate the autonomic nervous system such as beta-blockers, muscarinic

receptor inhibitors such as atropine and digoxin, and adenosine receptor activators such as adenosine.

(Lei et al., 2018, pp. 1879–1896).

45 **The correct answer is B.**

Rationales:

a. Hydrochlorothiazide has not been found to reduce cardiovascular disease risk.

b. Chlorthalidone has a long half-life and has been proven to reduce cardiovascular disease risk.

c. Furosemide has not been found to reduce cardiovascular risk.

d. Spironolactone has not been found to reduce cardiovascular risk.

(Whelton, 2018, p. e190).

46 **The correct answer is B.**

Rationales:

a. The latest guidelines recommend 150 minutes of moderate-intensity exercise to prevent cardiovascular disease, not 200 minutes.

b. The latest guidelines recommend 150 minutes of moderate-intensity exercise to prevent cardiovascular disease.

c. The latest guidelines recommend 150 minutes of moderate-intensity exercise to prevent cardiovascular disease, not 100 minutes.

d. The latest guidelines recommend 150 minutes of moderate-intensity exercise to prevent cardiovascular disease, not 75 minutes.

(Arnett et al., 2019).

47 **The correct answer is D.**

Rationales:

a. 3 months is insufficient. Twelve months is recommended as the minimum time a patient should be on dual antiplatelet therapy with a bare metal or drug-eluting stent placed for acute coronary syndrome.

b. 6 months is insufficient. Twelve months is recommended as the minimum time a patient should be on dual antiplatelet therapy with a bare metal or drug-eluting stent placed for acute coronary syndrome.

c. 9 months is insufficient. Twelve months is recommended as the minimum time a patient should be on dual antiplatelet therapy with a bare metal or drug-eluting stent placed for acute coronary syndrome.

d. The latest guidelines recommend patients who have had a bare metal or drug-eluting stent placed for acute coronary syndrome, be on dual antiplatelet therapy for at least 12 months.

(Levine et al., 2016, p. 1092).

48 **The correct answer is A.**

Rationales:

a. The latest recommendations state elective noncardiac surgery should be delayed 30 days for bare metal stents and optimally 6 months for drug-eluting stents.

b. The latest recommendations state elective noncardiac surgery should be delayed 30 days for bare metal stents and optimally 6 months for drug-eluting stents.

c. The latest recommendations state elective noncardiac surgery should be delayed 30 days for bare metal stents and optimally 6 months for drug-eluting stents.

d. The latest recommendations state elective noncardiac surgery should be delayed 30 days for bare metal stents and optimally 6 months for drug-eluting stents.

(Levine et al., 2016, p. 1100).

49 **The correct answer is C.**

Rationales:

a. The latest recommendations state elective noncardiac surgery should be delayed 30 days for bare metal stents and optimally 6 months for drug-eluting stents.

b. The latest recommendations state elective noncardiac surgery should be delayed 30 days for bare metal stents and optimally 6 months for drug-eluting stents.

c. The latest recommendations state elective noncardiac surgery should be delayed 30 days for bare metal stents and optimally 6 months for drug-eluting stents.

d. The latest recommendations state elective noncardiac surgery should be delayed 30 days for bare metal stents and optimally 6 months for drug-eluting stents.

(Levine et al., 2016, p. 1100).

Clinical Pearl

Patients with bare metal stents should avoid elective noncardiac surgery for 30 days post placement and patients with drug-eluting stents should avoid elective noncardiac surgery optimally for 6 months.

50 **The correct answer is A.**

Rationales:

a. In patients who have atrial fibrillation and a CHA2DS2-VASc score of 0, it is reasonable to omit antithrombotic therapy.

b. With a CHA2DS2-VASc score of 0, there is no need to start the patient on a direct oral anticoagulant.

c. With a CHA2DS2-VASc score of 0, there is no need to start the patient on a direct oral anticoagulant with aspirin.

d. With a CHA2DS2-VASc score of 0, there is no indication to perform an ablation.

(Craig et al., 2019, p. 13).

51 **The correct answer is B.**

Rationales:

a. An anterior MI would reveal ST elevations in leads V2 and V3.

b. A lateral MI would reveal ST elevations in leads I, aVL, V5, and V6.

c. An inferior MI would reveal ST elevations in leads II, III, and AvF.

d. A posterior MI would reveal ST depression in the septal and anterior leads (V1–V4) and the patient may have ST elevation in leads II, III, and AVF if an inferior MI is also present.

(Thaler, 2015, p. 241).

52 **The correct answer is C.**

Rationales:

a. The clopidogrel loading dose is 300 mg and the 75-mg dose is the daily recommended dose.

b. Prasugrel loading dose is 60 mg, not 180 mg.

c. Ticagrelor loading dose is 180 mg.

d. Ticagrelor 90 mg twice a day is the maintenance dose.

(O'Gara et al., 2016, p. e92).

53 **The correct answer is A.**

Rationales:

a. For patients having a STEMI who go to a PCI-capable hospital, first medical contact to device time is 90 minutes or less.

b. For patients having a STEMI who go to a PCI-capable hospital, first medical contact to device time is 90 minutes or less.

c. For patients having a STEMI who go to a PCI-capable hospital, first medical contact to device time is 90 minutes or less.

d. For patients having a STEMI who go to a PCI-capable hospital, first medical contact to device time is 90 minutes or less.

(O'Gara et al., 2016, p. e86).

54 **The correct answer is C.**

Rationales:

a. Heart failure with an ejection fraction less than or equal to 40% is considered reduced ejection fraction.

b. Heart failure with an ejection fraction of greater than or equal to 50 is considered preserved ejection fraction.

c. Heart failure with an ejection fraction between 41 and 49 is considered borderline ejection fraction.

d. A patient with acute decompensation has a reduced ejection fraction from baseline.

(Yancy, 2013, pp. 153–155).

55 **The correct answer is D.**

Rationales:

a. Patients in acute decompensated heart failure/pulmonary edema should receive a loop diuretic at least equal to or greater than their daily dose. The patient is receiving 80 mg daily; 20 mg IV is not adequate.

b. Patients in acute decompensated heart failure/pulmonary edema should receive a loop diuretic at least equal to or greater than their daily dose. The patient is receiving 80 mg daily; 40 mg IV is not adequate.

c. Patients in acute decompensated heart failure/pulmonary edema should receive a loop diuretic at least equal to or greater than their daily dose. The patient is receiving 80 mg daily; 60 mg IV is not adequate.

d. Patients in acute decompensated heart failure/pulmonary edema should receive a loop diuretic at least equal to or greater than their daily dose. The patient is receiving 80 mg daily; therefore, 80 mg IV is an adequate dose.

(Yancy, 2013, p. 194).

56 **The correct answer is C.**

Rationales:

a. ACE inhibitors are not usually associated with lower extremity edema.

b. Beta-blockers are not usually associated with lower extremity edema.

c. Dihydropyridines are associated with the side effect of lower extremity edema.

d. Alpha blockers are not usually associated with lower extremity edema.

(Arcangelo et al., 2017, pp. 298–299).

> **Clinical Pearl**
>
> Dihydropyridines may cause lower extremity edema in some patients.

57 **The correct answer is A.**

Rationales:

a. Nitrates are contraindicated in patients who have taken a phosphodiesterase type 5 inhibitor such as sildenafil.

b. Beta-blockers are not contraindicated with nitrates.

c. Morphine is not contraindicated with nitrates.

d. Heparin is not contraindicated with nitrates.

(Bhat et al., 2014, p. 102).

58 **The correct answer is D.**

Rationales:

a. Acute pulmonary embolism is associated with acute shortness of breath, hypoxemia, and sometimes chest discomfort.

b. Acute coronary syndrome is associated with chest pain that radiates to the neck and left arm and is associated with diaphoresis, shortness of breath, and nausea.

c. Pneumothorax is associated with shortness of breath, chest discomfort, and decreased breath sounds on the affected side.

d. Costochondritis is associated with chest pain, which is more prevalent on the affected side, and it is worse with movement and deep breathing. The patient will often complain of tenderness across the costochondral joints and sternoclavicular joint and rib tenderness.

(Bhat et al., 2014, p. 297).

59 **The correct answer is A.**

Rationales:

a. Digoxin toxicity is associated with bradycardia, hypotension, nausea, vomiting, diarrhea, lethargy, weakness, confusion, and seeing yellow halos around objects.

b. ACE inhibitor toxicity is associated with dizziness, hypotension, headache, hyperkalemia, abdominal pain, and elevated creatinine.

c. Beta-blocker toxicity is associated with bradycardia, dizziness, diarrhea, and heart failure exacerbation, but the patient does not see yellow halos around objects.

d. Calcium channel blocker toxicity is associated with bradycardia, dizziness, and diarrhea, but the patient does not see yellow halos around objects.

(Arcangelo et al., 2017, pp. 88–89).

60 **The correct answer is C.**

Rationales:

a. Atropine often doesn't work well in beta-blocker overdose due to the sympathetic blockade of the beta receptors by the beta-blocker.

b. Epinephrine will not work well in beta-blocker overdose due to the blockade of the beta receptors.

c. Glucagon is the drug of choice because it activates cyclic adenosine monophosphate (AMP) that increases the amount of calcium availability during depolarization, which augments contractility and HR.

d. Digoxin immune fab is ineffective in beta-blocker poisoning.

(Bhat et al., 2014, pp. 901–904).

References

Advanced Cardiac Life Support (2015). 16th ed. American Heart Association.

Arcangelo, V., et al. (2017). *Pharmacotherapeutics for advanced practice* (4th ed., p. 296). Philadelphia, PA: Wolters Kluwer.

Arnett, D., et al. (2019). 2019 ACC/AHA guideline on primary prevention of cardiovascular disease. *Journal of the American College of Cardiology, 74*(10), e177–e232.

Bhat, P., et al. (2014). *The Washington manual of medical therapeutics* (35th ed., p. 429). Philadelphia, PA: Wolters Kluwer.

Bickley, L. (2017). *Bates' guide to physical examination and history taking* (12th ed., p. 348). Philadelphia, PA: Wolters Kluwer.

Craig, T., et al. (2019). 2019 AHA/ACC/HRS focused update of the 2014 guideline for the management of patients with atrial fibrillation. *Journal of the American College of Cardiology, 13.* Prepress.

Gilbert, D. N., Eliopoulos, G. M., Chambers, H. F., & Saag, M. S. (2019). *The Sanford guide to antimicrobial therapy* 2019. Sperryville, VA: Antimicrobial Therapy, Inc.

Grundy, S., et al. (2019). 2018 Guideline on the management of blood cholesterol. *Journal of the American College of Cardiology, 73*(24), e324.

Hillis, L. D. (2011). 2011 ACCF/AHA guideline for coronary artery bypass graft surgery. *Journal of the American College of Cardiology, 58*(24), e149.

Kannam, J., & Gersh, B. (2019). Beta blockers in the management of stable ischemic heart disease. *UpToDate.*

Lei, M., et al. (2018). Modernized classification of cardiac antiarrhythmic drugs. *Circulation, 138,* 1879–1896.

Levine, G., et al. (2016). Guideline for percutaneous coronary intervention/DAPT focused update. *Journal American College of Cardiology, 68*(10), 1092.

Linden, H. (2019). Treatment of Lyme disease. *UpToDate.*

O'Gara, P., et al. (2016). Focused update of the 2012 guideline for the management of ST-elevation myocardial infarction. *Journal of the American College of Cardiology, 61*(4), e92.

Thaler, M. (2015). *The only EKG book you'll ever need* (p. 241). Philadelphia, PA: Wolters Kluwer.

Vaeskar, M., & Craig, T. (2012). ACE inhibitor induced angioedema. *Current Allergy Asthma Report, 12,* 72–78.

Whelton, P. (2018). 2017 Guideline for prevention, detection, evaluation and management of high blood pressure in adults. *Journal of the American College of Cardiology, 71*(19), e188.

Yancy, C. (2013). 2013 ACCF/AHA Guideline for the management of heart failure. *Journal of the American College of Cardiology, 62*(16), 153–155.

Yancy, C., et al. (2017). ACCF/AHA guideline for the management of heart failure/Focused update. *Journal of the American College of Cardiology, 62*(16), 155–194.

CHAPTER 5

Pulmonology

Brenda Engler, MSN, CRNP, AGACNP-BC and Elizabeth Wirth-Tomaszewski, DNP, CRNP, CCRN, ACNP-BC, ACNPC

Disease Questions

1 Auscultation of the chest can provide information about a possible differential diagnosis. How can crackles that indicate possible interstitial lung disease or pulmonary edema be described?

a. Gentle, rustling type sounds that are heard in the lung periphery throughout inspiration and softer during expiration

b. Discontinuous sounds that are brief, are nonmusical, and have a popping quality

c. Continuous sounds that are sonorous, are low-pitched, and often have a gurgling quality

d. Continuous sounds that may be heard on inspiration and/or expiration that are musical, are high-pitched, and may have a whistling quality

2 A 73-year-old nursing home resident presents to the emergency department with hypoxia after vomiting and aspirating gastric contents. What is the treatment for acute aspiration of gastric contents?

a. Supplemental oxygen; coughing and deep breathing; monitor for infection

b. Supplemental oxygen, piperacillin–tazobactam 4.5 g IV every 8 hours, and vancomycin per weight-based dosing

c. Supplemental oxygen and ampicillin–sulbactam 3 g IV every 6 hours

d. Supplemental oxygen, piperacillin–tazobactam 4.5 g IV every 8 hours, and fluconazole 400 mg IV daily

3 The pathophysiology that causes the hypoxia in acute pulmonary embolus can be described as:

a. Increased alveolar dead space

b. Bronchospasm secondary to decreased pulmonary blood flow

c. Left to right pulmonary shunting

d. Pulmonary edema secondary to pulmonary hypertension

4 A patient returns to the hospital following knee replacement surgery 2 weeks ago. The patient has been relatively sedentary since discharge. He states that he developed swelling of his entire left leg yesterday and now has developed shortness of breath. He was placed on nasal cannula oxygen, which improved his hypoxia, but he continues to have some tachypnea and tachycardia. You suspect a deep vein thrombosis and pulmonary embolus. You would expect which of the following blood gas results to support your diagnosis?

a. Decreased pH, increased pCO_2, low normal pO_2, normal bicarbonate

b. Decreased pH, normal pCO_2, low normal pO_2, decreased bicarbonate

c. Increased pH, decreased pCO_2, low normal pO_2, normal bicarbonate

d. Increased pH, normal pCO_2, low normal pO_2, increased bicarbonate

5 A patient is diagnosed with a saddle pulmonary embolus by computerized tomography. He has a blood pressure of 88/54, heart rate of 128, respiratory rate of 36, and pulse oximetry of 92% on nonrebreather oxygen. There are no noted contraindications for any possible therapies, and the patient states that he is agreeable with whatever treatment is deemed most appropriate. The following medication should be started immediately:

a. Unfractionated heparin infusion

b. Low molecular weight heparin subcutaneous daily

c. Intravenous alteplase bolus

d. Low molecular weight heparin subcutaneous twice daily

6 The adult-gerontology acute care nurse practitioner (AGACNP) is called to admit a patient with a small spontaneous primary pneumothorax for observation. When remembering the type of patients who are likely to develop a spontaneous primary pneumothorax, the AGACNP expects to be treating which of the following patients?

a. A 25-year-old tall thin male tobacco smoker with no other past medical history

b. A 47-year-old thin incarcerated woman with a history of pulmonary tuberculosis

c. A 64-year-old thin male tobacco smoker with a history of emphysema

d. A 35-year-old thin woman with a history of human immunodeficiency virus (HIV) and pneumocystis pneumonia

7 Assessment findings that are present for a patient with a pneumothorax include which of the following?

a. Decreased tactile fremitus, diminished breath sounds, dullness to percussion, and trachea midline

b. Increased tactile fremitus, diminished breath sounds, dullness to percussion, and trachea midline or towards the affected side

c. Increased tactile fremitus, coarse breath sounds, resonance to percussion, and trachea midline

d. Decreased tactile fremitus, diminished breath sounds, hyperresonance to percussion, and trachea midline or shifted away from the affected side

8 A rapid response is called for a patient with sudden onset of severe shortness of breath. The 38-year-old female with a past medical history of IV drug abuse was admitted with necrotizing pneumonia and has been on antibiotics and bronchodilators. She had an episode of coughing and then has become progressively more dyspneic. Her vital signs are heart rate 136, respiratory rate 42, blood pressure 86/44, and pulse oximeter of 88% on nonrebreather oxygen. Physical examination reveals trachea deviated to the right, hyperresonance to percussion on the left, and wheezing noted on auscultation with diminished breath sounds on the left. The first step in your treatment plan should be:

a. High-flow nasal cannula oxygen; nebulized inhaled bronchodilator; obtain chest radiograph

b. Noninvasive ventilation; crystalloid fluid bolus; prepare for possible need for vasopressors; obtain chest radiograph

c. Endotracheal intubation; start vasopressors; crystalloid fluid bolus; broaden antibiotic therapy; obtain chest radiograph after intubation

d. Needle decompression, small-bore chest tube placement to suction, obtain chest radiograph after procedures

9 A patient presents with increased shortness of breath after recently starting treatment for community-acquired pneumonia. He has face and mouth swelling without hives and is diagnosed with angioedema. When evaluating the medication list for a possible cause, which of the following drugs would be considered the most likely cause?

a. Azithromycin

b. Lisinopril

c. Furosemide

d. Famotidine

10 Patients with moderate persistent asthma have which of the following characteristics?

a. Symptoms ≤2 days per week, rescue inhaler use ≤2 days per week, nighttime awakenings ≤2 times per month, and no activity intolerance

b. Symptoms greater than 2 days per week but not daily, rescue inhaler use greater than 2 days per week but not daily and not more than once a day, nighttime awakenings 3–4 times per month, and minor activity intolerance

c. Symptoms daily, rescue inhaler use daily, nighttime awakenings greater than 1 time per week but not nightly, and some activity intolerance

d. Symptoms throughout the day, rescue inhaler use several times per day, nighttime awakenings often nightly, and significant activity intolerance

11 What is the first therapy for the treatment of an acute asthma attack?

a. Inhaled short-acting beta-adrenergic agonist

b. Inhaled long-acting beta-adrenergic agonist

c. Inhaled corticosteroid

d. Parenteral corticosteroid

12 A 28-year-old female patient is being treated for an acute asthma attack. The patient is receiving a continuous nebulized beta-adrenergic agonist and has been placed on noninvasive ventilation. She complains of continued shortness of breath despite treatment and feeling very tired. Her physical examination shows significant respiratory accessory muscle use and diminished breath sounds throughout with no wheezing. Her recent blood gas is as follows: pH 7.42, pCO_2 45, pO_2 102, and bicarbonate 25. The treatment step for this patient would be which of the following?

a. Continue noninvasive ventilation at current settings.

b. Increase expiratory positive airway pressure.

c. Increase the inspiratory positive airway pressure.

d. Prepare to place the patient on invasive mechanical ventilation.

13 A 56-year-old female is being admitted to the hospital with dyspnea. She states that this is the 2nd year that she has had a respiratory illness that has lasted several months. She had mucus production every day for over 4 months last year and has now had a productive cough for 3 months this year. Which of the following diagnoses can be added to this patient's medical history?

a. Emphysema

b. Asthma

c. Chronic bronchitis

d. Pneumonia

14 The typical chest x-ray (CXR) findings on a patient admitted with an exacerbation of emphysema can be described as:

a. Decreased vascular markings at the apices and hyperinflation with flattened diaphragms

b. Increased interstitial markings with normal diaphragms

c. Kerley B lines with blunted costophrenic angles

d. Diffuse patchy infiltrates noted bilaterally

15 The single most important intervention to slow the progression of chronic obstructive pulmonary disease (COPD) is:

a. Compliance with inhaled bronchodilator regimen

b. Use of inhaled corticosteroids

c. Exercise programs

d. Smoking cessation

16 A patient is hospitalized with an exacerbation of COPD by the medicine team and treatment was started with nasal cannula oxygen, inhaled bronchodilators, and antibiotics. Steroids are the fourth component of the treatment regimen. For a hospitalized patient with an acute exacerbation of COPD, the drug regimen for most patients is:

a. Inhaled budesonide nebulizer

b. Prednisone 30–40 mg oral daily for 5–10 days

c. Methylprednisolone 60 mg intravenous every 6 hours for 5–10 days

d. Methylprednisolone 1,000 mg intravenous daily for 3 days

17 A 64-year-old male presents to the hospital with worsening shortness of breath. He has limited his activities over the last several months as his shortness of breath makes it difficult to even climb a few stairs. His CXR shows hazy infiltrates over the lower lung zones, thickened pleura, and calcified plaques on the lateral chest walls and diaphragms. He states he has had several occupations over the years in construction and different types of factories. The preliminary diagnosis for this patient is:

a. Asbestosis

b. Pneumonia

c. Congestive heart failure

d. COPD

18 The AGACNP is notified by nursing staff of a patient complaining of a headache. Consistent with previously documented examination, the patient is slow to respond to questions and falls asleep when not stimulated. A dose of acetaminophen was reportedly minimally effective in relief of the headache a few hours ago. Review of laboratory tests is only notable for a carboxyhemoglobin level of 40% on 15 L of oxygen via a nonrebreather mask. Vital signs include heart rate 92, blood pressure 168/84, respiratory rate 24, and pulse oximeter 100%.

The next step in treatment would be which of the following?

a. Oxycodone 5 mg every 4 hours as needed for headache.

b. Titrate down the oxygen for goal pulse oximeter 88%–92% to treat hypercarbia.

c. Labetalol 20 mg IV now to treat hypertension as likely cause of headache.

d. Continue oxygen via nonrebreather mask.

19 Community-acquired pneumonia that requires hospitalization, but not admission to the intensive care unit, is a common diagnosis for the medicine team. The most appropriate antibiotic choice for a patient admitted to the medicine team to cover the diagnosis of community-acquired pneumonia without any risk factors for resistant organisms is:

a. Ceftriaxone

b. Ceftriaxone and azithromycin

c. Piperacillin–tazobactam

d. Cefepime and vancomycin

20 When deciding to admit patients to the hospital for community-acquired pneumonia, it is important to admit patients to prevent morbidity and mortality in patients who have higher severity of illness while preventing unnecessary hospital admissions. The CURB-65 can aid in the decision process. When calculating the CURB-65, the nurse practitioner notes which of the following components of the tool?

a. Confusion, urea (blood urea nitrogen [BUN]) greater than 20, respiratory rate greater than 30, blood pressure less than 90, and age greater than 65

b. Confusion, urea (BUN) greater than 30, respiratory rate greater than 20, blood pressure less than 100, and age greater than 65

c. Confusion, urea (BUN) greater than 30, respiratory rate greater than 30, blood pressure less than 100, and age greater than 65

d. Confusion, urea (BUN) greater than 30, respiratory rate greater than 20, blood pressure less than 90, and age greater than 65

21 A patient presents with cough, fever, chills, fatigue, anorexia, weight loss, and night sweats, and a diagnosis of tuberculosis is suspected. He had close contact with a person who is actively being treated for tuberculosis. While awaiting the sputum testing for mycobacterium tuberculosis, a purified protein derivative (PPD) screen was placed. When reading the PPD, you recall that an induration of what size is significant in this population?

a. 5 mm

b. 10 mm

c. 15 mm

d. 20 mm

22 Treatment for active tuberculosis is important to prevent the spread of the disease. Initial antibiotic therapy for active pulmonary tuberculosis should include:

a. Isoniazid and rifampin for 2 weeks

b. Isoniazid, cefepime, and vancomycin for 2 months

c. Isoniazid, rifampin, pyrazinamide, and ethambutol for 2 months

d. Isoniazid and rifampin for 4 months

23 The Light criteria are used to evaluate a pleural effusion. The AGACANP notes that the pleural fluid protein to serum protein ratio is greater than 0.5 and the pleural fluid lactate dehydrogenase (LDH) to serum LDH ratio is greater than 0.6. Using these diagnostic criteria, the likely cause of the pleural effusion would be:

a. Possible malignancy as the fluid is classified as transudate

b. Possible malignancy as the fluid is classified as exudate

c. Possible cirrhosis as the fluid is classified as transudate

d. Possible cirrhosis as the fluid is classified as exudate

24 A patient's pleural effusion was classified as a transudate with a pH of less than 7.2, and an empyema was diagnosed. The patient has been on antibiotics for 2 weeks that per sensitivities are appropriate to cover the organism present within the pleural drainage. A moderate-size loculated pleural effusion remains despite chest tube placement to drain the effusion. The next appropriate step for this patient would be which of the following?

a. More aggressive chest physiotherapy to assist in drainage of the pleural effusion.

b. Escalate antibiotic therapy to a more broad-spectrum choice to cover additional organisms.

c. Consult thoracic surgery for possible lung decortication.

d. Aggressive diuresis with scheduled furosemide to decrease the size of the pleural effusion.

25 A 48-year-old male was admitted to the hospital with progressive shortness of breath following a week-long illness of gastrointestinal symptoms of nausea and vomiting. He does have a history of esophagectomy for adenocarcinoma but has been doing well and eating a normal oral diet prior to the last week. A pleural effusion with infiltrate versus compressive atelectasis is noted on the CXR. A thoracentesis is completed with pleural fluid sent for testing. What is the best test of the pleural fluid to determine if the pleural effusion is parapneumonic due to aspiration pneumonia or a pleural effusion related to esophageal rupture?

a. Protein

b. Glucose

c. Red blood cells

d. Amylase

26 There are many different diseases that can cause interstitial lung disease. While the symptoms of progressive dyspnea on exertion and diffuse reticular infiltrates or ground-glass opacities are present in these patients, spirometry is an essential part of the diagnosis. What are the typical findings on the spirometry for a patient with interstitial lung disease?

a. Decreased forced expiratory volume in one second (FEV1)/forced vital capacity (FVC), normal or decreased FVC, decreased FEV1—obstructive pattern

b. Normal or increased FEV1/FVC, decreased FVC, normal or decreased FEV1—restrictive pattern

c. Decreased FEV1/FVC, decreased FVC, decreased FEV1—restrictive pattern

d. Normal or increased FEV1/FVC, decreased FVC, normal or decreased FEV1—obstructive pattern

27 When performing spirometry, the forced vital capacity is defined as which of the following?

a. The amount of gas exhaled at maximum speed after maximal inhalation

b. The amount of gas exhaled during a forceful breath within 1 second

c. The total amount of gas in the lungs at the end of maximal inhalation

d. The amount of gas in the lungs at the end of exhalation of a resting breath

28 Spirometry is ordered to classify the severity of chronic obstructive lung disease during preoperative testing on a patient. Patient has an FEV1 60%. Based on Global Initiative for Obstructive Lung Disease (GOLD) criteria, the AGACNP interprets the spirometry and place the patient in what classification?

a. Mild obstructive lung disease

b. Moderate obstructive lung disease

c. Severe obstructive lung disease

d. None of the above

29 A 29-year-old male presents with a moderate-size hemothorax following a motor vehicle crash with anterior rib 6–9 fractures. No other injuries were noted on his examination. Vital signs are heart rate 104, respiratory rate 22, blood pressure 118/54, and pulse oximetry 96% on 4 L/min nasal cannula oxygen. The next appropriate step for management of this patient would be which of the following?

a. Admit for observation of respiratory status and place chest tube if respiratory status worsens.

b. Place a small-bore chest tube in the 2nd intercostal space midclavicular line.

c. Place a small-bore chest tube in the 5th intercostal space midaxillary line.

d. Place a large-bore chest tube in the 5th intercostal space midaxillary line.

30 A patient is referred to pulmonary medicine for likely pulmonary hypertension. What is the best way to diagnose and quantify pulmonary hypertension prior to starting medical therapy?

a. Cardiac catheterization

b. Transthoracic echocardiogram

c. Transesophageal echocardiogram

d. Spirometry

31 A solitary pulmonary nodule of 1 cm is noted on a computed tomography (CT) of the chest that was completed as part of a workup for a trauma admission for a 27-year-old female nonsmoker. The nodule has distinct margins and appears calcified. The patient is stable to be discharged from a trauma perspective. What is the follow-up that should be recommended to the patient?

a. Repeat high-resolution CT in 3–6 months with follow-up with primary care provider for likely benign lesion

b. Repeat CT in 1 week with follow-up with primary care provider for likely malignant lesion

c. Referral to thoracic surgery for biopsy for likely malignant lesion

d. Repeat CT in 1 year with follow-up with primary care provider for likely malignant lesion

32 A patient complains of excessive fatigue and falling asleep during the day. He states that he never feels completely rested in the morning and has awakened at night at times due to snoring. His vital signs include heart rate 88, blood pressure 148/98, respiratory rate 16, pulse oximetry 96% on room air, and body mass index (BMI) of 48. What is the next step to treat this patient's symptoms?

a. Recommend over-the-counter diphenhydramine at bedtime to improve sleep.

b. Prescribe zolpidem to help with falling into a better sleep.

c. Prescribe temazepam to help with falling asleep and staying asleep.

d. Polysomnography and weight loss counseling.

33 A 33-year-old male presents with a 2-day history of hemoptysis. He also has lab data consistent with acute glomerulonephritis. He has been feeling unwell for several weeks, and has no sick contacts recently. Further lab data reveal a normocytic anemia, and his CXR reveals bilateral alveolar infiltrates. The AGACNP would order which of the following to confirm a diagnosis of Goodpasture syndrome?

a. Peripheral smear

b. Anti–glomerular basement membrane antibody

c. Iron panel

d. C reactive protein (CRP) and complements

Disease Answers/Rationales

1 **The correct answer is B.**

Rationales:

a. Vesicular breath sounds are gentle, rustling type sounds that are heard throughout inspiration and softer during expiration and are found throughout normal lung fields except over the suprasternal notch where bronchial breath sounds are noted.

b. Crackles are discontinuous, brief, nonmusical sounds that have a popping quality and may indicate possible interstitial lung disease or pulmonary edema.

c. Rhonchi are continuous, sonorous, low-pitched sounds that often have a gurgling quality and are due to rupture of fluid films in the larger airways due to excess secretions and abnormal airway collapsibility.

d. Wheezes are continuous, musical, high-pitched sounds that may be heard on inspiration and/or expiration and may have a whistling quality caused by airway narrowing to the point where airflow is limited. The airflow limitation causes airway walls to flutter producing the sound and can be caused by bronchospasm, excessive secretions, and mucosal edema.

(Papadakis & McPhee, 2018).

2 **The correct answer is A.**

Rationales:

a. Treatment of acute aspiration of gastric contents consists of simple nasal oxygen, airway maintenance, and treatment of respiratory failure. There's no evidence to suggest that antibiotics are required.

b. This option includes antibiotics appropriate for health care–associated pneumonia.

c. This option includes antibiotics appropriate for community-acquired pneumonia.

d. This option includes some antibiotics that are appropriate for immunocompromised hosts.

(Papadakis & McPhee, 2018, p. 317).

3 **The correct answer is A.**

Rationales:

a. Increased alveolar dead space leads to poor estimation through right to left shunting.

b. Bronchospasm is not associated with pulmonary embolism nor pulmonary blood flow.

c. Shunting occurs from right to left, not left to right.

d. Pulmonary hypertension causes pulmonary edema, as opposed to the reverse.

(Papadakis & McPhee, 2018, p. 306).

4 **The correct answer is C.**

Rationales:

a. Decreased pH, increased pCO_2, low normal pO_2, and normal bicarbonate indicate respiratory acidosis, which is commonly seen in air trapping and hypoventilation.

b. Decreased pH, normal pCO_2, low normal pO_2, and decreased bicarbonate indicate metabolic acidosis.

c. Increased pH, decreased pCO_2, low normal pO_2, and normal bicarbonate indicate respiratory alkalosis, which is commonly seen in pulmonary embolus as the patient increases the respiratory rate to attempt to compensate for hypoxemia related to the pulmonary embolus.

d. Increased pH, normal pCO_2, low normal pO_2, and increased bicarbonate indicate metabolic alkalosis.

(Papadakis & McPhee, 2018, p. 307).

5 **The correct answer is C.**

Rationales:

a. Unfractionated heparin infusion is one of the treatment options for low- to moderate-risk pulmonary embolus.

b. Low molecular weight heparin subcutaneous daily is used for prophylaxis dosing for deep vein thrombosis prevention.

c. Intravenous alteplase bolus is the treatment of choice for a pulmonary embolus that is considered severe or high risk, which is indicated by the tachycardia greater than 110, hypotension less than 100 systolic, and relative hypoxia on nonrebreather oxygen.

d. Low molecular weight heparin subcutaneous twice daily is a treatment option for low- to moderate-risk pulmonary embolus.

(Papadakis & McPhee, 2018, p. 309).

6 **The correct answer is A.**

Rationales:

a. A spontaneous primary pneumothorax is commonly seen in young thin males with no additional past medical history.

b. A patient with pulmonary tuberculosis has a risk for secondary pneumothorax, not primary pneumothorax.

c. A patient with emphysema has a risk for secondary pneumothorax, not primary pneumothorax.

d. A patient with pneumocystis pneumonia and HIV has a risk for secondary pneumothorax, not primary pneumothorax.

(Papadakis & McPhee, 2018, p. 317).

7 **The correct answer is D.**

Rationales:

a. Decreased tactile fremitus, diminished breath sounds, dullness to percussion, and midline trachea can be seen in a patient with a pleural effusion.

b. Increased tactile fremitus, diminished breath sounds, dullness to percussion, and trachea midline or towards the affected side can indicate pneumonia with lung consolidation and atelectasis. The trachea may shift towards the affected side as the alveoli collapse.

c. Increased tactile fremitus, coarse breath sounds, resonance to percussion, and trachea midline can be seen in conditions with secretions without dense consolidation or effusion such as viral pneumonia or COPD exacerbation.

d. Decreased tactile fremitus, diminished breath sounds, hyperresonance to percussion, and trachea midline or shifted away from the affected side indicate a pneumothorax. If the trachea is shifted away from the affected side, it indicates a tension pneumothorax.

(Papadakis & McPhee, 2018, p. 325).

8 **The correct answer is D.**

Rationales:

a. The high-flow nasal cannula can treat the hypoxia temporarily and nebulized inhaled bronchodilator can be used to treat the wheezing, but the tension pneumothorax should be diagnosed by the clinical examination and should be immediately treated as the patient is unstable with hypotension and hypoxemia and likely to decompensate quickly.

b. Noninvasive ventilation will likely worsen the symptoms of the tension pneumothorax by increasing the intrathoracic pressure. Crystalloids and vasopressors can be used to treat hypotension temporarily while supplies are gathered for emergent needle decompression and chest tube placement.

c. Endotracheal intubation and mechanical ventilation will likely worsen the symptoms of the tension pneumothorax by increasing the intrathoracic pressure. Crystalloids and vasopressors can be used to treat hypotension temporarily while supplies are gathered for emergent needle decompression and chest tube placement. If antibiotic therapy is already guided by cultures, then additional antibiotic therapy is not likely necessary.

d. Needle decompression and small-bore chest tube placement to suction is the treatment of choice for pneumothorax. If the patient also has known pleural effusions or fails to expand completely with the small-bore chest tube, a larger tube may be necessary.

(Papadakis & McPhee, 2018, p. 326).

9 **The correct answer is B.**

Rationales:

a. While the patient recently may have started the azithromycin for community-acquired pneumonia, it is not the most likely medication to cause angioedema. An allergic reaction would likely include hives.

b. Even though the lisinopril may be a chronic medication, angiotensin-converting inhibitors are the most likely cause of angioedema, which can happen months or years after starting the medication. The reaction can happen without any known inciting event or may be triggered by an infection or stress. Angioedema without hives is most commonly associated with angiotensin-converting enzyme inhibitor medications.

c. Furosemide is used to treat volume overload and may cause and allergic reaction for patients, especially those with sulfa allergies, but does not commonly cause angioedema.

d. Famotidine is one of the drugs that may be used as part of the treatment of angioedema.

(Papadakis & McPhee, 2018, p. 141).

10 **The correct answer is C.**

Rationales:

a. Patients with intermittent asthma have symptoms ≤2 days per week, rescue inhaler use ≤2 days per week, nighttime awakenings ≤2 times per month, and no activity intolerance.

b. Patients with mild persistent asthma have symptoms greater than 2 days per week but not daily, rescue inhaler use greater than 2 days per week but not daily and not more than once a day, nighttime awakenings 3–4 times per month, and minor activity intolerance.

c. Patients with moderate persistent asthma have symptoms daily, rescue inhaler use daily, nighttime awakenings greater than 1 time per week but not nightly, and some activity intolerance.

d. Patients with severe persistent asthma have symptoms throughout the day, rescue inhaler use several times per day, nighttime awakenings often nightly, and significant activity intolerance.

(Papadakis & McPhee, 2018, p. 256).

11 **The correct answer is A.**

Rationales:

a. Inhaled short-acting beta-adrenergic agonist is the first line in treatment for an acute asthma attack.

b. Long-acting beta-adrenergic agonist should not be used in an acute asthma attack, but may be added for long-term control in moderate persistent asthma.

c. Inhaled corticosteroid should not be used in the treatment of an acute asthma attack but can be started for long-term control in patients with mild persistent asthma.

d. Parenteral corticosteroid may be used as an adjunct in treatment in an acute asthma attack but should not be used as first-line therapy.

(Papadakis & McPhee, 2018, p. 265).

12 **The correct answer is D.**

Rationales:

a. While her arterial blood gas is normal, the patient has continued shortness of breath with signs of impending respiratory failure that include fatigue, accessory muscle use, minimal breath sounds, and high normal pCO_2. Patients with asthma and otherwise normal lung function should have low pCO_2 during an exacerbation. High pCO_2 is an ominous sign for impending respiratory failure.

b. Increasing expiratory positive airway pressure can help splint the airway open and increase oxygenation but will not improve the work of breathing.

c. Increasing the inspiratory positive airway pressure may slightly improve the work of breathing while preparing for intubation, but the patient would benefit more from invasive mechanical ventilation with the impending respiratory failure.

d. Intubation and placement on invasive mechanical ventilation is the appropriate next step for a patient with impending respiratory failure indicated by fatigue, accessory muscle use, minimal breath sounds, and high normal pCO_2. Patients with asthma and otherwise normal lung function should have low pCO_2 during an exacerbation.

(Papadakis & McPhee, 2018, p. 267).

13 **The correct answer is C.**

Rationales:

a. Emphysema has symptoms of exertional dyspnea, weight loss, and minimal cough.

b. Asthma has symptoms of wheezing with difficulty breathing, nonproductive cough, and chest tightness.

c. Chronic bronchitis is defined as productive cough for at least 3 months during each of 2 successive years. Since this patient now has had a productive cough for over 3 months for the 2nd year in a row, she can be diagnosed with chronic bronchitis.

d. Pneumonia is an acute infection that may have sputum production that has changed in color or consistency from baseline mucus production and does not usually extend the course over a period of years.

(Papadakis & McPhee, 2018, p. 269).

14 **The correct answer is A.**

Rationales:

a. Typical findings on a CXR for a patient admitted with an exacerbation of emphysema can be described as decreased vascular markings at the apices and hyperinflation with flattened diaphragms.

b. Increased interstitial markings with normal diaphragms may be seen in patients with interstitial lung disease.

c. Kerley B lines with blunted costophrenic angles is the typical finding on a patient admitted with pulmonary edema related to a congestive heart failure exacerbation.

d. Diffuse patchy infiltrates noted bilaterally is the typical finding on the CXR of a patient admitted with multilobar pneumonia.

(Papadakis & McPhee, 2018, p. 269).

15 **The correct answer is D.**

Rationales:

a. Bronchodilators have little impact on the disease course.

b. Use of inhaled corticosteroids has little impact on the disease course.

c. Exercise programs have little impact on the disease course.

d. Smoking cessation is the single most important intervention to slow the progression of COPD.

(Papadakis & McPhee, 2018, p. 273).

16 **The correct answer is B.**

Rationales:

a. Inhaled corticosteroids are not sufficient for the hospitalized patient.

b. Prednisone is generally sufficient for most patients, with a course as short as 5 days, or as long as 10 days.

c. Intravenous steroids are generally not required unless the patient is critically ill.

d. High-dose steroids are not indicated.

(Papadakis & McPhee, 2018, p. 273).

17 **The correct answer is A.**

Rationales:

a. Construction and factory work are risk factors when considering asbestosis. Pleural calcifications on CXR and progressive shortness of breath may be an indicator of asbestosis.

b. Pneumonia produces infiltrates, not calcified pleural plaques, on CXR.

c. Congestive heart failure appears as prominent pulmonary vasculature with Kerley B lines but does not produce calcified pleural plaques on CXR.

d. COPD appears to have flattened diaphragms and poor markings due to parenchymal deterioration.

(Papadakis & McPhee, 2018, p. 318).

18 **The correct answer is D.**

Rationales:

a. Treating the headache will not affect the elevated carboxyhemoglobin level, which is the root cause of the issue.

b. Carboxyhemoglobin is not a measure of carbon dioxide, rather carbon monoxide. This patient is not suffering from hypercarbia, and the decreased oxygen may be harmful.

c. The headache is likely caused by the elevated levels of carboxyhemoglobin, as opposed to hypertension.

d. Elevated levels of carboxyhemoglobin are treated with 100% oxygen via a nonrebreather mask. Hyperbaric oxygen can be considered as well in those with levels greater than 40%, those with metabolic acidosis, those over 50 years old, and/or those with neurologic deficits on examination.

(Papadakis & McPhee, 2018, p. 1595).

19 **The correct answer is B.**

Rationales:

a. Ceftriaxone alone is not sufficient treatment.

b. A macrolide and a beta-lactam are indicated.

c. Piperacillin–tazobactam is not needed for community-acquired pneumonia that does not require intensive care.

d. Cefepime and vancomycin are utilized in health care–acquired pneumonia.

(Papadakis & McPhee, 2018, p. 279).

20 **The correct answer is A.**

Rationales:

a. Confusion, BUN greater than 20, respiratory rate greater than 30, systolic blood pressure (SBP) lower than 90, and age greater than 65 all are valued at one point. If the score is 0–1, outpatient treatment may be considered. As the score rises, the treatment level escalates as well with intensive care being considered at a score of 4–5, due to mortality risk increasing to greater than 40%.

b. This option has the wrong values.

c. This option has the wrong values.

d. This option has the wrong values.

(Halter et al., 2017, p. 1964).

21 **The correct answer is A.**

Rationales:

a. A purified protein derivative (PPD) with an induration of 5 mm is significant in patients with known of suspected HIV infection, fibrotic lesions on chest radiograph consistent with past healed tuberculosis, or patients with recent close contact of patients with active tuberculosis.

b. A PPD with an induration of 10 mm is significant in patients who are injection drug users, residents of communal living, medically underserved high-risk minorities, and high-risk health conditions.

c. A PPD with an induration of 15 mm is significant in all patients who are not listed in any of the other higher-risk categories.

d. A PPD with an induration of 20 mm is not used as a category, as an induration of 15 mm is significant in all patients.

(Papadakis & McPhee, 2018, p. 291).

㉒ **The correct answer is C.**

Rationales:

a. Isoniazid and rifampin for 2 weeks is not an appropriate length of antibiotic therapy for tuberculosis. Tuberculosis requires a long duration of therapy, which puts patients at risk for noncompliance and spread of the illness.

b. Isoniazid, cefepime, and vancomycin for 2 months is an appropriate length of initial antibiotic therapy, but vancomycin and cefepime are not appropriate antibiotics to treat pulmonary tuberculosis.

c. Isoniazid, rifampin, pyrazinamide, and ethambutol for 2 months is the appropriate regimen of four antibiotics for the initial duration of 2 months. This treatment regimen then needs to be followed by an additional 4 months of double antibiotic therapy with isoniazid and rifampin.

d. Isoniazid and rifampin for 4 months is the appropriate follow-up antibiotic regimen following the initial 2 months of therapy. It is not effective therapy if the initial 2 months of the four-antibiotic regimen is not completed.

(Papadakis & McPhee, 2018, pp. 291–294).

㉓ **The correct answer is B.**

Rationales:

a. Using the Light criteria, if the pleural effusion was transudate, the pleural fluid protein to serum protein ratio would be less than 0.5 and the pleural fluid LDH to serum LDH ratio would be less than 0.6. The effusion noted in the question would be classified as exudate. Also, the fluid associated with possible malignancy is usually classified as exudate.

b. Using the Light criteria, the pleural effusion with the pleural fluid protein to serum protein ratio greater than 0.5 and the pleural fluid LDH to serum LDH ratio greater than 0.6 would be classified as exudate. One of the possible clinical diagnoses associated with an exudative effusion is malignancy.

c. Using the Light criteria, if the pleural effusion was transudate, the pleural fluid protein to serum protein ratio would be less than 0.5 and the pleural fluid LDH to serum LDH ratio would be less than 0.6. The effusion noted in the question would be classified as exudate. The pleural effusion associated with cirrhosis likely be classified as transudate.

d. Using the Light criteria, the pleural effusion with the pleural fluid protein to serum protein ratio greater than 0.5 and the pleural fluid LDH to serum LDH ratio greater than 0.6 would be classified as exudate. The diagnosis of cirrhosis would likely be related to a transudative effusion, not an exudative effusion.

(Light, 2013, p. 88).

㉔ **The correct answer is C.**

Rationales:

a. Chest physiotherapy will not affect a pleural effusion.

b. The antibiotic therapy is appropriate for the sensitivities. Escalating the antibiotics will not provide more effective coverage.

c. Thoracic surgery should be consulted for possible lung decortication versus video assisted thorascopic surgery.

d. Diuresis will not resolve the pleural effusion, as it is an empyema.

(Papadakis & McPhee, 2018, p. 325).

25 **The correct answer is D.**

Rationales:

a. Protein will be present in pleural fluid.

b. Glucose will be present in pleural fluid.

c. Multiple pathologies can cause red blood cells to spill into pleural fluid. This is not specific to aspiration ammonia or esophageal rupture.

d. Amylase is present in saliva, which can indicate a possible gastrointestinal source of the effusion, whether it be aspiration or esophageal rupture.

(Papadakis & McPhee, 2018, p. 324).

26 **The correct answer is C.**

Rationales:

a. These values are representative of a restrictive pattern, not an obstructive pattern.

b. FEV1/FVC would not be normal or increased in pulmonary fibrosis.

c. Interstitial lung disease causes a restrictive pattern with decreased FEV1/FVC, decreased FVC, and decreased FEV1.

d. FEV1/FVC would not be normal or increased in pulmonary fibrosis.

(Kasper et al., 2015, p. 1710).

27 **The correct answer is A.**

Rationales:

a. Forced vital capacity is defined as the amount of gas exhaled at maximum speed after maximal inhalation.

b. FEV1 is the amount of gas exhaled during a forceful breath within 1 second.

c. The total amount of gas in the lungs at the end or maximal inhalation is total lung capacity.

d. The amount of gas in the lungs at the end of exhalation of a resting breath is the functional residual capacity.

(Stockley & Cooper, 2018).

28 **The correct answer is B.**

Rationales:

a. Mild obstructive disease is classified as an FEV1 of greater than 80% predicted.

b. This patient's FEV1 is 60%, which is classified as moderate obstruction.

c. Severe obstruction is defined by FEV1 30%–50% predicted.

d. Answer B is correct.

(Stockley & Cooper, 2018).

29 **The correct answer is D.**

Rationales:

a. A moderate hemothorax should be evacuated to provide optimal lung expansion. Only small hemothoraces may be observed closely without a chest tube.

b. Small-bore chest tubes are not ideal for hemothoraces due to clotting. This location is optimal for pneumothorax due to the apical termination of the tube.

c. Small-bore chest tubes are not ideal for hemothoraces due to clotting, despite correct location.

d. A large-bore tube will facilitate draining of a moderate hemothorax.

(Papadakis & McPhee, 2018, p. 325).

30 **The correct answer is A.**

Rationales:

a. The best way to diagnose and quantify pulmonary hypertension prior to starting therapy is cardiac catheterization.

b. Transthoracic echocardiogram can be useful for screening for possible pulmonary hypertension, but a cardiac catheterization is the best way to confirm the diagnosis and quantify the degree of pulmonary hypertension prior to starting therapy.

c. Transesophageal echocardiograms will give better information on the valves but are not the best way to diagnose and classify pulmonary hypertension.

d. Spirometry is helpful in diagnosing restrictive or obstructive lung diseases but cannot be used to diagnose or quantify pulmonary hypertension.

(Papadakis & McPhee, 2018, p. 313).

31 **The correct answer is A.**

Rationales:

a. A high-resolution CT will provide more information at an interval that would allow for changes to be noted. This lesion is likely benign based on her age, nonsmoking status, distinct margins, and calcifications. Follow-up with her PCP is indicated.

b. Malignant lesions often have spiculated margins and peripheral halos. One week would not allow for enough time to capture changes on imaging.

c. Her lesion is likely benign.

d. Her lesion is likely benign.

(Papadakis & McPhee, 2018, p. 313).

32 **The correct answer is D.**

Rationales:

a. Although diphenhydramine may treat insomnia, this patient is exhibiting symptoms of obstructive sleep apnea (OSA). The root cause must be diagnosed and treated.

b. May be harmful in OSA by decreasing ventilation, and not treating the root cause.

c. May be harmful in OSA by decreasing ventilation, and not treating the root cause.

d. Polysomnography is indicated to determine the cause of his daytime sleepiness, and BMI reduction will assist with obesity hypoventilation.

(Papadakis & McPhee, 2018, p. 328).

33 **The correct answer is B.**

Rationales:

a. A peripheral smear will not confirm Goodpasture syndrome.

b. Linear IgG deposits will appear on glomeruli or on the membrane antibody in the serum when Goodpasture syndrome is present.

c. An iron panel will help diagnose the anemia, but not the Goodpasture syndrome.

d. CRP identifies inflammation, but is nonspecific.

(Papadakis & McPhee, 2018, p. 25).

References

Halter, J. B., Ouslander, J. G., Studenski, S., High, K. P., Asthana, S., Supiano, M. A., & Ritchie, C. (2017). *Hazzard's geriatric medicine and gerontology* (p. 1964). New York, NY: McGraw Hill Education.

Kasper, D. L., Fauci, A. S., Hauser, S. L., Longo, D. L., Jameson, J. L., & Loscalzo, J. (2015). *Harrison's principles of internal medicine* (19th ed., p. 1710). New York, NY: McGraw Hill Education.

Light, R. W. (2013). *Pleural diseases* (6th ed., p. 88). Philadelphia, PA: Wolters Kluwer. Retrieved from http://ebookcentral.proquest.com

Papadakis, M. A., & McPhee, S. J. (2018). *Current medical diagnosis and treatment* (58th ed.). New York, NY: McGraw Hill Education.

Stockley, J. A., & Cooper, B. G. (2018). Breathing out: forced exhalation, airflow limitation. In: D. Kaminsky, & C. Irvin (eds). *Pulmonary function testing. Respiratory medicine.* Cham, Switzerland: Humana Press. https://doi-org.ezproxy2.library.drexel.edu/10.1007/978-3-319-94159-2_6

CHAPTER 6

Gastroenterology

Kristen Scholz, MSN, CRNP, AGACNP

Disease Questions

1 A 34-year-old male presents to the emergency department with complaints of severe epigastric abdominal pain that worsens while lying flat. He finds some relief with sitting upright and leaning forward. His pain is associated with nausea, vomiting, and tachycardia. It developed abruptly after he returned home from a weekend trip that involved a significant amount of alcohol intake. The AGACNP suspects acute pancreatitis. What is the most efficient imaging to evaluate for necrotizing pancreatitis?

a. Plain radiographic films of the abdomen

b. Ultrasonography

c. Unenhanced computed tomography (CT)

d. Rapid bolus intravenous contrast-enhanced CT

2 In the setting of acute pancreatitis, which laboratory values will most likely be elevated despite the etiology?

a. Amylase and lipase

b. White blood cell (WBC)

c. Triglyceride level

d. Alanine aminotransferase (ALT)

3 Which scoring system is specific to the severity and mortality of acute pancreatitis?

a. Clinical Institute withdrawal assessment (CIWA)

b. Sequential organ failure assessment score (SOFA)

c. Ranson criteria

d. Prediction of Alcohol Withdrawal Severity Scale (PAWSS)

4 A 34-year-old male presents to the emergency department with complaints of severe epigastric abdominal pain that worsens while lying flat. He finds some relief with sitting upright and leaning forward. His pain is associated with nausea, vomiting and tachycardia. His lipase level is significantly elevated, and contrast CT of the abdomen and pelvis is showing an edematous pancreas. He is admitted to your service for further management and care. He is noted to be marginally hypotensive on your examination. What is the initial treatment therapy to be started?

a. Normal saline (NS) at 100 mL/hr

b. Crystalloid infusion of 20 mL/kg over 1 hour followed by infusion rates up to 250 mL/hr for the next 24–28 hours to maintain mean arterial pressure (MAP) > 65 mm Hg and urine output > 0.5 mL/kg/hr

c. Addition of vasopressors

d. Prophylactic antibiotic therapy covering gram-negative organisms

5 Jaundice will occur secondary to accumulation of what?

a. Bilirubin

b. Blood urea nitrogen

c. Ammonia

d. Potassium

6 The adult-gerontology acute care nurse practitioner (AGACNP) is caring for a 56-year-old male with a history of cirrhosis. He is admitted with acute on chronic liver failure. He presented with fever, abdominal pain, ascites, and rebound tenderness. His blood cultures are positive for gram-negative bacteria on preliminary results. There is no apparent source of infection on traditional imaging. What is the next most appropriate diagnostic approach?

a. Repeat CT scan of the abdomen; something was likely missed

b. Magnetic resonance cholangiopancreatography (MRCP)

c. Diagnostic paracentesis

d. Ultrasound

7 What is the pathophysiology of the formation of ascites?

a. Hyperbilirubinemia

b. Hyperkalemia

c. Jaundice

d. Sodium retention

8 The AGACNP is caring for a 56-year-old male with a past medical history of cirrhosis. He had tense ascites on examination and is now status post paracentesis. The interventional radiology team reported that they removed 6.5 L of fluid from the patient's abdomen. What is the next appropriation action from the provider?

a. Administer albumin.

b. Observe.

c. Administer lactulose.

d. Administer rifaximin.

9 What is the most measurable toxin related to hepatic encephalopathy?

a. Blood urea nitrogen

b. Ammonia

c. Aspartate aminotransferase (AST)

d. Alanine aminotransferase

10 A 58-year-old male with a history of alcoholic liver cirrhosis presents to the emergency room with recurrent hematemesis. He has had banding of varices in the past. Despite these procedures, he continues to have variceal bleeding noted on endoscopy. What may be the next appropriate procedure for this patient?

a. Transjugular intrahepatic portosystemic shunt (TIPS)

b. Colonoscopy

c. Endoscopic retrograde cholangiopancreatography (ERCP)

d. MRCP

11 The AGACNP is caring for a 39-year-old female with alcoholic cirrhosis. She is admitted with abdominal distention, and pain. Her Model for End-Stage Liver Disease (MELD) score is calculated to be 19. What is the MELD score a predictor of?

a. Likelihood of alcohol withdrawal

b. Three-month mortality risk in patients with cirrhosis

c. Sepsis and septic shock

d. Severity of acute pancreatitis

12 The AGACNP is caring for a patient who has had a lengthy hospitalization for neuroleptic malignant syndrome secondary to abrupt aripiprazole (Abilify) cessation. He has been receiving benzatropine, a medication with anticholinergic properties. He is noted to have elevated tube feeding residuals by the nursing staff. CT scan imaging is suspicious for pseudo-obstruction, also known as Ogilvie syndrome. The colonic dilation is noted to be 8.5 cm. What is the appropriate management?

a. Colonoscopy decompression

b. Neostigmine administration

c. Removal of precipitants and conservative decompression with rectal tube

d. Administration of methylnaltrexone

13 The AGACNP is caring for a 27-year-old female with a sudden onset of right upper quadrant abdominal pain that radiates to the epigastrium, which occurred after eating fried chicken. Right upper quadrant ultrasound shows gallbladder wall thickening, pericholecystic fluid, and positive Murphy sign. What is the most likely diagnosis?

a. Diverticulitis

b. Acute cholecystitis

c. Ischemic hepatitis

d. Ulcerative colitis

14 What is the most appropriate imaging to evaluate whether or not acute cholecystitis is secondary to an obstructed cystic duct?

a. ERCP

b. MRCP

c. Colonoscopy

d. Hepatobiliary iminodiacetic acid (HIDA) scan

15 What is the etiology of ischemic hepatitis?

a. An acute fall in cardiac output

b. Viral illness

c. Portal hypertension

d. Excessive alcohol intake

16 A clinic patient with no history of esophageal stricture that has been seen in the past and treated for gastroesophageal reflux disease (GERD) returns to the clinic with worsening odynophagia despite *compliance* with your previously prescribed PPI regimen. What diagnostic testing should they be referred for?

a. Barium contrast esophagram

b. HIDA scan

c. Upper endoscopy

d. Colonoscopy

17 The AGACNP receives an esophagogastroduodenoscopy (EGD) report from a gastroenterologist. The report describes the presence of orange gastric-type epithelium extending upward from the stomach into the esophagus in a circumferential fashion. What is the most likely diagnosis?

a. Barrett esophagus

b. Granulomatous gastritis

c. Peptic ulcer disease

d. Varices

18 The AGACNP is caring for a 46-year-old male in the intensive care unit admitted for sepsis with a persistent fever. A clear source of infection has not been identified. Ultrasound of the right upper quadrant reveals a thick-walled gallbladder with longitudinal distention to 5.5 cm, with pericholecystic fluid present. There are no notable gallstones. What is the most accurate diagnosis given in these findings?

a. Pyelonephritis

b. *Clostridioides difficile* infection

c. Diverticulosis

d. Acalculous cholecystitis

19 The AGACNP is seeing a 52-year-old male in the emergency department with chronic end-stage renal disease (ESRD) on peritoneal dialysis. He presents to the emergency room with generalized abdominal pain, fever, nausea, and vomiting. He expresses to you that he noticed cloudiness to the fluid (effluent) coming out during the draining stage of the dialysis treatment. He is very guarded on abdominal examination. What is the most likely diagnosis?

a. Acute gastroenteritis

b. Peritoneal dialysis–related peritonitis

c. Acute gallstone pancreatitis

d. Acute appendicitis

20 What is the recommended treatment for nonperforated appendicitis?

a. Observation

b. Intravenous fluids (IVFs)

c. Antibiotics

d. Timely appendectomy either open or laparoscopically

21 What is the mechanism of pill-induced esophagitis?

a. Direct prolonged mucosal contact

b. Dysphagia

c. Reflux of gastric contents into the esophagus

d. Candida infection

22 The AGACNP is caring for a patient with a known history of cirrhosis. She presents with hematemesis. She is currently hemodynamically stable. The emergency department started the patient on a pantoprazole drip. What other medication should you start the patient on at this time?

a. Clarithromycin 500 mg orally twice daily and amoxicillin 1 g orally twice daily

b. Octreotide

c. Glucocorticoids

d. Mesalamine

23 A patient with a known history of alcoholic liver cirrhosis has been stabilized over the past 12–24 hours with transfusions of packed red blood cells (PRBCs) and fresh frozen plasma (FFP) along with pantoprazole and octreotide drips. What is the next step in the diagnostic treatment plan if esophageal varices are suspected?

a. TIPS

b. Transfer to a tertiary facility for liver transplant evaluation

c. Emergent endoscopy

d. No intervention; the patient has been stabilized

24 The AGACNP is caring for a patient who has had dyspepsia. She is now status post EGD, and the gastric mucosal biopsies are positive for *Helicobacter pylori*. What is the appropriate eradication therapy?

a. Pantoprazole 40 mg by mouth twice daily

b. Ceftriaxone

c. Octreotide

d. Standard triple therapy with proton pump inhibitor twice daily, clarithromycin 500 mg orally twice daily, and amoxicillin 1 g orally twice daily

25 The AGACNP is admitting a patient with a recent knee surgery approximately 2 weeks ago. He presents to the emergency department with dyspepsia and coffee-ground emesis. He states that he has been taking naproxen regularly since his knee surgery for pain management because he didn't want to take the oxycodone/APAP that was prescribed. EGD shows gastritis. What is the most likely etiology and treatment?

a. Pill-induced esophagitis with addition of proton pump inhibitor

b. Nonsteroidal anti-inflammatory drug (NSAID)-induced gastritis requiring discontinuation of offending agent and addition of daily proton pump inhibitor

c. Viral gastroenteritis with observation

d. *H. pylori* infection; obtain biopsies

26 The AGACNP is caring for a patient with known history of Crohn disease who is admitted to the hospital for treatment of a flare-up. The patient is febrile and ill appearing and continues to have bloody diarrhea despite active treatment, and she has abdominal distention and tenderness. The abdominal examination does not show peritoneal signs. She is hypotensive. CT of the abdomen with contrast is showing colonic distention. What are the radiographic criteria for diagnosis of toxic megacolon?

a. Colonic distention less than 6 cm

b. Colonic distention greater than 4.5 cm

c. Colonic distention greater than 6 cm

d. Colonic distention greater than 3 cm

27 A patient with toxic megacolon has failed decompression, glucocorticoid treatment, and infliximab treatment, What is the next step in the treatment plan?

a. Subtotal colectomy

b. Increasing glucocorticoid dosing

c. Replacing the rectal tube

d. Adding total parenteral nutrition (TPN)

28 What is the normal pressure gradient within the portal system?

a. 6–8 mm Hg

b. 10–12 mm Hg

c. 2–6 mm Hg

d. 15 mm Hg

29 The AGACNP is seeing a patient admitted for alcoholic hepatitis. She is found to have a discriminant function of greater than 32. How does this change your treatment plan?

a. Addition of glucocorticoids

b. Addition of lactulose and rifaximin

c. Addition of antibiotics for spontaneous bacterial peritonitis (SBP) prophylaxis

d. Addition of peginterferon

30 How is hepatitis A contracted?

a. Exposure to infected blood

b. Fecal–oral route

c. Sexual intercourse and injection drugs

d. Mother-to-child transmission

31 The AGACNP is assessing hepatitis B serologies of a patient. Positive anti-HBs will signify which of the following?

a. Acute infection

b. Chronic hepatitis B virus (HBV) infection

c. Occult HBV infection

d. Vaccination or immunity

32 Persistence of HBsAg for more than 6 months after the acute phase of illness signifies which of the following?

a. Vaccination or immunity

b. Chronic hepatitis B

c. Acute infection

d. Occult infection

c. Glomerular nephritis

d. Contrast nephropathy

33 What is the incubation period for hepatitis C?

a. 2–3 weeks

b. 6–7 weeks

c. 10–12 weeks

d. 1–2 weeks

34 The AGACNP is evaluating a young nurse who has suffered a needlestick injury while working. She states that her patient has a history of hepatitis C. She is very concerned and asks how hepatitis C is treated. What is the treatment for hepatitis C?

a. Observation as it is a viral illness

b. Broad-spectrum antibiotics

c. Antiretroviral agents

d. Peginterferon

35 What is the standard approach to assessing the level of inflammation and fibrosis of the liver in nonalcoholic fatty liver disease (NAFLD)?

a. Ranson criteria

b. MELD score

c. Liver biopsy

d. Exploratory laparotomy

36 A 67-year-old male with advanced liver disease secondary to alcohol abuse is becoming progressively more hypotensive. His creatinine is steadily rising each day. He has progressed to oliguria. The nephrology team has ruled out all traditional causes of renal failure. What is the likely diagnosis?

a. Hepatorenal syndrome

b. Acute tubular necrosis (ATN)

37 A patient recently completed an antibiotic course for health care–acquired pneumonia. She is returning to the hospital for evaluation of ongoing diarrhea, weakness, fever, and a leukocytosis of 21,000 and a new onset of acute kidney injury with a serum creatinine of 1.8 mg/dL. What infectious etiology should you be highly suspicious of?

a. Viral gastroenteritis

b. Diverticulitis

c. Acute pancreatitis

d. Severe *C. difficile* infection

38 The AGACNP is caring for a patient who recently completed an antibiotic course for health care–acquired pneumonia. She is returning to the hospital for evaluation of ongoing diarrhea, weakness, fever and a leukocytosis of 21,000 and a new onset of acute kidney injury with a serum creatinine of 1.8 mg/dL. There is a high suspicion that this patient has a *C. difficile* infection. What is the next appropriate clinical action?

a. Send a stool specimen for *C. difficile* and initiate empiric antibiotic coverage.

b. Send a viral stool panel.

c. Perform a colonoscopy.

d. Insert a rectal tube.

39 What is the treatment for an initial episode of nonsevere *C. difficile* infection?

a. Vancomycin pulse-tapered regimen

b. Fecal microbiota transplantation

c. Oral vancomycin followed by rifaximin

d. Oral vancomycin 125 mg four times per day for 10 days

40 The AGACNP is caring for a patient who is s/p CABG ×3 Post-op day 5. He has had bleeding complications in the immediate postoperative period. He is complaining of abdominal distension, nausea, and inability to tolerate oral intake. The nursing staff states that he had an episode of vomiting this morning. The AGACNP is concerned for a postoperative ileus. What radiographic imaging is most appropriate?

a. Abdominal CT

b. Plain abdominal films

c. Endoscopy

d. Colonoscopy

41 What radiographic sign distinguishes an ileus from a small bowel obstruction?

a. Dilated loops of bowel throughout the bowel

b. Free air

c. A transition point

d. Liquid stool in the colon

42 What is the pathogenesis behind coagulopathy in liver disease?

a. Destruction of hemoglobin

b. Platelet dysfunction

c. Increased production of bilirubin

d. Decreased production of coagulation factors at the level of the hepatocyte

43 Charcot triad in conjunction with abnormal liver tests is suspicious for what acute process?

a. Acute cholangitis

b. Cholecystitis

c. Diverticulitis

d. Appendicitis

44 Individuals with severe and fulminant ulcerative colitis are at risk for what life-threatening process?

a. Diarrhea

b. Toxic megacolon and perforation

c. Abdominal cramping

d. Fatigue

45 What is the initial treatment for ulcerative colitis?

a. Budesonide

b. 7–10 days of oral antibiotics to cover gram-negative rods and anaerobes

c. Oral glucocorticoids and mesalamine

d. Pantoprazole

46 The AGACNP is caring for a patient who has an ongoing workup for abdominal pain and diarrhea. Colonoscopy reveals mucosal changes that reveal a cobblestone pattern. What is the most likely diagnosis?

a. Ulcerative colitis

b. Diverticulosis

c. Adenocarcinoma

d. Crohn disease

47 The AGACNP is working at a human immunodeficiency virus (HIV) clinic and is seeing a patient with complaints of progressive odynophagia. She describes feeling like she has "cotton mouth," and describes that foods don't taste the same, along with pain while swallowing. Given these symptoms, what should the AGACNP be concerned for in this patient population?

a. Candida esophagitis

b. GERD

c. Barrett esophagus

d. Pill-induced esophagitis

48 Predominant elevation in unconjugated (indirect) bilirubin is caused by which of the following?

a. Overproduction, impaired uptake, abnormalities of conjugation

b. Hepatocellular disease, impaired canalicular excretion of bilirubin, or biliary obstruction

c. Trauma or muscle compression

d. Hypovolemia

49 Hemochromatosis is an autosomal recessive disease caused, in most cases, by what gene mutation?

a. *CF* gene

b. Trisomy 21

c. The *HFE* gene on chromosome 6

d. FBN1 mutation

50 The human homeostatic iron regulator (HFE) protein is thought to play an important role in what process?

a. Sensation of iron stores by duodenal crypt cells

b. Production of clotting factors

c. Platelet aggregation

d. Hemoglobin transport

Disease Answers/Rationales

1 The correct answer is D.

Rationales:

a. Plain radiographic films may show gallstones only if calcified, or may show a gas-filled segment of the transverse colon abruptly ending at the area of pancreatic inflammation. However, they are nonspecific.

b. Ultrasonography may identify stones in the gallbladder. However, this study is often limited by bowel gas.

c. Unenhanced CT will show an enlarged pancreas and differentiate pancreatitis from other intra-abdominal pathology. However, it will not identify areas of necrosis.

d. Contrast-enhanced CT is of value in evaluating the severity of pancreatitis along with identifying edematous versus necrotizing disease and delineating the severity of necrosis. The presence of a fluid collection within the pancreas correlates with an increased mortality rate.

(Papadakis & McPhee, 2014, pp. 691–692).

2 The correct answer is A.

Rationales:

a. Serum amylase and lipase are elevated within 24 hours in 90% of cases of acute pancreatitis. Usually, they are more than three times the upper limit of normal. The lipase will remain elevated longer than the amylase and is slightly more accurate in the diagnosis of acute pancreatitis.

b. The WBC will often be elevated in acute pancreatitis. However, it can be elevated in a multitude of abdominal pathologies and infectious states and is not specific to acute pancreatitis.

c. Triglyceride levels will be elevated in cases of acute pancreatitis that are specifically related to hypertriglyceridemia. These patients will likely have fasting triglyceride levels greater than 1,000 mg/dL.

d. The ALT may be elevated in addition to lipase and amylase in the setting of pancreatitis from a biliary cause.

(Papadakis & McPhee, 2014, pp. 690–691).

3 The correct answer is C.

Rationales:

a. The CIWA score is a widely used scale to evaluate the severity of alcohol withdrawal syndrome.

(Stuppaeck et al., 1994).

b. The SOFA score is an assessment score that facilitates identification of patients who are at risk of dying from sepsis.

(Seymour et al., 2016).

c. The Ranson criteria are one of the earliest scoring systems for severity of acute pancreatitis. They consist of 11 factors, 5 of which are assessed at admission and the remaining 6 are assessed within 48 hours. The first five factors assessed on admission are age > 55, WBC > 16, blood glucose >200 mg/dL, serum LDH >350 units/L, and aspartate aminotransferase >250 units/L. The following six factors are evaluated at 48 hours: hematocrit drop of more than 10 percentage points, blood urea nitrogen rise greater than 5 mg/dL, arterial PO_2 of less than 60 mm Hg, serum calcium less than 8 mg/dL, base deficit over 4 mEq/L, and estimated fluid sequestration of greater than 6 L. Mortality rates correlate with the number of criteria present.

(Ranson et al., 1974;
Papadakis & McPhee, 2014, pp. 690–691).

d. The PAWSS is a screening tool to evaluate the risk of development of alcohol withdrawal syndrome prior to initiation of symptoms. The maximum score is 10. A score of greater than or equal to 4 suggests high risk for moderate to severe alcohol withdrawal syndrome.

(Maldonado et al., 2015).

4 The correct answer is B.

Rationales:

a. Severe pancreatitis is associated with intravascular volume depletion through capillary leak resulting in hypovolemia. Crystalloid infusion is warranted. However, more aggressive fluid rates are necessary to prevent additional pancreatic necrosis.

b. Severe pancreatitis is associated with loss of intravascular volume and hypovolemia secondary to capillary leak that can lead to additional pancreatic necrosis. Aggressive crystalloid resuscitation is recommended early in the course.

c. Crystalloid resuscitation is the initial therapy of choice. Addition of vasopressors may be necessary in severe cases where hypovolemic shock is apparent. All vasoconstrictive medications can decrease splanchnic blood flow and could worsen pancreatic necrosis. Careful addition and titration is recommended.

d. One third of patients with necrotizing pancreatitis develop infections in the necrotic area of the pancreas. The pathogens are most likely gram-negative organisms. These infections are associated with significantly increased mortality. However, prophylactic antibiotic therapy has not been shown to decrease mortality rates in severe pancreatitis and is not recommended on initiate of therapy.

(Marino, 2014, pp. 724–725).

5 The correct answer is A.

Rationales:

a. Jaundice or icterus results from an accumulation of bilirubin. Bilirubin is a product of heme metabolism within the body tissues. Abnormalities occur in the formation, transport, metabolism, or excretion of bilirubin causing increased levels or hyperbilirubinemia. Normal total serum bilirubin levels are 0.2–1.2 mg/dL. Jaundice typically occurs when serum bilirubin levels are around 3 mg/dL.

(Papadakis & McPhee, 2014, p. 641).

b. Blood urea nitrogen is used in assessing kidney function. It is an end product of protein metabolism.

(Papadakis & McPhee, 2014, pp. 867–868).

c. Ammonia is primarily produced in the gastrointestinal tract (GI) tract. It is produced by enterocytes from bacterial catabolism of nitrogen. Elevation is typically a consequence of liver dysfunction.

(Ong et al., 2003).

d. Hyperkalemia is defined by a serum potassium level of greater than 5 mEq/L. This may result in peaked T waves and widened QRS complexes and result in life-threatening dysrhythmias.

(Papadakis & McPhee, 2014, p. 846).

6 **The correct answer is C.**

Rationales:

a. SBP is defined as an ascitic fluid infection without an evident intra-abdominal treatable source. Repeat CT scan will likely not give any new information.

(Such & Runyon, 1998).

b. MRCP provides accurate measurement of the bile and pancreatic ducts in 95% of examination associated anatomic variants, such as pancreatic divisum and choledochal cysts, and pancreatic duct disruptions.

(Reinold & Bret, 1996).

c. A positive diagnostic paracentesis will show an absolute neutrophil count greater than or equal to 250 cells/mm³, which is indicative of infection. Initiation of antibiotic therapy is warranted.

(Marino, 2014, p. 727).

d. Transabdominal ultrasonography is most often used to obtain images of the hepatobiliary, urogenital, and pelvic structures. Its utility for imaging the alimentary GI tract is less well established principally because of technical difficulties in obtaining quality images of the region.

(Nylund et al., 2017).

7 **The correct answer is D.**

Rationales:

a. Plasma elevation of predominantly unconjugated bilirubin is due to the overproduction of bilirubin, impaired bilirubin uptake by the liver, or abnormalities of bilirubin conjugation. Elevations in bilirubin can cause jaundice, which can typically be clinically detected with serum bilirubin greater than 2 mg/dL.

(Reisman, Gips, Lavelle, & Wilson, 1996).

b. Hyperkalemia can cause muscle weakness, and cardiac arrhythmia.

(Acker, Johnson, Palevsky, & Greenberg, 1998).

c. Jaundice is often used interchangeably with hyperbilirubinemia. However, a careful clinical examination cannot detect jaundice until the serum bilirubin is greater than 2 mg/dL, twice the normal limit.

(Reisman et al., 1996).

d. In patients with cirrhosis, ascites is a result of sodium retention by the kidneys in response to activation of the renin–angiotensin–aldosterone system. Typical management of ascites is aimed at reducing sodium retention.

8 **The correct answer is A.**

Rationales:

a. Patients with tense ascites can receive immediate relief from large-volume paracentesis. Typically, up to 5 L of volume can be removed without hemodynamic compromise. For every additional liter removed, 8.5 mg/kg of albumin should be administered.

(Bernardi, Caraceni, & Navickis, 2017).

b. Patients with tense ascites can receive immediate relief from large-volume paracentesis. Typically up to 5 L of volume can be removed without hemodynamic compromise. For every additional liter removed, 8.5 mg/kg of albumin should be administered for every additional liter removed.

(Bernardi et al., 2017).

c. Treatment of hepatic encephalopathy includes lowering the ammonia level with medications such as lactulose and rifaximin. Polyethylene glycol appears to be effective after recent study.

(Rahimi, Singal, Cuthbert, & Rockey, 2014).

d. Treatment of hepatic encephalopathy includes lowering the ammonia level with medications such as lactulose and rifaximin. Polyethylene glycol appears to be effective after recent study.

(Rahimi, Singal, Cuthbert, & Rockey, 2014).

9 **The correct answer is B.**

Rationales:

a. Blood urea nitrogen is an index of assessing kidney function. It is synthesized in the liver and is an end product of protein metabolism.

(Papadakis & McPhee, 2014, p. 867).

b. Ammonia is the most readily available marker of hepatic encephalopathy. However, the diagnosis is made based on the detection of characteristic cognitive impairment, psychomotor deficits, and asterixis in the absence of structural brain disease.

(Ong et al., 2003).

c. AST is present in the liver and other organs including cardiac muscle, skeletal muscle, kidney, and brain.

(Kwo, Cohen, & Lim, 2017).

d. ALT is present primarily in the liver and thus is more specific to liver injury and disease processes.

(Kwo et al., 2017).

> **Clinical Pearl**
>
> Alcoholic hepatitis is usually characterized by fever, right upper quadrant pain, hepatomegaly, and jaundice. The condition is usually reversible with abstinence. If the patient is encephalopathic, steroids may improve short-term mortality in those with discriminant function index of 32 or greater, or a MELD score of 18 or greater.

10 **The correct answer is A.**

Rationales:

a. The TIPS procedure is a stent insertion via the internal jugular vein between a branch of the hepatic vein and the portal vein to decrease overall portal hypertension.

(Papadakis & McPhee, 2014, p. 667).

b. Colonoscopy is used both diagnostically and therapeutically and permits examination and treatment of the rectum, the colon, and a portion of the terminal ileum.

(Rex et al., 2015).

c. ERCP is an endoscopic procedure in which an endoscope is guided into the duodenum allowing for instruments to be passed into the bile ducts and pancreatic ducts.

(Chutkan et al., 2006).

d. MRCP provides accurate measurement of the bile and pancreatic ducts in 95% of examination associated anatomic variants, such as pancreatic divisum and choledochal cysts and pancreatic duct disruptions.

(Reinold & Bret, 1996).

11 **The correct answer is B.**

Rationales:

a. The CIWA score is a widely used scale to evaluate the severity of alcohol withdrawal syndrome.

(Stuppaeck et al., 1994).

b. The original MELD score is a prospectively developed and validated chronic liver disease severity scoring system that uses patients' laboratory values for serum bilirubin, serum creatinine, and the INR to predict 3-month survival.

(Freeman et al., 2002).

c. The SOFA score is an assessment score that facilitates identification of patients who are at risk of dying from sepsis.

(Seymour et al., 2016).

d. The Ranson criteria are one of the earliest scoring systems for severity of acute pancreatitis. They consist of 11 factors, 5 of which are assessed at admission and the remaining 6 are assessed within 48 hours. The first five factors assessed on admission are age > 55, WBC > 16, blood glucose >200 mg/dL, serum LDH >350 units/L, and aspartate aminotransferase >250 units/L. The following six factors are evaluated at 48 hours: Hct drop of more than 10 percentage points, blood urea nitrogen rise greater than 5 mg/dL, arterial PO_2 of less than 60 mm Hg, serum calcium less than 8 mg/dL, base deficit over 4 mEq/L, and estimated fluid sequestration of greater than 6 L. Mortality rates correlate with the number of criteria present.

(Ranson et al., 1974).

12 **The correct answer is C.**
Rationales:

a. Colonoscopy decompression is reserved for patients who have failed both conservative management and neostigmine therapy or have a contraindication to neostigmine.

(Pereira et al., 2015).

b. In patients with cecal diameter greater than 12 cm who have failed 24–48 hours of conservative management, pharmacological therapy with neostigmine is warranted.

(Valle & Godoy, 2014).

c. In absence of significant pain and extreme colonic distention (greater than 12 cm) supportive management of Ogilvie syndrome is warranted. This includes treatment of the underlying disease process, discontinuation of medications that can cause decreased colonic motility, bowel rest, decompression with nasogastric tube (NGT) and rectal tube attached to gravity, and encouragement of physical activity.

(Eisen et al., 2002).

d. In patients whose acute colonic pseudo-obstruction may be precipitated by opiates, administration of subcutaneous methylnaltrexone is warranted.

(Weinstock & Chang, 2011).

13 **The correct answer is B.**
Rationales:

a. Acute diverticulitis is suspected in patients with lower abdominal pain, typically in the left lower quadrant. In the absence of complications, acute uncomplicated diverticulitis can be treated nonoperatively.

(Buchs et al., 2013).

b. An acute attack can be associated with a fatty meal. Right upper quadrant pain is typical as well as localized pain to the epigastrium and hypochondrium. Ultrasonography is often obtained first and will show stones if present. It will show signs suggestive of cholecystitis such as gallbladder wall thickening, pericholecystic fluid, and sonographic Murphy sign.

(Papadakis & McPhee, 2014, p. 684).

c. Ischemic hepatitis refers to diffuse hepatic injury resulting from acute hypoperfusion. It is usually first detected because of elevation of liver function tests. Patients may occasionally have symptoms including nausea, vomiting, anorexia, malaise, and right upper quadrant pain.

(Lightsey & Rockey, 2017).

d. Patients with ulcerative colitis usually present with diarrhea, which may be associated with blood. Bowel movements are frequent and small in volume as a result of rectal inflammation. Associated symptoms include colicky abdominal pain, urgency, tenesmus, and incontinence.

(Silverberg et al., 2005).

14 **The correct answer is D.**

Rationales:

a. ERCP is an endoscopic procedure in which an endoscope is guided into the duodenum allowing for instruments to be passed into the bile ducts and pancreatic ducts.

(Chutkan et al., 2006).

b. MRCP provides accurate measurement of the bile and pancreatic ducts in 95% of examination associated anatomic variants, such as pancreatic divisum and choledochal cysts and pancreatic duct disruptions.

(Reinold & Bret, 1996).

c. Colonoscopy is used both diagnostically and therapeutically and permits examination and treatment of the rectum, the colon, and a portion of the terminal ileum.

(Rex et al., 2015).

d. Hepatobiliary imaging, also known as HIDA scan, is useful in demonstrating an obstructed cystic duct, which is oftentimes the cause of acute cholecystitis.

(Papadakis & McPhee, 2014, p. 684).

15 **The correct answer is A.**

Rationales:

a. The hallmark sign of ischemic hepatitis is a rapid elevation of serum aminotransferase levels, greater than 5,000 units/L and an early rise in the serum lactate dehydrogenase (LDH) level. It is typically a result of an acute fall in the cardiac output, likely secondary to acute myocardial infarction, shock states

(hemorrhagic, septic), or arrhythmia. The mortality rate is usually high and secondary to the underlying disease process.

(Papadakis & McPhee, 2014, p. 678).

b. Several viruses have been associated with acute liver failure, including hepatitis A, B, C, D, and E. In addition, acute liver failure can be seen with herpes simplex virus, varicella–zoster virus, Epstein-Barr virus, adenovirus, and cytomegalovirus.

(Lee et al., 2008).

c. Portal hypertension develops when there is resistance to portal blood flow and is aggravated by increased portal collateral flow. The resistance most often occurs within the liver as in the setting of cirrhosis.

(Garcia-Pagan, Gracia-Sancho, & Bosch, 2012).

d. Excessive alcohol consumption is associated with a range of hepatic manifestations, including alcoholic fatty liver, alcoholic hepatitis, and cirrhosis.

(Jinjuvadia & Liangpunsakul, 2015).

16 **The correct answer is C.**

Rationales:

a. A barium contrast esophagram would be performed prior to an EGD in a patient with a history of proximal esophageal lesion or known complex stricture. Blind intubation of the proximal esophagus during endoscopy may be associated with a risk of perforation. However, performing a barium study prior to EGD has not demonstrated decreased rates of endoscopic complications or improved outcomes.

(American Gastroenterological Association medical position statement on management of oropharyngeal dysphagia, 1999, p. 452).

b. Hepatobiliary imaging, also known as HIDA scan, is useful is demonstrating an obstructed cystic duct, which is oftentimes the cause of acute cholecystitis.

(Papadakis & McPhee, 2014, p. 684).

c. Upper endoscopy is excellent for documenting the type and extent of tissue damage in GERD and identifying other lesions that may mimic the symptoms of GERD.

(Papadakis & McPhee, 2014, p. 576).

d. Colonoscopy is used both diagnostically and therapeutically and permits examination and treatment of the rectum, the colon, and a portion of the terminal ileum.

(Rex et al., 2015).

17 **The correct answer is A.**

Rationales:

a. Barrett esophagus is a condition in which the squamous epithelium of the esophagus is replaced by metaplastic columnar epithelium. It is present in 10% of patients with chronic reflux. There are three types of columnar epithelium identified. They are gastric cardiac, gastric fundus, and specialized intestinal metaplasia. Only the latter is believed to carry an increased risk of neoplasia.

(Papadakis & McPhee, 2014, pp. 576–577).

b. A granuloma is an organized aggregation of combined histiocytic, lymphocytic, and plasmacytic infiltrate (granulomatous infiltration). When the organized collection of cells is identified in the stomach, it is referred to as granulomatous gastritis.

(Maeng et al., 2004).

c. A peptic ulcer is a defect in the gastric or duodenal mucosa that extends through the muscularis mucosa into the deeper layers of the wall.

(Sandler et al., 2002).

d. Esophageal varices are dilated submucosal veins that develop in patients with underlying portal hypertension and may result in serious upper gastrointestinal bleeding.

(Papadakis & McPhee, 2014, pp. 583–586).

18 **The correct answer is D.**

Rationales:

a. Symptoms and signs of pyelonephritis classically include fever, chills, flank pain, and costovertebral angle tenderness and nausea and vomiting.

(Fairley et al., 1971).

b. Patients with an acute *C. difficile* infection may develop signs of systemic toxicity. Proposed criteria for severe *C. difficile* infection are a WBC count of greater than 15,000 cells/mL and a serum creatinine of greater than or equal to 1.5 mg/dL.

(McDonald et al., 2018).

c. Diverticulosis is defined by the presence of diverticula in the colon. Diverticulosis may be symptomatic or asymptomatic.

(Everhart & Ruhl, 2009).

d. Acalculous cholecystitis is an acute necroinflammatory disease of the gallbladder. It results from gallbladder stasis and ischemia that causes a local inflammatory response in the gallbladder. Clinical presentation may often only be presence of an unexplained fever. There may also be a palpable mass in the right upper quadrant and less often jaundice. Ultrasound may show a 3.5–4 mm or more, thick-walled gallbladder that is distended longitudinally greater than 5 cm.

(Ryu, Ryu, & Kim, 2003).

19 **The correct answer is B.**

Rationales:

a. Acute gastroenteritis is defined as diarrheal disease of rapid onset that last less than 2 weeks and may be accompanied by nausea, vomiting, fever, and abdominal pain.

(Hall et al., 2011).

b. The most common symptoms of peritonitis among the peritoneal dialysis patients are abdominal pain and cloudy peritoneal effluent. Other symptoms include fever, nausea, and diarrhea.

(Oliveira et al., 2012).

c. In patients with gallstone pancreatitis, the pain is well localized and the onset of pain is rapid, reaching maximum intensity in 10–20 minutes. The pain persists for several hours to days and may be partially relieved by sitting up or bending forward.

(Banks & Freeman, 2006).

d. Acute appendicitis has a typical constellation of symptoms that include right lower quadrant abdominal pain, anorexia, nausea, and vomiting. The onset of abdominal pain is usually the first symptom.

(Lee, Walsh, & Ho, 2001).

> **Clinical Pearl**
>
> Shock liver can be caused by decreased cardiac output due to several etiologies. The hallmark is transaminitis, followed by a marked increase in LDH. If the related cause of the hypoperfusion is right-sided heart failure, known as congestive hepatopathy, elevated bilirubin levels and jaundice may be noted.

20 **The correct answer is D.**

Rationales:

a. A meta-analysis of 11 nonrandomized studies showed that a short in hospital delay of 12–24 hours before surgery was not associated with an increased risk of perforation. However, delaying appendectomy for greater than 48 hours was associated with increased surgical site infections and other complications.

(United Kingdom National Surgical Research Collaborative; Bhangu, 2014).

b. IVF are a part of the treatment plan for appendicitis. However, the current standard treatment for appendicitis is appendectomy.

(Baird et al., 2017).

c. Antibiotics can be used to augment rather than replace surgical intervention.

(Baird et al., 2017).

d. Nonperforated appendicitis, also referred to as simple appendicitis or uncomplicated appendicitis, refers to acute appendicitis without radiographic signs of perforation. For adults, timely appendectomy is recommended.

(Baird et al., 2017).

21 **The correct answer is A.**

Rationales:

a. A number of different medications may injure the esophagus, presumably through direct prolonged mucosal contact. The most common medications to cause injury are NSAIDs, potassium chloride pills, quinidine, zalcitabine, zidovudine, alendronate, and risedronate, emipronium bromide, vitamin C, and antibiotics. Hospitalized patients are at high risk as they are often supine. Symptoms include severe retrosternal chest pain, odynophagia, and dysphagia beginning several hours after pill ingestion.

(Papadakis & McPhee, 2014, p. 580).

b. Dysphagia is a subjective sensation of difficulty or abnormality of swallowing. It can be due to a structural or motility abnormality in the passage of solids or liquids from the oral cavity to the stomach.

(Aziz et al., 2016).

c. GERD is a condition that develops when the reflux of stomach contents causes troublesome symptoms/complications.

(Vakil et al., 2006).

d. Oropharyngeal candidiasis is a common local infection seen in infants; older adults; those who wear dentures; patients treated with antibiotics, chemotherapy, and radiation; and those with cellular immune deficiency states, such as acquired immune deficiency syndrome (AIDS). The most common symptoms that occur are a cottony feeling in the mouth, loss of taste, and pain during eating or swallowing.

(Sangeorazn et al., 1994).

22 **The correct answer is B.**

Rationales:

a. These specific antibiotics are typically used in the eradication of *H. pylori*. Combination regimens that use two or three antibiotics with a proton pump inhibitor or bismuth are required to achieve adequate rates of eradication.

(Papadakis & McPhee, 2014, pp. 594–595).

b. Octreotide reduces splanchnic and hepatic blood flow and portal pressures in cirrhotic patients.

(Papadakis & McPhee, 2014, pp. 583–584).

c. Disease severity and mortality risk in patients with alcoholic hepatitis may be estimated using the Maddrey discriminant function. Patients with a DF of greater than 32 have a high short-term mortality and may benefit from treatment with glucocorticoids.

(Maddrey et al., 1978).

d. This medication is used in the treatment of ulcerative colitis. Patients with severe ulcerative colitis should be treated with oral glucocorticoids and a combination of high-dose 5-aminosalicylic acid such as mesalamine.

(Mowat et al., 2011).

23 **The correct answer is C.**

Rationales:

a. The TIPS procedure is a stent insertion via the internal jugular vein between a branch of the hepatic vein and the portal vein to decrease overall portal hypertension.

(Papadakis & McPhee, 2014, p. 667).

b. In the setting of acute liver failure, early transfer to a transplantation center is essential. Patients with stage 3 or 4 encephalopathy should be intubated. The head of the bed should be elevated 30°. CPP monitoring may be necessary in order to keep the intracranial pressure below 20 mm Hg and the cerebral perfusion pressure above 70 mm Hg.

(Papadakis & McPhee, 2014, pp. 652–653).

c. Emergent endoscopy is performed after the patient's hemodynamic status has been optimized. Endoscopy is performed to exclude other causes of upper GI bleeding. Acute endoscopic treatment of varices is performed with banding or sclerotherapy.

(Papadakis & McPhee, 2014, p. 584).

d. Emergent endoscopy is performed after the patient's hemodynamic status has been optimized. Endoscopy is performed to exclude other causes of upper GI bleeding. Acute endoscopic treatment of varices is performed with banding or sclerotherapy.

(Papadakis & McPhee, 2014, p. 584).

24 **The correct answer is D.**

Rationales:

a. Pantoprazole is a proton pump inhibitor and is a typical treatment for patients admitted to the hospital with acute upper GI bleeding.

(Dorward et al., 2006).

b. Ceftriaxone is a broad-spectrum antibiotic used in the treatment and prophylaxis of SBP. Most cases of SBP are due to gut bacteria such as *Escherichia coli* and *Klebsiella*. However, streptococcal and infrequently staphylococcal infections can occur. As a result, relatively broad-spectrum therapy is warranted. The antibiotic choice should take local resistant patterns into account.

(Ge & Runyon, 2015).

c. Octreotide reduces splanchnic and hepatic blood flow and portal pressures in cirrhotic patients.

(Papadakis & McPhee, 2014, pp. 583–584).

d. Eradication of *H. pylori* has proven to be difficult. Combination regimens that use two or three antibiotics with a proton pump inhibitor or bismuth are required to achieve adequate rates of eradication.

(Papadakis & McPhee, 2014, pp. 594–595).

25 **The correct answer is B.**

Rationales:

a. A number of different medications may injure the esophagus, presumably through direct prolonged mucosal contact. NSAIDs are one of the top culprit medications. However, injury typically occurs in the esophagus. Symptoms include severe retrosternal chest pain, odynophagia, and dysphagia beginning several hours after pill ingestion.

(Papadakis & McPhee, 2014, p. 580).

b. In patients with NSAID-induced ulcers, the offending agents should be discontinued whenever possible. Both gastric and duodenal ulcers respond quickly to therapy with H2-receptor antagonists or proton pump inhibitor.

(Papadakis & McPhee, 2014, p. 596).

c. Acute gastroenteritis is defined as diarrheal disease of rapid onset that last less than 2 weeks and may be accompanied by nausea, vomiting, fever, and abdominal pain.

(Hall et al., 2011).

d. *H. pylori* is a chronic bacterial infection associated with peptic ulcer disease. The sensitivity and specificity of biopsy urease testing is approximately 90%–95%.

(Chey & Wong, 2007).

26 **The correct answer is C.**

Rationales:

a. The diagnosis of toxic megacolon should be suspected in all patients presenting with abdominal distension and acute or chronic diarrhea. Toxic megacolon is diagnosed based on clinical signs of systemic toxicity combined with radiographic evidence of colonic distension greater than 6 cm in diameter.

(Autenrieth & Baumgart, 2012).

b. The diagnosis of toxic megacolon should be suspected in all patients presenting with abdominal distension and acute or chronic diarrhea. Toxic megacolon is diagnosed based on clinical signs of systemic toxicity combined with radiographic evidence of colonic distension greater than 6 cm in diameter.

(Autenrieth & Baumgart, 2012).

c. The diagnosis of toxic megacolon should be suspected in all patients presenting with abdominal distension and acute or chronic diarrhea. Toxic megacolon is diagnosed based on clinical signs of systemic toxicity combined with radiographic evidence of colonic distension greater than 6 cm in diameter.

(Autenrieth & Baumgart, 2012).

d. Abdominal CT is more reliable in evaluating both the length and severity of colitis and the presence of colonic dilation than plain abdominal films. CT may even distinguish toxic megacolon from severe acute colitis.

(Imbriaco & Balthazar, 2001).

27 **The correct answer is A.**

Rationales:

a. Patients who fail to respond to one of the second-line agents after another 3 days require surgery without delay. Subtotal colectomy with end-ileostomy is the procedure of choice for urgent or emergent surgery for toxic megacolon.

(Danovitch, 1989).

b. Patients who do not respond to intravenous glucocorticoids within 3 days should receive either infliximab or cyclosporine as a second-line therapy.

(Dassopoulos et al., 2013).

c. Patients who fail to respond to conservative management and one of the second-line agents after another 3 days require surgery without delay. Subtotal colectomy with end-ileostomy is the procedure of choice for urgent or emergent surgery for toxic megacolon.

(Danovitch, 1989).

d. TPN is of limited value in patients with severe inflammatory bowel disease from any cause. It may be necessary for provision of nutrient to patients in whom it cannot otherwise be tolerated enterally, but it offers no proven benefit in terms of avoiding surgery or decreasing hospital stay in patients with acute colitis due to ulcerative colitis.

(Dickinson et al., 1980).

28 **The correct answer is C.**

Rationales:

a. Under normal circumstances, the pressure gradient between the portal vein and inferior vena cava is 2–6 mm Hg.

b. Under normal circumstances, the pressure gradient between the portal vein and inferior vena cava is 2–6 mm Hg.

c. Under normal circumstances the pressure gradient between the portal vein and inferior vena cava is 2–6 mm Hg.

d. When the gradient exceeds 10–12 mm Hg, significant portal hypertension exists. Esophageal varices are the most common cause of gastrointestinal bleeding secondary to portal hypertension.

(Papadakis & McPhee, 2014, p. 583).

29 **The correct answer is A.**

Rationales:

a. Disease severity and mortality risk in patients with alcoholic hepatitis may be estimated using the Maddrey discriminant function. Patients with a DF of greater than 32 have a high

short-term mortality and may benefit from treatment with glucocorticoids.

(Maddrey et al., 1978).

b. Treatment of hepatic encephalopathy includes lowering the ammonia level with medications such as lactulose and rifaxamin. Polyethylene glycol appears to be effective after recent study.

(Rahimi, Singal, Cuthbert, & Rockey, 2014).

c. Broad-spectrum antibiotics are used in the treatment and prophylaxis of SBP. Most cases of SBP are due to gut bacteria such as *E. coli* and *Klebsiella*. However, streptococcal and infrequently staphylococcal infections can occur. As a result, relatively broad-spectrum therapy is warranted. The antibiotic choice should take local resistant patterns into account.

(Ge & Runyon, 2015).

d. Treatment of patients with acute hepatitis C with peginterferon significantly decreases the risk of chronic hepatitis C. Typically, those infected with HCV genotype 1 require a 24-week course of treatment. If HCV RNA is undetectable at 4 weeks, a 12-week course is sufficient.

(Papadakis & McPhee, 2014, p. 650).

Clinical Pearl

Cholangitis should be suspected in those with right upper quadrant tenderness, jaundice, fever followed by hypothermia, gram-negative bacteremia, and septic shock.

---

30 **The correct answer is B.**

Rationales:

a. Transmission of HCV is primarily through exposure to infected blood.

(Frank et al., 2000).

b. Hepatitis A virus is transmitted by the fecal–oral route, and its spread is favored by crowding and poor sanitation. Common sources of outbreak may result from contaminated water or food.

(Papadakis & McPhee, 2014, pp. 644–645).

c. The predominant mode of HBV transmission varies in different geographical areas. Mother-to-child is the predominant mode of transmission in high-prevalence areas. In comparison, horizontal transmission, particularly in early childhood, accounts for most cases of chronic HBV infection in intermediate-prevalence areas, while unprotected sexual intercourse and injection drug use in adults are the major routes of spread in low-prevalence areas.

(Kim et al., 2002).

d. The predominant mode of HBV transmission varies in different geographical areas. Mother-to-child is the predominant mode of transmission in high-prevalence areas. In comparison, horizontal transmission, particularly in early childhood, accounts for most cases of chronic HBV infection in intermediate-prevalence areas, while unprotected sexual intercourse and injection drug use in adults are the major routes of spread in low-prevalence areas.

(Kim et al., 2002).

31 **The correct answer is D.**

Rationales:

a. HBsAg is the hallmark serological marker of HBV infection. It appears 1–10 weeks after an acute exposure to HBV.

(Liaw et al., 1991).

b. Persistence of HBsAG for more than 6 months implies chronic infection.

(Chu, Liaw, Pao, & Huang, 1989).

c. Occult HBV infection is defined as the presence of detectable HBV DNA by polymerase chain reaction in patients who are negative for HBsAG.

(Chaudhuri et al., 2004).

d. Specific antibody to HBsAg appears in most individuals after clearance of HBsAg after successful vaccination against hepatitis B.

(Papadakis & McPhee, 2014, pp. 647–648).

32 **The correct answer is B.**

Rationales:

a. Specific antibody to HBsAg appears in most individuals after clearance of HBsAg after successful vaccination against hepatitis B.

(Papadakis & McPhee, 2014, pp. 647–648).

b. The appearance of HBsAg in the serum is the first evidence of infection, appearing before biochemical evidence of liver disease and persisting throughout the clinical illness. Persistence of HBsAg more than 6 months after the acute illness signifies chronic hepatitis B.

(Papadakis & McPhee, 2014, p. 647).

c. HBsAg is the hallmark serological marker of HBV infection. It appears 1–10 weeks after an acute exposure to HBV.

(Liaw et al., 1991).

d. Occult HBV infection is defined as the presence of detectable HBV DNA by polymerase chain reaction in patients who are negative for HBsAG.

(Chaudhuri et al., 2004).

33 **The correct answer is B.**

Rationales:

a. The incubation period for hepatitis C averages 6–7 weeks and is oftentimes asymptomatic or mild illness with waxing and waning aminotransferase elevations.

b. The incubation period for hepatitis C averages 6–7 weeks and is oftentimes asymptomatic or mild illness with waxing and waning aminotransferase elevations.

c. The incubation period for hepatitis C averages 6–7 weeks and is oftentimes asymptomatic

or mild illness with waxing and waning
aminotransferase elevations.

d. The incubation period for hepatitis C averages
6–7 weeks and is oftentimes asymptomatic
or mild illness with waxing and waning
aminotransferase elevations.

(Papadakis & McPhee, 2014, pp. 649–650).

34 **The correct answer is D.**

Rationales:

a. Treatment of patients with acute hepatitis C with
peginterferon significantly decreases the risk
of chronic hepatitis C. Typically, those infected
with HCV genotype 1 require a 24-week course
of treatment. If HCV RNA is undetectable at
4 weeks, a 12-week course is sufficient.

b. Hepatitis B is a viral etiology.

c. Antiretroviral agents are used in the treatment
of HIV. Epidemiological data have demonstrated
that potent three-drug antiretroviral therapy
regimens, which were introduced in 1996, have
led to remarkable declines in morbidity and
mortality among HIV patients.

d. Treatment of patients with acute hepatitis C
with peginterferon significantly decreases
the risk of chronic hepatitis C. Typically,
those infected with HCV genotype 1 require a
24-week course of treatment. If HCV RNA is
undetectable at 4 weeks, a 12-week course is
sufficient.

(Papadakis & McPhee, 2014, p. 650).

35 **The correct answer is C.**

Rationales:

a. The Ranson criteria constitute one of the
earliest scoring systems for severity of acute
pancreatitis. It consists of 11 factors, 5 of
which are assessed at admission and the
remaining 6 are assessed within 48 hours. The
first five factors assessed on admission are age
> 55, WBC > 16, blood glucose >200 mg/

dL, serum LDH > 350 units/L, and aspartate
aminotransferase >250 units/L. The following
six factors are evaluated at 48 hours: Hct drop
of more than 10 percentage points, blood urea
nitrogen rise greater than 5 mg/dL, arterial
PO_2 of less than 60 mm Hg, serum calcium less
than 8 mg/dL, base deficit over 4 mEq/L, and
estimated fluid sequestration of greater
than 6 L. Mortality rates correlate with the
number of criteria present.

(Ranson et al., 1974).

b. The original MELD score is a prospectively
developed and validated chronic liver disease
severity scoring system that uses patients'
laboratory values for serum bilirubin, serum
creatinine, and the INR to predict 3-month
survival.

(Freeman et al., 2002).

c. Percutaneous liver biopsy is diagnostic and is
the standard approach to assessing the degree
of inflammation and fibrosis. The risk of the
procedure must be balanced with the benefits of
the information that it will give.

(Papadakis & McPhee, 2014, p. 664).

d. Exploratory laparotomy is not the standard
approach in assessing NAFLD.

(Papadakis & McPhee, 2014, p. 664).

36 **The correct answer is A.**

Rationales:

a. Hepatorenal syndrome develops in those
patients who have advanced liver disease due
to cirrhosis, alcoholic hepatitis, acute liver
failure, and metastatic disease. Hepatorenal
syndrome typically occurs when there is
a decrease in renal perfusion induced by
worsening hepatic injury. Vasodilation in the
splanchnic circulation is triggered by worsening
portal hypertension (HTN). This plays a role
in the hemodynamic changes that occur in
hepatorenal syndrome.

(Gines, Guevara, Arroyo, & Rodes, 2003).

b. ATN can occur with prolonged severe ischemia. This can result in histological changes, including necrosis, with denuding of the epithelium and occlusion of the tubular lumen by casts and cell debris.

(Langenberg et al., 2006).

c. Glomerular disease syndromes are typically classified based upon the pattern of urinary abnormalities, the existence of systemic features, and the degree of renal dysfunction. In glomerular nephritis, inflammation within the glomerulus leads to the passage of not only plasma proteins but also inflammatory cells and RBCs into the renal tubule.

(Vinen & Oliveira, 2003).

d. Contrast nephropathy is a generally reversible form of acute kidney injury that occurs soon after the administration of radiocontrast media.

(Weisbord & Palevsky, 2005).

37 **The correct answer is D.**

Rationales:

a. Acute gastroenteritis is defined as diarrheal disease of rapid onset that lasts less than 2 weeks and may be accompanied by nausea, vomiting, fever, and abdominal pain. Oftentimes it is a viral source and is self-limiting.

(Hall et al., 2011).

b. Acute diverticulitis is suspected in patients with lower abdominal pain, typically in the left lower quadrant. In the absence of complications, acute uncomplicated diverticulitis can be treated nonoperatively.

(Buchs et al., 2013).

c. Most patients with acute pancreatitis have acute onset of persistent, severe epigastric abdominal pain.

(Swaroop, Chari, & Clain, 2004).

d. Patients with an acute *C. difficile* infection may develop signs of systemic toxicity. Proposed

criteria for severe *C. difficile* infection are a WBC count of greater than 15,000 cells/mL and a serum creatinine of greater than or equal to 1.5 mg/dL.

(McDonald et al., 2018).

38 **The correct answer is A.**

Rationales:

a. Treatment is warranted for patients with typical manifestations of *C. difficile* infection and a positive diagnostic laboratory assay. In addition, empiric treatment is reasonable in the setting of high clinical suspicion, particularly for those that may have severe or fulminant colitis, while assays are pending.

(Surawicz et al., 2013).

b. Some laboratories have access to multiplex stool tests, with which molecular tests for a panel of many different viral pathogens can be performed. This can be performed simultaneously with *C. difficile* testing. However, if there is suspicion for *C. difficile*, empiric treatment should not be delayed.

(Binnicker, 2015).

c. Colonoscopy is used both diagnostically and therapeutically and permits examination and treatment of the rectum, the colon, and a portion of the terminal ileum. This can be done to rule out other causes. However, it should not delay empiric antibiotic treatment.

(Rex et al., 2015).

d. This can be done simultaneously. However, it should not proceed starting antibiotic therapy.

39 **The correct answer is D.**

Rationales:

a. Recurrent *C. difficile* infection (CDI) is defined by resolution of CDI symptoms while on appropriate therapy, followed by reappearance of symptoms within 2–8 weeks after treatment has been stopped. For patients with a first recurrence of CDI who were treated with vancomycin, pulse-tapered dosing of oral vancomycin is recommended.

(McDonald et al., 2018).

b. For patients with multiple recurrences who have received appropriate antibiotic treatment for at least three CDIs, fecal microbiota transplantation is recommended.

(Hota et al., 2017).

c. There are no rigorous studies regarding the approach to management for patients with more than one episode of recurrent *C. difficile*. Vancomycin followed by rifaximin may be effective for the treatment of recurrent CDI.

(Johnson et al., 2007).

d. Antibiotics for treatment of nonsevere *C. difficile* infection include oral vancomycin or oral fidaxomicin.

(McDonald et al., 2018).

> ● **Clinical Pearl**
>
> Acute pancreatitis is often quantified by use of the Ranson criteria, assessing upon admission and again 48 hours later. Mortality rates correlate reliably with the number of criteria present.

40 **The correct answer is B.**

Rationales:

a. Abdominal CT can be used if plain films are inconclusive. However, it is not the initial imaging study.

(Frager et al., 1995).

b. Plain abdominal films are often the first diagnostic imaging obtained for the evaluation of abdominal distention, nausea, or pain. Supine and upright films may show dilated loops of bowel in patients with postoperative ileus.

(Frager et al., 1995).

c. Upper endoscopy is excellent for documenting the type and extent of tissue damage in GERD and identifying other lesions that may mimic the symptoms of GERD. It is not necessary for the diagnosis of ileus.

(Papadakis & McPhee, 2014, p. 576).

d. Colonoscopy is used both diagnostically and therapeutically and permits examination and treatment of the rectum, the colon, and a portion of the terminal ileum.

(Rex et al., 2015).

41 **The correct answer is C.**

Rationales:

a. A diagnosis of bowel obstruction can be made by the finding of dilated proximal bowel with distal collapsed bowel

(Markogiannakis et al., 2007).

b. The appearance of pneumoperitoneum on plain films depends on the location of the air and patient positioning. Air outside the GI can be located freely in the peritoneal cavity (i.e., free air). This is a sign of gastrointestinal perforation.

(Furukawa et al., 2005).

c. Plain abdominal films are often the first diagnostic imaging obtained for the evaluation of abdominal distention, nausea, or pain. Supine and upright films may show dilated loops of bowel in patients with postoperative ileus. With an ileus, there should be demonstration of air in the colon and rectum without a transition zone to suggest obstruction.

(Frager et al., 1995).

d. A diagnosis of bowel obstruction can be made by the finding of dilated proximal bowel with distal collapsed bowel. There may be residual stool in the colon. However, this is not a definitive diagnostic finding.

(Markogiannakis et al., 2007).

The correct answer is D.

Rationales:

a. This is known as hemolysis. When hemolysis is present, laboratory studies show increased levels of LDH along with reduced haptoglobin often accompanied by increases in indirect bilirubin and clinical jaundice.

(Mohandas & Schrier, 1989, p. 391).

b. Platelets are produced within the bone marrow. The hepatocyte is the site of production of almost all of the numbered coagulation factors including fibrinogen, thrombin, and factors V, VII, IX, X, and XI.

(Marks, 2013).

c. Plasma elevation of predominantly unconjugated (indirect) bilirubin may be due to overproduction of bilirubin, impaired bilirubin uptake by the liver, or abnormalities of bilirubin conjugation. Examples include hemolysis, extravasation of blood into tissue, and dyserythropoiesis.

(Papadakis & McPhee, 2014, pp. 641–642).

d. The hepatocyte is the site of production of almost all of the numbered coagulation factors including fibrinogen, thrombin, and factors V, VII, IX, X, and XI.

(Marks, 2013).

43 **The correct answer is A.**

Rationales:

a. The classic presentation of acute cholangitis is fever, abdominal pain, and jaundice. This is also known as Charcot triad. Fifty to seventy-five percent of patients with acute cholangitis will have all three findings.

b. The classic presentation of acute cholangitis is fever, abdominal pain, and jaundice. This is also known as Charcot triad. Fifty to seventy-five percent of patients with acute cholangitis will have all three findings.

c. The classic presentation of acute cholangitis is fever, abdominal pain, and jaundice. This is also known as Charcot triad. Fifty to seventy-five percent of patients with acute cholangitis will have all three findings.

d. The classic presentation of acute cholangitis is fever, abdominal pain, and jaundice. This is also known as Charcot triad. Fifty to seventy-five percent of patients with acute cholangitis will have all three findings.

(Saik, Greenburg, Farris, & Peskin, 1975).

 The correct answer is B.

Rationales:

a. Diarrhea is a typical feature. However, it is not necessarily a life-threatening complication of the disease process.

b. Fulminant colitis refers to a subgroup of patients with severe ulcerative colitis who have more than 10 stools per day, continuous bleeding, abdominal pain, distention, and acute/severe toxic symptoms. These patients are at high risk of progressing to toxic megacolon and bowel perforation.

c. Abdominal cramping is a clinical feature of ulcerative colitis. However, it is not a life-threatening complication of the disease process.

d. Fatigue is a clinical feature of ulcerative colitis. However, it is not a life-threatening complication of the disease process.

(Danovitch, 1989).

45 **The correct answer is C.**

Rationales:

a. Budesonide is recommended as first-line treatment of mild Crohn disease.

(Sanborn, 2014).

b. This is a typical treatment plan for the outpatient management of diverticulitis.

(Kellum et al., 1992).

c. Patients with severe ulcerative colitis should be treated with oral glucocorticoids and a combination of high-dose 5-aminosalicylic acids such as mesalamine.

(Mowat et al., 2011).

d. Pantoprazole is a proton pump inhibitor and is a typical treatment for patients admitted to the hospital with acute upper GI bleeding.

(Dorward et al., 2006).

46 **The correct answer is D.**

Rationales:

a. Endoscopic findings of ulcerative are nonspecific. Biopsies are necessary to establish the chronicity of inflammation and to exclude other causes of colitis.

b. Colonoscopy has no role in establishing the diagnosis of acute diverticulitis, as the inflammation is peridiverticular. Endoscopic evaluation of the colon should be avoided in the acute setting fur due to the risk of perforation or exacerbation of the existing inflammation. After the complete resolution of symptoms associated with acute diverticulitis, a colonoscopy is performed.

(Jacobs, 2007).

c. Colorectal cancer may appear mass-like, nodular, ulcerated, or plaque-like.

(Connell et al., 1994).

d. Colonoscopy with intubation of the terminal ileum is used to establish the diagnosis of ileocolonic Crohn disease. Endoscopic features include focal ulcerations adjacent to areas of normal-appearing mucosa along with polypoid mucosal changes that give a cobblestone appearance.

(Wayne, 1977).

47 **The correct answer is A.**

Rationales:

a. Oropharyngeal candidiasis is a common local infection seen in infants; older adults; those who wear dentures; patients treated with antibiotics, chemotherapy, and radiation; and those with cellular immune deficiency states, such as AIDS. The most common symptoms that occur are a cottony feeling in the mouth, loss of taste, and pain during eating or swallowing.

(Sangeorazn et al., 1994).

b. Gastroesophageal reflux is a condition that develops when the reflux of stomach contents causes troublesome symptoms or complications. It is not specific to the immunocompromised patient.

(Vakil et al., 2006).

c. Barrett esophagus is a condition in which the squamous epithelium of the esophagus is replaced by metaplastic columnar epithelium. It is present in 10% of patients with chronic reflux. There are three types of columnar epithelium identified. They are gastric cardiac, gastric fundus, and specialized intestinal metaplasia. Only the latter is believed to carry an increased risk of neoplasia.

(Papadakis & McPhee, 2014, pp. 576–577).

d. A number of different medications may injure the esophagus, presumably through direct prolonged mucosal contact. The most common medications to cause injury are NSAIDs, potassium chloride pills, quinidine, zalcitabine, zidovudine, alendronate, and risedronate, emipronium bromide, vitamin C, and antibiotics. Hospitalized patients are at high risk as they are often supine. Symptoms include severe retrosternal chest pain, odynophagia, and dysphagia beginning several hours after pill ingestion.

(Papadakis & McPhee, 2014, p. 580).

48 **The correct answer is A.**

Rationales:

a. Plasma elevation of predominantly unconjugated (indirect) bilirubin may be due to overproduction of bilirubin, impaired bilirubin uptake by the liver, or abnormalities of bilirubin conjugation. Examples include hemolysis, extravasation of blood into tissue, and dyserythropoiesis.

(Papadakis & McPhee, 2014, pp. 641–642).

b. Plasma elevation of conjugated bilirubin may be due to hepatocellular disease, impaired canalicular excretion of bilirubin, or biliary obstruction.

(Sticova & Jirsa, 2013).

c. Plasma elevation of predominantly unconjugated (indirect) bilirubin may be due to overproduction of bilirubin, impaired bilirubin uptake by the liver, or abnormalities of bilirubin conjugation. Examples include hemolysis, extravasation of blood into tissue, and dyserythropoiesis.

(Papadakis & McPhee, 2014, pp. 641–642).

d. Plasma elevation of predominantly unconjugated (indirect) bilirubin may be due to overproduction of bilirubin, impaired bilirubin uptake by the liver, or abnormalities of bilirubin conjugation. Examples include hemolysis, extravasation of blood into tissue, and dyserythropoiesis.

(Papadakis & McPhee, 2014, pp. 641–642).

49 **The correct answer is C.**

Rationales:

a. Hemochromatosis is an autosomal recessive disease caused in most cases by the mutation in the *HFE* gene on chromosome 6.

b. Hemochromatosis is an autosomal recessive disease caused in most cases by the mutation in the *HFE* gene on chromosome 6.

c. Hemochromatosis is an autosomal recessive disease caused in most cases by the mutation in the *HFE* gene on chromosome 6.

d. Hemochromatosis is an autosomal recessive disease caused in most cases by the mutation in the *HFE* gene on chromosome 6.

(Papadakis & McPhee, 2014, p. 673).

50 **The correct answer is A.**

Rationales:

a. The HFE protein is thought to play an important role in the process by which duodenal crypt cells sense body iron stores, leading in turn to increased iron absorption from the duodenum. A decrease in the synthesis or expression of hepcidin, the principle iron regulatory hormone, is thought to be a key pathogenic factor in all forms of hemochromatosis.

b. The HFE protein is thought to play an important role in the process by which duodenal crypt cells sense body iron stores, leading in turn to increased iron absorption from the duodenum. A decrease in the synthesis or expression of hepcidin, the principle iron regulatory hormone, is thought to be a key pathogenic factor in all forms of hemochromatosis.

c. The HFE protein is thought to play an important role in the process by which duodenal crypt cells sense body iron stores, leading in turn to increased iron absorption from the duodenum. A decrease in the synthesis or expression of hepcidin, the principle iron regulatory hormone, is thought to be a key pathogenic factor in all forms of hemochromatosis.

d. The HFE protein is thought to play an important role in the process by which duodenal crypt cells sense body iron stores, leading in turn to increased iron absorption from the duodenum. A decrease in the synthesis or expression of hepcidin, the principle iron regulatory hormone, is thought to be a key pathogenic factor in all forms of hemochromatosis.

(Papadakis & McPhee, 2014, p. 673).

References

Acker, C. G., Johnson, J. P., Palevsky, P. M., & Greenberg, A. (1998). Hyperkalemia in hospitalized patients: Causes, adequacy of treatment, and results of an attempt to improve physician compliance with published therapy guidelines. *Archives of Internal Medicine, 158,* 917.

American Gastroenterological Association medical position statement on management of oropharyngeal dysphagia. (1999). *Gastroenterology, 116,* 452.

Autenrieth, D. M., & Baumgart, D. C. (2012). Toxic megacolon. *Inflammatory Bowel Diseases, 18,* 584.

Aziz, Q., Fass, R., Gyawali, C. P., et al. (2016). Functional esophageal disorders. *Gastroenterology.* pii: S0016-5085(16)00178-5.

Baird, D. L. H., Simillis, C., Kontovounisios, C., et al. (2017) Acute appendicitis. *BMJ, 357,* j1703.

Banks, P. A., & Freeman, M. L. (2006). Practice Parameters Committee of the American College of Gastroenterology. Practice guidelines in acute pancreatitis. *The American Journal of Gastroenterology, 101,* 2379.

Bernardi, M., Caraceni, P., & Navickis, R. J. (2017). Does the evidence support a survival benefit of albumin infusion in patients with cirrhosis undergoing large volume paracentesis? *Expert Review of Gastroenterology & Hepatology, 11,* 191.

Binnicker, M. J. (2015). Multiplex molecular panels for diagnosis of gastrointestinal infection: Performance, result interpretation and cost effectiveness. *Journal of Clinical Microbiology, 53,* 3723.

Buchs, N. C., Konrad-Mugnier, B., Jannot, A. S., et al. (2013). Assessment of recurrence and complications following uncomplicated diverticulitis. *The British Journal of Surgery, 100,* 976.

Chaudhuri, V., Tayal, R., Nayak, B., et al. (2004). Occult hepatitis B virus infection in chronic liver disease: Full length genome and analysis of mutant surface promoter. *Gastroenterology, 127,* 1356.

Chey, W. D., Wong, B. C.; Practice Parameters Committee of the American College of Gastroenterology. (2007). American College of Gastroenterology guidelines on the management of *Helicobacter pylori* infection. *The American Journal of Gastroenterology, 102,* 1808.

Chu, C. M., Liaw, Y. F., Pao, C. C., & Huang, M. J. (1989). The etiology of acute hepatitis superimposed upon previously unrecognized asymptomatic HBsAG carriers. *Hepatology, 9,* 452.

Chutkan, R. K., Ahmad, A. S., Cohen, J., et al. (2006). ERCP core curriculum. *Gastrointestinal Endoscopy, 63,* 361.

Connell, W. R., Sheffield, J. P., Kamm, M. A., et al. (1994). Lower gastrointestinal malignancy in Crohn's disease. *Gut, 35*(3), 47.

Danovitch, S. H. (1989). Fulminant colitis and toxic megacolon. *Gastroenterology Clinics of North America, 18,* 73.

Dassopoulos, T., Sultan, S., Falck-Ytter, Y. T., et al. (2013). American Gastroenterological Association Institute technical review on the use of thiopurines, methotrexate, and anti-TNF-alpha biologic drugs for the induction and maintenance of remission in the inflammatory Crohn's disease. *Gastroenterology, 145,* 1464.

Dickinson, R. J., Ashton, M. G., Axon, A. T., et al. (1980). Controlled trial of intravenous hyperalimentation and total bowel rest as an adjunct to the routine therapy of acute colitis. *Gastroenterology, 79,* 1199.

Dorward, S., Sreedharan, A., Leontiadis, G. I., et al. (2006). Proton pump inhibitor treatment initiated prior to the endoscopic diagnosis in upper gastrointestinal bleeding. *Cochrane Database of Systematic Reviews,* CD005415.

Eisen, G. M., Baron, T. H., Dominitz, J. A., et al. (2002). Acute colonic pseudo-obstruction. *Gastrointestinal Endoscopy, 56,* 789.

Everhart, J. E., & Ruhl, C. E. (2009). Burden of digestive diseases in the United States part II: Lower gastrointestinal diseases. *Gastroenterology, 136,* 741.

Fairley, K. F., Carson, N. E., Gutch, R. C., et al. (1971). Site of infection in acute urinary tract infection in general practice. *Lancet, 2,* 615.

Frager, D., Medwid, S. W., Baer, J. W., et al. (1995). Distinction between post-operative ileus and mechanical small bowel obstruction: Value of CT compared with clinical and other radiographic findings. *AJR American Journal of Roentgenology, 164,* 891.

Frank, C., Mohamed, M. K., Strictland, G. T., et al. (2000). The role of parenteral antischistosomal therapy in the spread of hepatitis C virus in Egypt. *Lancet, 355,* 887.

Freeman, R. B., Jr., Wiesner, R. H., Harper, A., et al. (2002). The new liver allocation system: Moving toward evidence-based transplant policy. *Liver Transplantation, 8,* 851.

Furukawa, A., Sakoda, M., Yamasaki, M., et al. (2005). Gastrointestinal tract perforation: CT diagnosis of presence, site, and cause. *Abdominal Imaging, 30,* 524.

Garcia-Pagan, J. C., Gracia-Sancho, J., & Bosch, J. (2012). Functional aspects on the pathophysiology of portal hypertension in cirrhosis. *Journal of Hepatology, 57,* 458.

Ge, P. S., & Runyon, B. A. (2015). Preventing future infections in cirrhosis: A battle cry for stewardship. *Clinical Gastroenterology and Hepatology, 13,* 760.

Gines, P., Guevara, M., Arroyo, V., & Rodes, J. (2003). Hepatorenal syndrome. *Lancet, 362,* 1819.

Hall, A. J., Rosenthal, M., Gregoricus, N., et al. (2011). Incidence of acute gastroenteritis and role of norovirus, Georgia, USA, 2004–2005. *Emerging Infectious Diseases, 17,* 7.

Hota, S. S., Sales, V., Tomlinson, G., et al. (2017). Oral Vancomycin followed by fecal transplantation Versus

Tapering oral Vancomycin treatment for recurrent *Clostridium difficile* Infection: An open label, randomized controlled trial. *Clinical Infectious Diseases, 64*, 265.

Imbriaco, M., Balthazar, E. J. (2001). Toxic megacolon: role of CT in evaluation and detection of complications. *Clinical Imaging, 25*, 349.

Jacobs, D. O. (2007). Clinical practice. Diverticulitis. *New England Journal of Medicine, 357*, 2057.

Jinjuvadia, R., Liangpunsakul, S. (2015). Translational research and evolving hepatitis treatment consortium. Trends in alcoholic hepatitis–related hospitalizations, financial burden, and mortality in the United States. *Journal of Clinical Gastroenterology, 49*, 506.

Johnson, S., Schriever, C., Galang, M., et al. (2007). Interruption of recurrent *Clostridium difficile*-associated diarrhea episodes by serial therapy with vancomycin and rifaximin. *Clinical Infectious Diseases, 44*, 846.

Kellum, J. M., Sugerman, H. J., Coppa, G. F., et al. (1992). Randomized prospective comparison of cefoxitine and gentamicin-clindamycin in the treatment of acute colonic diverticulitis. *Clinical Therapeutics, 14*, 376.

Kim, W. R., Ishitani, M. B., Dickson, E. R., et al. (2002). Rising burden of hepatitis B in the United States: Should the other virus be forgotten? *Hepatology, 36*, 222A.

Kwo, P. Y., Cohen, S. M., & Lim, J. K. (2017). ACG Clinical Guideline: Evaluation of abnormal liver chemistries. *The American Journal of Gastroenterology, 112*, 18.

Langenberg, C., Wan, L., Egi, M., et al. (2006). Renal blood flow in experimental septic acute renal failure. *Kidney International, 69*, 1996.

Lee, S. L., Walsh, A. J., & Ho, H. S. (2001). Computed tomography and ultrasonography do not improve and may delay the diagnosis and treatment of appendicitis. *Archives of Surgery, 136*, 556.

Lee, W. M., Squires, R. H., Jr., Nyberg, S. L., et al. (2008). Acute liver failure: Summary of a workshop. *Hepatology, 47*, 1401.

Liaw, Y. F., Sheen, I. S., Chen, T. J., et al. (1991). Incidence, determinants and significance of delayed clearance of serum HBsAg in chronic hepatitis B virus infection: A prospective study. *Hepatology, 13*, 627.

Lightsey, J. M., & Rockey, D. C. (2017). Current concepts in ischemic hepatitis. *Current Opinion in Gastroenterology, 33*, 158.

Maddrey, W. C., Bointnott, J. K., Bedine, M. S., et al. (1978). Corticosteroid therapy of alcoholic hepatitis. *Gastroenterology, 75*, 193.

Maeng, L., Lee, A., Choi, K., et al. (2004). Granulomatous gastritis: A clinicopathologic analysis of 18 biopsy cases. *The American Journal of Surgical Pathology, 28*, 941.

Maldonado, J. R., Sher, Y., Das, S., et al. (2015). Prospective validation study of the Prediction of Alcohol Withdrawal Severity Scale (PAWSS) in medically ill inpatients: A new scale for the Prediction of Complicated Alcohol Withdrawal Syndrome. *Alcohol, 50*, 509.

Marino, P. L. (2014). *Marinos the ICU book.* Philadelphia, PA: Wolters Kluwer Health/Lippincott Williams & Wilkins.

Markogiannakis, H., Messaris, E., Dardamanis, D., et al. (2007). Acute mechanical bowel obstruction: Clinical presentation, etiology, management and outcome. *World Journal of Gastroenterology, 13*, 432.

Marks, P. W. (2013). Hematologic manifestations of liver disease. *Seminars in Hematology, 50*, 216.

McDonald, L. C., Gerding, D. N., Johnson, S., et al. (2018). Clinical practice guidelines for *Clostridium difficile* infection in adults and children: 2017 update by the Infectious Diseases Society of America and Society for Healthcare Epidemiology of America. *Clinical Infectious Diseases, 66*, e1.

Mohandas, N., & Schrier, S. L. (1989). Mechanism of red cell destruction in hemolytic anemias. In W. C. Mentzer, & G. M. Wagner (Eds.), *The hereditary hemolytic anemias* (p. 391). New York, NY: Churchill Livingstone.

Mowat, C., Cole, A., Windsor, A., et al. (2011). Guidelines for the management of inflammatory bowel disease is adults. *Gut, 60*, 571.

Nylund, K., Maconi, G., Hollerwerger, A., et al. (2017). EFSUMB recommendations and guidelines for gastrointestinal ultrasound. *Ultraschall in der Medizin, 38*, 273.

Oliveira, L. G., Luengo, J., Caramori, J. C., et al. (2012). Peritonitis in recent years: Clinical findings and predictors of treatment response of 170 episodes at single Brazilian center. *International Urology and Nephrology, 44*, 1529.

Ong, J. P., Aggarwal, A., Krieger, D., et al. (2003). Correlation between ammonia levels and the severity of hepatic encephalopathy. *The American Journal of Medicine, 114*, 188.

Papadakis, M. A., & McPhee, S. J. (2014). *Current medical diagnosis and treatment* (53rd ed.). New York, NY: McGraw-Hill.

Pereira, P., Djeudi, F., Leduc, P., et al. (2015). Ogilvie's syndrome-acute colonic pseudo-obstruction. *Journal of Visceral Surgery, 152*, 99.

Rahimi, R. S., Singal, A. G., Cuthbert, J. A., & Rockey, D. C. (2014). Lactulose vs. polyethylene glycol 3350-electrolyte solution for treatment of overt hepatic encephalopathy: The HELP randomized clinical trial. *JAMA Internal Medicine, 174*, 1727.

Ranson, J. H., Rifkind, K. M., Roses, D. F., et al. (1974). Prognostic signs and the role of operative management in acute pancreatitis. *Surgery, Gynecology & Obstetrics, 139*, 69.

Reinold, C., & Bret, P. M. (1996). Current status of MR cholangiopancreatography. *AJR American Journal of Roentgenology, 166*, 1285.

Reisman, Y., Gips, C. H., Lavelle, S. M., & Wilson, J. H. (1996). Clinical presentation of (subclinical) jaundice-the Euricterus project in The Netherlands, United Dutch Hospitals and Euricterus Project Management Group. *Hepato-Gastroenterology, 43,* 1190.

Rex, D. K., Schoenfeld, P. S., Cohen, J., et al. (2015). Quality indicators for colonoscopy. *Gastrointestinal Endoscopy, 81,* 31.

Ryu, J. K., Ryu, K. H., & Kim, K. H. (2003). Clinical features of acute acalculus cholecystitis. *Journal of Clinical Gastroenterology, 36,* 166.

Saik, R. P., Greenburg, A. G., Farris, J. M., & Peskin, G. W. (1975). Spectrum of cholangitis. *The American Journal of Surgery, 130,* 143.

Sanborn, W. J. (2014). Crohn's disease evaluation and treatment: Clinical decision tool. *Gastroenterology, 147,* 702.

Sandler, R. S., Everhart, J. E., Donowitz, M., et al. (2002). The burden of selected digestive diseases in the United States. *Gastroenterology, 122,* 1500.

Sangeorazn, J. A., Bradley, S. F., He, X., et al. (1994). Epidemiology of oral candidiasis in HIV-infected patients: Colonization, infection, treatment, and emergence of fluconazole resistance. *The American Journal of Medicine, 97,* 339.

Seymour, C. W., Liu, V. X., Iwashyna, T. J., et al. (2016). Assessment of clinical criteria for sepsis: For the Third International Consensus Definitions of Sepsis and Septic Shock (Sepsis-3). *JAMA, 315,* 775.

Silverberg, M. S., Satsangi, J., Ahmad, T., et al. (2005). Toward an integrated clinical, molecular and serological classification of inflammatory bowel disease: Report of a Working Party of the 2005 Montreal World Congress of Gastroenterology. *Canadian Journal of Gastroenterology, 19*(Suppl A), 5A.

Sticova, E., & Jirsa, M. (2013). New insights in bilirubin metabolism and their clinical implications. *World Journal of Gastroenterology, 19,* 6398.

Stuppaeck, C. H., Barnes, C., et al. (1994). Assessment of alcohol withdrawal syndrome-validity and reliability of the translated and modified Clinical Institute withdrawal assessment for alcohol scale (CIWA-A). *Addiction, 84,* 1353.

Such, J., & Runyon, B. A. (1998). Spontaneous bacterial peritonitis. *Clinical Infectious Diseases, 27,* 669.

Surawicz, C. M., Brandt, L. J., Binion, D. G., et al. (2013). Guidelines for diagnosis, treatment, and prevention, of *Clostridium difficile* infections. *The American Journal of Gastroenterology, 108,* 478.

Swaroop, V. S., Chari, S. T., & Clain, J. E. (2004). Sever acute pancreatitis. *JAMA, 291,* 2865.

United Kingdom National Surgical Research Collaborative; Bhangu, A. (2014). Safety of short, in-hospital delays before surgery for acute appendicitis: Multicentre cohort study, systematic review, and meta-analysis. *Annals of Surgery, 259,* 894.

Vakil, N., Van Zanten, S. V., Kahrilas, P., et al. (2006). The Montreal definition and classification of gastroesophageal reflux disease: A global evidence-based consensus. *The American Journal of Gastroenterology, 101,* 1900.

Valle, R. G., & Godoy, F. L. (2014). Neostigmine for acute colonic pseudo-obstruction: A meta-analysis. *Annals of Medicine and Surgery (London), 3,* 60.

Vinen, C. S., & Oliveira, D. B. (2003). Acute glomerulonephritis. *Postgraduate Medical Journal, 79,* 206.

Wayne, J. D. (1977). The role of colonoscopy in the differential diagnosis of inflammatory bowel disease. *Gatrointestinal Endoscopy, 23,* 150.

Weinstock, L. B., & Chang, A. C. (2011). Methylnaltrexone for treatment of acute colonic pseudo-obstruction. *Journal of Clinical Gastroenterology, 45,* 883.

Weisbord, S. D., & Palevsky, P. M. (2005). Radiocontrast-induced acute renal failure. *Journal of Intensive Care Medicine, 20,* 63.

CHAPTER 7

Genitourinary

Binu Shajimon, DrNP

Disease Questions

1 The adult-gerontology acute care nurse practitioner (AGACNP) is examining a 38-year-old male in the emergency department. He was found unresponsive by his friend after a drug overdose and not discovered for several hours. On admission, his blood urea nitrogen (BUN) is 42, creatinine level is 4.6 mg/dL, and potassium is 4.8. Urinalysis revealed pH of 7, white blood cell (WBC)+3, and blood 2+, but the microscopic evaluation reveals only 0–2 red blood cell (RBC)/high-power field (HPF). Which of the following is the likely cause of hematuria and acute renal failure in this patient?

a. Acute glomerulonephritis

b. Nephrotic syndrome

c. Rhabdomyolysis

d. Acute interstitial nephritis

2 A 60-year-old bus driver with a 30-pack-year history of cigarette smoking presents to the emergency department with complaint of increased frequency of urination and nocturia but denies gross hematuria. Physical examination reveals an enlarged prostate. Urinalysis with microscopy revealed pale yellow urine with pH of 6.5, blood 1+, nitrite and ketones negative, WBC 1 HPF, and RBC 6 HPF. Based on this patient's history, symptoms, and urinalysis findings, which one of the following is the most appropriate next step?

a. Advise that his enlarged prostate is causing microscopic hematuria, obtain renal ultrasound, and follow up in 3 months.

b. Obtain BUN and creatinine levels, perform computed tomographic urography, and refer for cystoscopy.

c. Treat with an antibiotic for urinary tract infection (UTI) and repeat the urinalysis and culture.

d. Repeat urinalysis in 6 months and perform urine cytology to evaluate for bladder cancer.

3 A 58-year-old Hispanic male has been treated for chronic bacterial prostatitis (CBP). The patient with CBP usually presents with:

a. Prostatic pain lasting at least 3 months without consistent culture results.

b. Persistent pain associated with urination or ejaculation or lower urinary tract symptoms related to voiding or storage.

c. Recurrent UTIs with the same organism identified on repeated cultures.

d. No history of prostate pain, but leukocytes or bacteria have been found incidentally on workup for other conditions.

4 The risk factors for acute bacterial prostatitis include all of the following EXCEPT:

a. Intraprostatic ductal reflux.

b. Erectile dysfunction.

c. Unprotected anal intercourse.

d. Transurethral surgery.

5 A 45-year-old woman checks into the hospital with complaints of weight gain, irregular menstrual cycles, and increased hair growth on her chin and upper lip. She has also noticed areas of dark, velvety patches in her armpit area. What would NOT be an indicated treatment for this patient's condition?

a. Weight loss

b. Oral contraceptive pill (OCP)

c. Estrogen supplements

d. Spironolactone

6 A 20-year-old male comes to the emergency department with excruciating pain in his scrotum and abdomen along with nausea and vomiting that started about an hour ago. Upon physical examination, you find swelling in his scrotum and high-riding left testicle. Vital signs:

temperature is 100.2°F, BP is 132/95, and HR is 72. Urine testing came back negative, but the cremasteric reflex was absent on the left side but present on the right side. What is the most appropriate treatment indicated in this diagnosis?

a. Orchiopexy

b. Manual detorsion

c. Supportive care

d. Tamsulosin

7 After encountering a woman who presents with suprapubic pain, urinary frequency and urgency, and dysuria, the AGACNP decides to perform a urinary analysis. Vital signs are normal, and she denies fever or chills. Her urinalysis is positive for leukocyte esterase and nitrates. She is diagnosed with acute cystitis due to an infection with *Escherichia coli*. What is a common risk factor associated with acute cystitis?

a. Smoking

b. Family history of cystitis

c. Female sex

d. Cyclophosphamide

8 A 65-year-old woman who has had multiple children via vaginal deliveries comes to the clinic with the complaint of "pee leaking" every time she coughs or sneezes. She denies other complaints, and her vitals are within normal limits. She denies pain and just wants to know if this is normal for her age. The AGACNP recommends Kegel exercises to help strengthen her pelvic floor muscles. Why is she experiencing these symptoms?

a. Detrusor overactivity

b. Detrusor underactivity

c. Urethral hypermobility or intrinsic sphincter deficiency

d. Bladder outlet obstruction

9 A 65-year-old African American male with no past medical history comes to the emergency room complaining of difficulty stopping and starting urine stream, dysuria, and increased frequency of urination. His vitals are normal, but his prostatic-specific antigen (PSA) levels are high. Digital rectal examination findings indicate a smooth, elastic enlargement of the lateral and middle lobes of his prostate. What is the diagnosis?

a. Benign prostatic hyperplasia (BPH)

b. Prostatic adenocarcinoma

c. Acute cystitis

d. Prostatitis

10 A 30-year-old white female with a history of hepatitis B presents with a chief complaint of frothy urine. A 24-hour urine is performed, which is positive for fatty casts and 5 g of protein/day. Serum labs reveal low albumin levels in her blood. What is the most likely diagnosis?

a. Diabetic glomerulonephropathy

b. Alport syndrome

c. Minimal change disease

d. Membranous nephropathy

11 A 50-year-old man diagnosed with autosomal dominant polycystic kidney disease (ADPKD) comes to the clinic for a follow-up. He has flank pain, blood in his urine, and multiple renal cysts revealed on ultrasound. His vitals are as follows: BP 145/100, 98.7°F, and 15 RR. What other conditions is this diagnosis NOT usually associated with?

a. Mitral valve prolapse

b. Berry aneurysm

c. Polycystic kidney disease

d. Hepatic cysts

12 A 65-year-old hospitalized male currently ordered neomycin on the floor has developed acute kidney injury on hospital Day 7. He has now developed oliguria and has a high FeNa, and urinalysis shows granular casts. What is this patient most at risk for in this stage of his diagnosis?

a. Hyperkalemia

b. Hypokalemia

c. Metabolic alkalosis

d. Insulin resistance

13 A 52-year-old woman comes to the clinic with complaints of amenorrhea for about 1 year. Her vitals are within normal limits, and she admits to hot flashes, sleep disturbances, and vaginal dryness. What clinical value is most indicative of the most likely diagnosis?

a. High estrogen levels

b. High FSH (follicle-stimulating hormone)

c. Low gonadotropin-releasing hormone (GnRH)

d. Decreased androgens

14 The AGACNP is evaluating a 65-year-old man who presents with worsening lower extremity edema. He has a history of type 2 diabetes, diabetic neuropathy, hypertension, and degenerative joint disease. On physical examination, he has a blood pressure of 160/90 mm Hg. His albumin/creatinine ratio is 165. His creatinine is 1.3 mg/dL. Which of the following medications would be prescribed for treating this patient with proteinuria?

a. Amlodipine

b. Lisinopril

c. Diltiazem

d. Terazosin

15 A 42-year-old woman presents to the emergency room with complaints of pelvic pain, bleeding, dysmenorrhea, dyspareunia, and constipation. Upon examination, her uterus does not seem to be enlarged but she seems to have "chocolate (blood-filled) ovarian cysts" noted on ultrasound. What is the treatment indicated for this diagnosis?

a. Aminoglycosides

b. Hysterectomy

c. Clindamycin

d. Nonsteroidal anti-inflamatory drugs (NsAIDs)

Disease Answers/Rationales

1 **The correct answer is C.**

Rationales:

a. In acute glomerulonephritis RBCs and/or RBC casts are usually seen in the urine.

b. Nephrotic syndrome in adults wouldn't cause hematuria.

c. The patient's history and the clinical picture fit the criteria for rhabdomyolysis and muscle damage causing the acute kidney failure. The diagnosis of rhabdomyolysis can be confirmed by creatine kinase (CK), which is the most reliable and sensitive indicator of muscle injury.

d. In acute interstitial nephritis, WBCs, urine eosinophils, and/or white cell casts are usually seen in the urine.

(Mishra & Dave, 2013, p. 86; Petejova & Martinek, 2014, p. 224).

2 **The correct answer is B.**

Rationales:

a. It should not be assumed that BPH is the explanation for hematuria, particularly in the high-risk population for urologic malignancy—men, smokers, and those older than 35 years. Renal ultrasonography is less sensitive (50% sensitive and 95% specific) in detecting urothelial lesions, small renal masses, and urinary calculi and does not reliably produce diagnostic certainty. Thus, it may lead to indeterminate findings that result in additional imaging and costs.

b. Microscopic hematuria may result from completely benign causes to potentially invasive malignancy. The American Urological Association (AUA) defines asymptomatic microscopic hematuria as three or more RBCs per HPF in a properly collected specimen in the absence of obvious causes such as infection, menstruation, vigorous exercise, medical renal disease, viral illness, trauma, or a recent urologic procedure. Also, the risk of urologic malignancy is increased in men, persons older than 35 years, and persons with a history of smoking; thus, obtaining BUN and creatinine levels, performing computed tomographic urography, and referring for cystoscopy is the most appropriate course of action. A serum creatinine level should be obtained to screen for medical renal disease and to evaluate renal function before performing a contrast-enhanced radiology test. The upper urinary tract is best evaluated with multiphasic computed tomography urography, which identifies hydronephrosis, urinary calculi, and renal and ureteral lesions. The lower urinary tract is best evaluated with cystoscopy for urethral stricture disease, BPH, and bladder masses.

c. In patients with microscopic hematuria, treating empirically with antibiotics could delay treatment of potentially curable diseases.

d. The AUA does not recommend repeating urinalysis with microscopy before the workup, especially in patients who smoke, because tobacco use is a risk factor for urothelial cancer.

(Grossfeld et al., 2013, p. 1145; Schrier, 2007; Sharp, Barnes, & Erickson, 2013, pp. 747–754).

3 **The correct answer is C.**

Rationales:

a. In chronic nonbacterial prostatitis (CNP)/ chronic pelvic pain syndrome (CPPS), the patient presents with prostatic pain lasting at least 3 months without consistent culture results. CNP/CPPS presents similarly to CBP, but it is much more common and urine culture results are negative or inconsistent.

b. Chronic prostatitis presents as persistent pain associated with urination or ejaculation or lower urinary tract symptoms related to voiding or storage.

c. CBP presents as recurrent UTIs with the same organism identified on repeated cultures.

d. Asymptomatic inflammatory prostatitis—No history of prostate pain, but leukocytes or bacteria have been found incidentally on workup for other conditions.

(Le & Schaeffer, 2009, pp. 527–536; Rees, Abrahams, Doble, & Cooper, 2015, pp. 509–525; Weidner & Anderson, 2008, pp. 91–95).

> **Clinical Pearl**
>
> Acute bacterial prostatitis is acute bacterial infection of the prostate. Chronic bacterial prostatitis is recurrent urinary tract infection caused by the same organism, secondary to chronic bacterial infection of the prostate.

4 **The correct answer is B.**

Rationales:

a. Acute prostatitis presents as an acute UTI. Associated predisposing risk factors include bladder outlet obstruction secondary to BPH or an immunosuppressed state resulting in intraprostatic ductal reflux. It is caused by the same type of bacteria that causes UTIs, as well as sexually transmitted diseases.

b. Erectile dysfunction is not a risk factor for acute bacterial prostatitis, but persons diagnosed with histological prostatitis suffer from erectile dysfunction to a more severe degree than do those without prostatitis.

c. Meatal inoculation may occur during unprotected anal intercourse, instrumentation, and prolonged catheterization cause ascending urethral infection in younger men, which leads to acute bacterial prostatitis typically presents as an acute onset of fever, chills, malaise, dysuria, and perineal or rectal pain.

d. Acute bacterial prostatitis can be a complication of previous instrumentation, such as cystoscopy or prostate needle biopsy.

(Deem, Rhee, & Piesman 2019, January 4; Mcdougal, Wein, Kavoussi, Partin, & Peters, 2016, pp. 91–95).

5 **The correct answer is C.**

Rationales:

a. Weight loss is a primary recommendation for polycystic ovarian syndrome (PCOS) and can lead to cycle regulation by decreasing peripheral estrone formation.

b. OCP can prevent endometrial hyperplasia due to unopposed estrogen.

c. This patient presents classically for PCOS, in which she has enlarged, bilateral cystic ovaries (unruptured follicles) that can lead to insulin resistance (acanthosis nigricans), hirsutism, anovulation, and decreased fertility in women. There is an increased risk of endometrial cancer due to unopposed estrogen, and estrogen supplements would not be indicated as they would enhance this effect. There are three major goals for treatment of PCOS: control irregular menses, treat hirsutism, and manage infertility. Control of menses can be accomplished by the use of OCP, progesterone withdrawal, lifestyle modifications and weight loss, and metformin. Hirsutism can be treated by decreasing testosterone action and production, OCP, lifestyle modifications, metformin, and hair removal methods. Finally, infertility can be managed by lifestyle changes, metformin, insulin sensitization, clomiphene citrate, gonadotrophs, GnRH analogs, aromatase inhibitors, surgical approaches, and in vitro maturation of oocytes.

d. Spironolactone can be indicated to treat the symptoms of hirsutism found in PCOS.

(Sabatini, 2011; Williams, Rami Mortada, & Porter, 2016, pp. 106–113).

6 **The correct answer is A.**

Rationales:

a. This patient's symptoms all lead to signs of testicular torsion, in which the testicle rotates around the spermatic cord and impedes blood flow. Typical findings include extreme pain, a high-riding testis, and an absent cremasteric reflex on the affected side, which are all noted in this patient. Treatment is usually surgical correction (orchiopexy) within 6 hours, if available. If not done, the testis can be left nonviable and can lead to impaired fertility.

b. Manual detorsion can be indicated in the diagnosis of testicular torsion, but only if surgical correction is unavailable within the time frame of 6 hours.

c. Testicular torsion is a surgical emergency and will not resolve with supportive care.

d. Tamsulosin is an alpha-1 inhibitor indicated in the treatment of BPH and is not recommended for testicular torsion.

(Ogunyem, Weiker, & Abel, 2019, February 2; Ringdahl & Teague, 2013, pp. 1739–1743).

7 **The correct answer is C.**

Rationales:

a. Smoking is not a specific risk factor for acute cystitis.

b. Acute cystitis is not a genetically associated diagnosis, and family history is not usually pertinent.

c. Females have a higher risk of acute cystitis due to a shorter urethra, which makes the likelihood for infection higher compared to males. Other risk factors for acute cystitis include sexual intercourse (honeymoon cystitis), indwelling catheter, diabetes mellitus, and impaired bladder emptying. "The definition of acute uncomplicated cystitis implies an uncomplicated UTI in a premenopausal, nonpregnant woman with no known urologic abnormalities or comorbidities."

d. Cyclophosphamide is not a specific risk factor for acute cystitis but can be important for other diagnoses including transitional cell carcinoma, which can be sequelae of chronic cystitis.

(Colgan & Williams, 2011, pp. 771–776; Moreno et al., 2008b, pp. 2529–2534; Yamamoto, Higuchi, & Nojima, 2010, pp. 450–456).

8 **The correct answer is C.**

Rationales:

a. Detrusor overactivity would lead to a diagnosis of urgency incontinence, which would present with a leak with an urge to void immediately and is usually associated with a UTI. This woman's leaking with increased intra-abdominal pressure and risk factor of vaginal deliveries leads more toward the diagnosis of stress incontinence.

b. Detrusor underactivity is associated with overflow incontinence, which is associated with incomplete emptying leading to a leak with overfilling. This can be associated with polyuria, obstruction, or a neurogenic bladder. An increased postvoid residual would be seen on catheterization or ultrasound. This patient's symptoms lean more toward stress incontinence.

c. This woman is experiencing stress incontinence due to outlet incompetence (urethral hypermobility or intrinsic sphincter deficiency), which leads to a leak of urine associated with increased intra-abdominal pressure (i.e., sneezing, coughing, lifting). Risk factors for stress incontinence include obesity, vaginal delivery, or prostate surgery. Indicated treatment includes Kegel exercises to strengthen the muscles of the pelvic floor or weight loss.

d. Bladder outlet obstruction is associated with overflow incontinence, which is associated with incomplete emptying leading to a leak with overfilling. This can be associated with polyuria, obstruction, or a neurogenic bladder. An increased postvoid residual would be seen on catheterization or ultrasound. This patient's symptoms lean more toward stress incontinence.

(Mcdougal et al., 2016, pp. 27–315; Shaw, 2004, pp. 27–31).

9 **The correct answer is A.**

Rationales:

a. This is a classic presentation for BPH. Hyperplasia of the prostate can lead to distention and hypertrophy of the bladder and obstruction, which can lead to the urinary symptoms that this man presents with. Treatment includes α_1-antagonists and 5α-reductase inhibitors.

b. Prostatic adenocarcinoma is also common in men >50 years of age and would present with a high PSA level, but it arises most often in the posterior lobe and can also be diagnosed with high prostatic acid phosphatase (PAP) levels. BPH is not premalignant and does not lead to prostatic adenocarcinoma.

c. Acute cystitis would normally present with suprapubic pain, dysuria, urinary frequency, and urgency. Risk factors include female gender (shorter urethra), sexual intercourse, an indwelling catheter, diabetes, or impaired bladder emptying. UA would also show leukocyte esterase and nitrates. A high PSA would be atypical.

d. Prostatitis could also present with dysuria, frequency, and urgency, but the prostate would be warm, tender, and enlarged and a bacterial infection would be present. A high PSA would be atypical.

(Dubey, Kapoor, & Muruganandham, 2007; Epperly & Moore, 2013, pp. 3657–3664; Lee, 2017, p. 15).

10 **The correct answer is D.**

Rationales:

a. Although diabetic glomerulonephropathy is characterized as a nephrotic syndrome, this woman does not present with any signs of diabetes (polyuria, polydipsia, and polyphagia) and Kimmelstiel–Wilson lesions are not indicated on light microscopy. This condition is also not usually associated with a history of systemic lupus erythematosus (SLE).

b. Alport syndrome is a nephritic syndrome caused by a mutation in type 4 collagen and will typically lead to symptoms that include eye problems, glomerulonephritis, sensorineural deafness, and RBC casts in the urine, none of which are indicated in this scenario.

c. Minimal change disease is also characterized as a nephrotic syndrome, but it is usually common in children who are recovering from a recent infection. Membranous nephropathy is more likely in this woman's case.

d. The fatty casts, high proteinuria, hypoalbuminemia, and frothy urine all lead to a diagnosis of nephrotic syndrome. A history of hepatitis is a common secondary cause associated with membranous nephropathy, a subset of nephrotic syndrome, and is the most likely diagnosis of all the choices listed. It is also associated with SLE, drugs, infections, or solid tumors or may be primarily due to antibodies against the PLA2 receptor.

(Alsaad & Herzenberg, 2007, pp. 18–26; Genetics Home Reference, 2013; Lai et al., 1991, pp. 1457–1463; Madaio & Harrington, 2001, p. 25).

11 **The correct answer is C.**

Rationales:

a. Mitral valve prolapse is commonly associated with ADPKD.

b. Berry aneurysm is commonly associated with ADPKD.

c. PCOS is not usually associated with ADPKD.

d. Hepatic cysts are commonly associated with ADPKD.

(Gabow et al., 1992, pp. 1311–1319; Haque & Moatasim, 2008, pp. 84–90; Harris & Torres, 2018, July 19; Srivastava & Patel, 2014, pp. 303–307).

12 **The correct answer is A.**

Rationales:

a. This patient who has been hospitalized for 1 week with a history of aminoglycoside use and presents with oliguria and granular casts in his urine most likely has acute tubular necrosis (ATN), which is an intrinsic subset of acute kidney injury. The three phases of ATN include the inciting event (i.e., neomycin), maintenance phase (oliguria, 1–3 weeks), and the recovery phase. He is currently in the maintenance phase of ATN and is most at risk for hyperkalemia of all the options listed.

b. The patient could experience hypokalemia and other electrolyte wasting during the recovery phase of ATN, but he is currently in the maintenance phase as to which hyperkalemia is more likely.

c. During the maintenance phase of ATN, metabolic acidosis, not alkalosis, is a common complication.

d. Insulin resistance is not associated with ATN.

(Liango & Jaber, 2019; Mahboob Rahman, Shad, & Smith, 2012, pp. 631–639; Renal and Urology News, 2019, January 16).

Clinical Pearl

UTIs identified in males should trigger investigation into possible STIs in those who are sexually active.

13 **The correct answer is B.**

Rationales:

a. Menopause is mainly a diagnosis due to a loss of ovarian follicles due to age and would lead to low estrogen levels.

b. This woman is most likely experiencing the physiologic changes that accompany menopause due to an age-related decline in the number of ovarian follicles and a subsequent decline in estrogen levels. The loss of estrogen would lead to a loss of inhibin and negative feedback from Sertoli cells, and therefore high FSH levels, which are most indicative of menopause. The American Association of Clinical Endocrinologists suggests that an FSH level >40 IU/L confirms the diagnosis of menopause along with the accompanying history and physical examination.

c. Low estrogen levels lead to a loss of negative feedback and thus high GnRH levels.

d. Menopause allows for increased peripheral conversion of estrogen (estrone) into androgens and thus leads to symptoms such as hirsutism.

(Chaplin, 2016, pp. 27–32; Conrad, 2018; Coope, 1984, pp. 888–890).

14 **The correct answer is B.**

Rationales:

a. Dihydropyridine calcium channel blockers (CCBs) may worsen edema as peripheral edema is one of the common side effects of CCBs as a class.

b. Lisinopril is an ACE inhibitor, which is the first line of treatment for proteinuria. Given that the patient has diabetic retinopathy, neuropathy, an elevated blood pressure, and microalbuminuria (on the basis of his albumin/creatinine ratio), ACE inhibitor is the appropriate choice of drug for this patient as it reduces microalbuminuria or clinical proteinuria and retard the progression toward end-stage renal failure. It will also lower systemic blood pressure.

c. Nondihydropyridine CCBs may worsen edema as peripheral edema is one of the common side effects of CCBs as a class.

d. Terazosin would be a good choice if BPH were present; however, it's not the best choice for hypertension.

(Basi, Fesler, Mimran, & Lewis, 2008, pp. S194–S201; Jafar et al., 2003, p. 244; Van Buren & Toto, 2011, pp. 28–41).

Clinical Pearl

Priapism is a medical emergency, requiring emergent urologic consultation.

15 **The correct answer is D.**

Rationales:

a. Endometriosis is not a diagnosis due to a bacterial infection, and thus antibiotics would not be an effective treatment option.

b. Hysterectomy is not indicated in the treatment of endometriosis as opposed to other uterine conditions including adenomyosis.

c. Endometriosis is not a diagnosis due to a bacterial infection, and thus antibiotics would not be an effective treatment option.

d. This woman's symptoms most likely point toward a diagnosis of endometriosis, in which endometrial glands and stroma are present outside of the endometrial cavity, including the ovaries (the most common site) as seen in this patient. Of all the options listed, NSAIDs are the only option that is indicated in the diagnosis. Other treatment options include nutritional therapy, OCP, GnRH agonist, or surgical treatment.

(Becker, 2015, pp. 17–21; Mandai et al., 2012; Obstetrics and Gynecology Reports, pp. 16–24).

References

Alsaad, K. O., & Herzenberg, A. M. (2007). Distinguishing diabetic nephropathy from other causes of glomerulosclerosis: An update. *Journal of Clinical Pathology*, 60(1), 18–26. doi: 10.1136/jcp.2005.035592

Basi, S., Fesler, P., Mimran, A., & Lewis, J. B. (2008). Microalbuminuria in type 2 diabetes and hypertension: A marker, treatment target, or innocent bystander? *Diabetes Care*, 31(Suppl 2), S194–S201. doi: 10.2337/dc08-s249

Becker, C. (2015). Diagnosis and management of endometriosis. *Prescriber*, 26(20), 17–21. doi: 10.1002/psb.1398

Chaplin, S. (2016). NICE guideline: Diagnosis and management of the menopause. *Prescriber*, 27(1), 27–32. https://doi.org/10.1002/psb.1427

Colgan, R., & Williams, M. (2011). Diagnosis and treatment of acute uncomplicated cystitis. *American Family Physician*, 84(7), 771–776.

Conrad, M. (2018). *Menopause symptoms and signs: Causes.* Retrieved September 11, 2019, from https://www.emedicinehealth.com/menopause/symptom.htm

Coope, J. (1984). Menopause: Diagnosis and treatment. *BMJ*, 289(6449), 888–890. doi: 10.1136/bmj.289.6449.888

Dubey, D., Kapoor, R., & Muruganandham, K. (2007). Acute urinary retention in benign prostatic hyperplasia: Risk factors and current management. *Indian Journal of Urology*, 23(4), 347. doi: 10.4103/0970-1591.35050

Epperly, T. D., & Moore, K. E. (2013). Health issues in men: Part I. Common genitourinary disorders. *American Family Physician*, 61(12), 3657–3664. Retrieved from https://www.aafp.org/afp/2000/0615/p3657.html

Gabow, P. A., Johnson, A. M., Kaehny, W. D., Kimberling, W. J., Lezotte, D. C., Duley, I. T., & Jones, R. H. (1992). Factors affecting the progression of renal disease in autosomal-dominant polycystic kidney disease. *Kidney International*, 41(5), 1311–1319. https://doi.org/10.1038/ki.1992.195

Grossfeld, G. D., Wolf, S., Litwin, M. S., Hricak, H., Shuler, C. L., Agerter, D. C., & Carroll, P. (2013). Asymptomatic microscopic hematuria in adults: Summary of the AUA best practice policy recommendations. *American Family Physician*, 63(6), 1145. Retrieved from https://www.aafp.org/afp/2001/0315/p1145.html

Harris, P. C., & Torres, V. E. (2018, July 19). Polycystic kidney disease, autosomal dominant. Retrieved September 11, 2019, from https://www.ncbi.nlm.nih.gov/books/NBK1246/

Jafar, T. H., Stark, P. C., Schmid, C. H., Landa, M., Maschio, G., de Jong, P. E., … Levey, A. S. (2003). Progression of chronic kidney disease: The role of blood pressure control, proteinuria, and angiotensin-converting enzyme inhibition: A patient-level meta-analysis. *Annals of Internal Medicine*, 139(4), 244. https://doi.org/10.7326/0003-4819-139-4-200308190-00006

Le, B. V., & Schaeffer, A. J. (2009). Genitourinary pain syndromes, prostatitis, and lower urinary tract symptoms. *Urologic Clinics of North America*, 36(4), 527–536. https://doi.org/10.1016/j.ucl.2009.08.005

Lee, S. W. (2017). Chronic prostatitis/chronic pelvic pain syndrome and male bladder pain syndrome/interstitial cystitis: How are they related? *Urogenital Tract Infection*, *12*(1), 15. https://doi.org/10.14777/uti.2017.12.1.15

Liango, O., & Jaber, B. L. (2019). *UpToDate*. Retrieved September 11, 2019, from https://www.uptodate.com/contents/nonoliguric-versus-oliguric-acute-kidney-injury

Mandai, M., Suzuki, A., Matsumura, N., Baba, T., Yamaguchi, K., Hamanishi, J., … Konishi, I. (2012). Clinical management of ovarian endometriotic cyst (chocolate cyst): Diagnosis, medical treatment, and minimally invasive surgery. *Current Obstetrics and Gynecology Reports*, *1*(1), 16–24. doi: 10.1007/s13669-011-0002-3

Mcdougal, W. S., Wein, A. J., Kavoussi, L. R., Partin, A. W., & Peters, C. (2016). *Campbell-Walsh urology eleventh edition review*. Philadelphia, PA: Elsevier.

Mishra, A., & Dave, N. (2013). Acute renal failure due to rhabdomyolysis following a seizure. *Journal of Family Medicine and Primary Care*, *2*(1), 86. doi:10.4103/2249-4863.109962

Ogunyem, O. I., Weiker, M., & Abel, E. J. (February 2, 2019). *Testicular torsion treatment & management: Approach considerations, surgical detorsion*. Retrieved September 11, 2019, from https://emedicine.medscape.com/article/2036003-treatment

Rees, J., Abrahams, M., Doble, A., & Cooper, A. (2015). Diagnosis and treatment of chronic bacterial prostatitis and chronic prostatitis/chronic pelvic pain syndrome: A consensus guideline. *BJU International*, *116*(4), 509–525. https://doi.org/10.1111/bju.13101

Ringdahl, E. N., & Teague, L. (2013). Testicular torsion. *American Family Physician*, *74*(10), 1739–1743. Retrieved from https://www.aafp.org/afp/2006/1115/p1739.html

Sabatini, R. (2011). *Polycystic ovarian syndrome: An enigmatic endrocrinological disorder*. New York, NY: Nova Biomedical Books.

Schrier, R. W. (2007). *Diseases of the kidney & urinary tract*. Philadelphia, PA: Wolters Kluwer Health/Lippincott Williams & Wilkins.

Sharp, V. J., Barnes, K. T., & Erickson, B. A. (2013). Assessment of asymptomatic microscopic hematuria in adults. *American Family Physician*, *88*(11), 747–754.

Shaw, C. (2004). Stress urinary incontinence in women. *Primary Health Care*, *14*(5), 27–31. https://doi.org/10.7748/phc2004.06.14.5.27.c507

Van Buren, P. N., & Toto, R. (2011). Hypertension in diabetic nephropathy: Epidemiology, mechanisms, and management. *Advances in Chronic Kidney Disease*, *18*(1), 28–41. doi: 10.1053/j.ackd.2010.10.003

Weidner, W., & Anderson, R. U. (2008). Evaluation of acute and chronic bacterial prostatitis and diagnostic management of chronic prostatitis/chronic pelvic pain syndrome with special reference to infection/inflammation. *International Journal of Antimicrobial Agents*, *31*(1), 91–95. https://doi.org/10.1016/j.ijantimicag.2007.07.044

Wein, A. J., Kavoussi, L. R., Partin, A. W., & Peters, C. A. (2014). *Inflammatory and pain conditions of the male genitourinary tract: Prostatitis and related pain conditions, orchitis, and epididymitis*. Philadelphia, PA: Elsevier.

Williams, T., Mortada, R., & Porter, S. (2016). Diagnosis and treatment of polycystic ovary syndrome. *American Family Physician*, *94*(2), 106–113. Retrieved from https://www.aafp.org/afp/2016/0715/p106.html

Yamamoto, S., Higuchi, Y., & Nojima, M. (2010). Current therapy of acute uncomplicated cystitis. *International Journal of Urology*, *17*(5), 450–456. doi: 10.1111/j.1442-2042.2010.02500.x

CHAPTER 8

Nephrology

Rachel A. Schroy, DNP

Disease Questions

1 Septic shock, dehydration, ruptured abdominal aneurysm, and acute congestive heart failure are examples of which classification of acute kidney injury (AKI) causes?

a. Postrenal disorders

b. Prerenal disorders

c. Intrinsic renal disorders

d. Extrinsic renal disorders

2 What is the pathogenesis of acute tubular necrosis (ATN) in AKI?

a. It is an obstruction in the lumen of renal tubules from sloughed cells of the epithelial cells lining the renal tubules, which were initially damaged from inflammation.

b. It is injury sustained after a lack of decreased perfusion to the kidneys.

c. It is inflammation to the renal interstitium commonly caused by a hypersensitivity reaction from penicillins.

d. It is injury that occurs secondary to an obstruction distal to the renal parenchyma.

3 In the United States, what two chronic conditions are the main cause for chronic kidney disease (CKD)?

a. Hyperlipidemia and hypertension

b. Hypertension and diabetes mellitus

c. Peripheral vascular disease and lupus

d. Diabetes mellitus and cirrhosis

4 A 45-year-old male is found to have worsening CKD. Over the last 3 months, his new average glomerular filtration rate (GFR) is 28 mL/min/1.73 m. Based on the National Kidney Foundation guidelines, what stage is his CKD?

a. Stage II

b. Stage III

c. Stage IV

d. Stage V

5 A 54-year-old male with CKD and poorly controlled hypertension presents to the emergency room with his wife. His wife reports that over the last 1–2 weeks, the patient has been confused and irritable, has been experiencing increased fatigue and decreased appetite with episodes of nausea/vomiting, has had complaints of a metallic taste in his mouth, and has had itching all over but with no rash. What do you expect the diagnosis to be?

a. Uremic syndrome

b. Atopic dermatitis

c. Scabies

d. Urinary tract infection

6 Common electrolyte derangements seen in end-stage CKD are:

a. Hyperkalemia, hypophosphatemia, and hypercalcemia

b. Hypokalemia, hypophosphatemia, and hypocalcemia

c. Hyperkalemia, hyperphosphatemia, and hypocalcemia

d. Hypokalemia, hyperphosphatemia, and hypercalcemia

7 According to the Kidney Disease Improving Global Outcomes (KDIGO) criteria for defining AKI, all of the following define AKI EXCEPT:

a. An increase in serum creatinine within a 48-hour period of at least 0.3 mg/dL

b. A decrease in urine output within a 6-hour period of at least 0.5 mL/kg/hr

c. An increase in serum creatinine from baseline within a 7-day period of at least 1.5 mg/dL

d. An increase of blood urea nitrogen (BUN) within a 48-hour period of at least 20 mmol/L

8 A 72-year-old female is admitted with severe sepsis secondary to pneumonia. Laboratory and clinical findings show that she has developed AKI stage II according to the KDIGO criteria. Her home medications are furosemide 40 mg by mouth daily, ibuprofen 400 mg by mouth twice daily as needed for pain or fever, and lisinopril 10 mg by mouth daily. Which of her home medications should be stopped at this time due to her new AKI?

a. Furosemide

b. Ibuprofen

c. Lisinopril

d. All of the above

9 A 68-year-old male African American truck driver with a history of insulin-dependent diabetes and CKD stage II presents to the emergency room with acute-onset shortness of breath, tachypnea, tachycardia, and refractory hypoxemia. The provider has ordered a stat CT angiography to rule out pulmonary embolism. The provider knows that the patient has a high risk of developing what after the CT study?

a. Acute pyelonephritis

b. Contrast-induced AKI

c. CKD stage VI

d. Acute congestive heart failure

10 For patients who require IV iodinated contrast agents for a procedure and who are at high risk of developing contrast-induced AKI, what is the most effective preventative treatment?

a. IV furosemide 40 mg twice daily for 24 hours postprocedure

b. *N*-acetylcysteine (NAC) 1,200 mg daily for 24 hours postprocedure

c. Isotonic saline at 150 mL/hr started at least 3 hours before procedure and continued for at least 6 hours postprocedure

d. Methylprednisolone sodium succinate 1 g IV for 3 days postprocedure

11 A 55-year-old female with history of CKD stage IV, diabetes mellitus, hypertension, and hyperlipidemia presents with septic shock secondary to community-acquired pneumonia and is noted to have an increase in her serum creatinine greater than 0.5 mg/dL when her baseline serum creatinine is 4.3 mg/dL. Over the last 24 hours, the patient's urine output decreased to less than 0.2 mL/kg/hr despite fluid resuscitation and improved hemodynamics with vasopressors. What do you anticipate will be implemented next in her plan of care?

a. Continuous renal replacement therapy through hemofiltration

b. Low-dose dopamine infusion

c. Intermittent hemodialysis therapy

d. Furosemide infusion

12 A 49-year-old female with CKD stage VI who receives hemodialysis three times a week and is anuric otherwise. What medication do you expect to see as part of her home mediation regiment to help control one of her chronic electrolyte imbalances?

a. Furosemide

b. Calcium acetate

c. Potassium chloride

d. Spironolactone

13 A 44-year-old male with a history of alcoholic cirrhosis and ascites admitted with severe sepsis secondary to spontaneous bacterial peritonitis (SBP) and with an increased model end-stage liver disease (MELD) score now 33. It is noted that since admission 3 days ago, the patient's creatinine has doubled and is now 2.6 mg/dL. What diagnosis are you adding to his list of hospital problems?

a. CKD stage III

b. Intrinsic AKI

c. Hepatorenal syndrome

d. Postrenal AKI

14 A 55-year-old female presented with malaise and increased generalized weakness. Laboratory findings showed a serum potassium (K+) of 6.8 mEq/L, and the patient had peaked T waves on ECG. The patient was given 10 mL IV of 10% calcium gluconate, 10 units IV of regular insulin, 50 mL IV of 50% dextrose, and 30 g oral sodium polystyrene sulfonate. Which medication will facilitate the removal of excess K+?

a. 10% calcium gluconate

b. Regular insulin

c. 50% dextrose

d. Sodium polystyrene sulfonate

15 What is the major advantage of using continuous renal replacement therapy (CRRT) over intermittent hemodialysis?

a. It removes life-threatening solutes twice as fast compared to intermittent hemodialysis.

b. It causes less trauma to the red blood cells.

c. It is less likely to cause hemodynamic instability because it is a more gradual process.

d. It can remove a larger amount of fluid volume in a shorter period of time compared to intermittent hemodialysis.

16 What is the definition of hypernatremia?

   a. Serum sodium greater than 140 mEq/L

   b. Urine osmolality greater than 300 mOsm/kg

   c. Serum sodium greater than 145 mEq/L

   d. Serum osmolality greater than 300 mOsm/kg H_2O

17 A 61-year-old male arborist with a history of congestive heart failure who takes furosemide at home and whose dose was recently doubled 2 weeks ago. The patient presents with complaints of increased fatigue, weakness, decreased urine output despite medication compliance, and episodes of dizziness to the point that he feels unsafe to do his job. The patient is found to have a systolic blood pressure of 90 and serum sodium (Na+) of 157 $mOsm/kg$ H_2O. How do you plan on managing his hypernatremia?

   a. Fluid resuscitate him with 1–2 L normal saline 0.9%, and then replace the remainder of the patient's free water deficit with 0.45% saline over the next 24–48 hours.

   b. Administer furosemide 40 mg and monitor Na+ levels.

   c. Fluid resuscitate patient with hypotonic saline with goal to correct hypernatremia in 2–4 hours.

   d. Start hypotonic saline with goal to correct free water deficit in 48 hours.

18 A 26-year-old female admitted with a traumatic brain injury after falling down a flight of stairs while intoxicated. The patient is intubated and sedated; the overnight team reports that her urine output increased dramatically over the last 12 hours, and she is now net negative 3.5 L without receiving any diuretics. She also has a Na+ level of 159 this morning. What is her new diagnosis and what is your initial management plan?

   a. Nephrogenic diabetes insipidus (DI). Start hydrocortisone 100 mg every 8 hours and start isotonic saline.

   b. Central DI. Check serum and urine osmolarity, start desmopressin 2 μg subcutaneously every 12 hours, and correct the hypernatremia at a rate of 0.5 mEq/L per hour or less.

   c. Nephrogenic DI. Every hour adjust intravenous fluid (IVF) resuscitation to match urinary output.

   d. Central DI. Check serum and urine osmolarity and start 5% dextrose with water at a rate of 250 mL/hr.

19 What is a hallmark finding for DI?

   a. Concentrated urine and hypotonic plasma

   b. Concentrated urine and hypertonic plasma

   c. Dilute urine and hypotonic plasma

   d. Dilute urine and hypertonic plasma

20 A 46-year-old male is admitted with increased confusion and has a history of chronic alcohol abuse. The patient's wife reports that he drinks at least a case of beer a day and his last drink was day of admission, and she denies any change in his drinking habits. Patient was found to have an ethanol level of 220 and a serum sodium of 114 mEq/L. What is the patient's primary diagnosis and reason for confusion?

   a. Delirium tremens

   b. Alcohol intoxication

   c. Beer potomania

   d. Psychogenic polydipsia

21 What is a common cause of a patient developing hyponatremia during hospital admission?

   a. Use of hypotonic IVFs

   b. Sodium-restrictive diets

   c. Use of spironolactone diuretics

   d. Use of normal saline 0.9% for fluid resuscitation

22 A patient with chronic hyponatremia is admitted with severe hyponatremia. As you manage this patient's hyponatremia, you are aware that the patient is at a greater risk for developing which complication from the treatment compared to someone with acute hyponatremia?

a. Severe hypernatremia

b. Central pontine myelinolysis

c. Hyperchloremia

d. Acute kidney injury

23 What is the pathophysiology of the life-threatening encephalopathy that can occur with hypotonic hyponatremia?

a. Destruction of the myelin sheath layer over the cerebral nerve cells resulting in decreased ability of the nerve cells to transfer signals to each other

b. Acute cerebral atrophy as due to severe dehydration

c. Cerebral edema causing increased intracranial pressure and possible brain stem herniation

d. Central nervous system dysfunction due to increased levels of noxious agents of gastric origin

24 A 32-year-old female, who was admitted with sepsis secondary to pneumonia, had the following laboratory findings this morning: creatinine 0.8 mg/dL, magnesium 0.8 mEq/L, potassium 3 mEq/L, and ionized calcium 1 mmol/L. With your understanding of electrolyte disorders, which treatment plan would you do first?

a. Treat the hypomagnesemia.

b. Treat the hypocalcemia.

c. Treat the hyperkalemia.

d. Treat the hypokalemia.

25 You have a 27-year-old trauma patient who required a large eight units of packed red blood cells (PRBCs) as well as other blood products for resuscitation and who also sustained an AKI. What electrolyte abnormalities are concerned that he may develop postresuscitation?

a. Hypermagnesemia and hyperkalemia

b. Hypocalcemia and hypokalemia

c. Hypercalcemia and hypomagnesemia

d. Hypocalcemia and hyperkalemia

26 A patient is admitted with severe hypomagnesemia, and you start the patient on telemetry monitoring because you are concerned about the patient developing which cardiac rhythm?

a. Bradycardia

b. Torsades de pointes

c. Supraventricular tachycardia

d. Atrial fibrillation

27 A 47-year-old female admitted with severe sepsis secondary to hospital-acquired pneumonia has a history of chronic obstructive pulmonary disease (COPD) and CKD stage IV. The patient is having increased work of breathing and hypoxia requiring intubation this morning. Her morning laboratory findings were Na+ 131 mEq/L, K+ 4.8 mEq/L, and creatinine 2.8 mg/dL. Which neuromuscular blocker will you be sure NOT to use on this patient?

a. Succinylcholine

b. Rocuronium

c. Vecuronium

d. Cisatracurium

28 What is the most common extrarenal cause for hypokalemia?

a. Prescribed B2-agonist bronchodilators

b. Metabolic alkalosis

c. Severe diarrhea

d. Metabolic acidosis

29 A 35-year-old male recently diagnosed with acute lymphoblastic leukemia was admitted yesterday for monitoring after receiving his first dose of chemotherapy. This morning, his laboratory findings show a new AKI, slight hyperkalemia, and hyperphosphatemia. As the provider, what life-threatening diagnosis are you concerned he is developing?

a. Chronic kidney disease

b. Tumor lysis syndrome (TLS)

c. Disseminated intravascular coagulation (DIC)

d. Acute pancreatitis

30 An 80-year-old female septic patient with serum laboratory finds of sodium 131 mEq/L, albumin level 1.8 g/dL, potassium 3.2 mEq/L, creatinine 2.4 mg/dL, calcium 6.5 mg/dL, and ionized calcium 4.8 mg/dL. What factor is causing the discrepancy in calcium levels?

a. Acute kidney injury

b. Hyponatremia

c. Hypokalemia

d. Hypoalbuminemia

Disease Answers/Rationales

1 The correct answer is B.

Rationales:

a. Postrenal disorders causing AKI are obstructive in nature and are distal to the renal parenchyma. All the examples in this question do not cause obstruction distal to the kidneys.

b. Prerenal disorders causing AKI decrease blood flow to the renal parenchyma. The examples in this question would all cause a decrease in blood flow to the kidneys.

c. Intrinsic renal disorders are true kidney diseases causing AKI.

d. Extrinsic renal disorders are not an actual classification for causes of AKI.

(Makris & Spanou, 2016, pp. 85–98; Marino, 2014, pp. 636–637).

2 The correct answer is A.

Rationales:

a. ATN occurs when sloughed epithelial cell in the renal tubules, which were initially injured by inflammatory changes, cause obstruction on the luminal side of the glomerulus resulting in decreased GFR.

b. This answer is a description of prerenal disorders causing AKI. ATN is a renal disorder causing AKI.

c. Acute interstitial nephritis (AIN) is an inflammatory injury to the renal interstitium commonly caused by a drug hypersensitivity or viral infection.

d. This answer is a description of a postrenal disorder causing AKI. ATN is a renal disorder causing AKI.

(Marino, 2014, pp. 636–637).

3 The correct answer is B.

Rationales:

a. Hyperlipidemia is not one of the main causes of CKD.

b. Hypertension and diabetes mellitus account for over 70% of the cases of late-stage CKD in the United States.

c. Peripheral vascular disease and lupus are not the two leading causes of CKD in the United States.

d. Diabetes mellitus and cirrhosis are not the leading causes of CKD in the United States.

(Papadakis & McPhee, 2019).

4 The correct answer is C.

Rationales:

a. According to the National Kidney Foundation, CKD stage II has a GFR of 60–89 mL/min/1.73 m.

b. According to the National Kidney Foundation, the GFR range for CKD stage III is 30–59 mL/min/1.73 m.

c. According to the National Kidney Foundation, the GFR range for CKD stage IV is 15–29 mL/min/1.73 m.

d. According to the National Kidney Foundation, the GFR range for CKD stage V is less than 15 mL/min/1.73 m.

(Papadakis & McPhee, 2019).

5 The correct answer is A.

Rationales:

a. Uremic syndrome results from the accumulation of metabolic waste products in the body that are not be excreted due to advanced CKD. Common symptoms of uremic syndrome are listed in the question.

b. Atopic dermatitis is commonly seen with an itchy rash that is scaly and with red plagues, usually affecting the face, neck, knees, elbows, and trunk. Atopic dermatitis does not cause neurologic or gastrointestinal symptoms.

c. Scabies is an infestation of *Sarcoptes scabiei*, which usually spares the head and neck of the host. The pruritic lesions seen with scabies are excoriations with small vesicles and burrows.

d. A urinary tract infection is a bacterial infection in the urinary tract, usually occurring in women of this age group, and does not cause pruritus or a metallic taste in the mouth.

(Papadakis & McPhee, 2019).

6 The correct answer is C.

Rationales:

a. Hypophosphatemia and hypercalcemia are not seen in end-stage CKD.

b. Hypokalemia and hypophosphatemia are not seen in end-stage CKD.

c. Hyperkalemia, hyperphosphatemia, and hypocalcemia are common electrolyte derangements seen in end-stage CKD.

d. Hypokalemia and hypercalcemia are not seen in end-stage CKD.

(Papadakis & McPhee, 2019).

7 The correct answer is D.

Rationales:

a. According to the KDIGO criteria, AKI is an increase in serum creatinine $\geq$0.3 mg/dL within a 48-hour period.

b. According to KDIGO, AKI is defined as a decrease in urinary output within a 6-hour period of at least 0.5 mL/kg/hr.

c. According to KDIGO, AKI is defined as an increase in serum creatinine $\geq$1.5 times the patient's baseline, which occurs over a 7-day period.

d. The KDIGO criteria do not take into account the change in BUN when defining AKI.

(Makris & Spanou, 2016, pp. 85–98).

8 **The correct answer is D.**

Rationales:

a. In the initial management of AKI, the provider should stop all nephrotoxic drugs and promote adequate volume for renal perfusion. This would mean stopping furosemide because it's a loop diuretic.

b. In the initial management of AKI, the provider should stop all nephrotoxic drugs, which would include any nonsteroidal anti-inflammatory drugs (NSAIDs).

c. In the initial management of AKI, the provider should stop all nephrotoxic drugs, which would include any ACE inhibitors.

d. In the initial management of AKI, the provider should stop all nephrotoxic drugs, promote adequate volume for renal perfusion, and treat the underlying cause. All her home medications would need to be discontinued at this time due to the reasons discussed above.

(Acute Kidney Injury Work Group, 2012, pp. 1–141; Marino, 2014, pp. 639–641).

Clinical Pearl

Medication reconciliation and review are paramount in patients who develop AKI, particularly if this occurred after admission.

9 **The correct answer is B.**

Rationales:

a. Acute pyelonephritis is a bacterial infection which causes inflammation to the kidneys. It is not a complication from receiving intravenous (IV) iodinated contrast agents.

b. Contrast induced AKI is seen within 72 hours after receiving IV iodinated contrast agents and the risk is greater in people with chronic renal insufficiency, multiorgan failure, or in the setting of the use of other nephrotoxic agents.

c. Developing CKD VI after exposure to IV iodinated contrast agents is not a common complication. Most contrast induced AKI resolves in a few weeks.

d. Acute congestive heart failure is not a complication of being exposed to IV iodinated contrast agents.

(Marino, 2014, pp. 640-641; Papadakis & McPhee, 2019).

10 **The correct answer is C.**

Rationales:

a. Furosemide does not improve renal function in AKI.

b. The use of NAC in preventing contrast-induced AKI has mixed results. Successful use of NAC for prevention of contrast-induced AKI would be at higher doses than the answer given, such as 1,200 mg twice daily for 48 hours.

c. Intravenous hydration is the most effective preventative measure for contrast-induced AKI, and it is recommended that at least 300–500 mL of isotonic saline should be infused prior to an emergency procedure.

d. Methylprednisolone sodium succinate is not used in the prevention or treatment of contrast-induced AKI.

(Marino, 2014, pp. 640–641).

11 **The correct answer is A.**

Rationales:

a. In the setting of hemodynamic instability, the slower process of hemofiltration causes less hemodynamic compromise and is more ideal in patients that are already in a shock state.

b. Low-dose dopamine does not improve renal function in the setting of AKI.

c. Intermittent hemodialysis will have increased risk for causing hypotension given the large amount of blood needed to run through the dialysis chamber at one time.

d. Furosemide does not improve renal function in the setting of AKI, and it does not increase urine output when a patient is oliguric due to AKI.

(Marino, 2014, pp. 640–646).

12 **The correct answer is B.**

Rationales:

a. Due to her chronic state of CKD stage VI and being anuric, furosemide will have no effect on improving her urine output or electrolyte abnormalities.

b. Calcium acetate is a phosphate binder taken three times a day around mealtime to help reduce the dietary phosphate absorption in patients with end-stage renal disease.

c. Patients with end-stage renal disease should not be on potassium supplements due to the high risk of fatal hyperkalemia from poor, or no, ability to excrete it renally.

d. Due to the patient's end-stage renal disease, diuretics will have no effect on improving urine output, and in the setting of spironolactone use, there is a risk of causing hyperkalemia because it is a potassium-sparing diuretic.

(Papadakis & McPhee, 2019).

13 **The correct answer is C.**

Rationales:

a. The patient has no prior history of CKD, and CKD is a progressive decline in renal function over years, not acutely over a few days.

b. In the setting of advanced cirrhosis and severe sepsis, this decline in renal function would be considered a prerenal AKI.

c. Hepatorenal syndrome occurs due to advanced cirrhosis causing alterations in circulation, which result in vasoconstriction to the kidneys.

d. In the setting of advanced cirrhosis and severe sepsis, this decline in renal function would be considered a prerenal AKI.

(Marino, 2014, p. 729; Papadakis & McPhee, 2019).

14 **The correct answer is D.**

Rationales:

a. Calcium opposes the depolarization produced by hyperkalemia on the myocardial cells, but it has no role in reducing serum K+.

b. Regular insulin activates the sodium–potassium exchange pump on the skeletal muscle cells, which drives extracellular K+ into the cells. The effects of insulin are temporary, so other measures need to be started to facilitate removal of excess K+.

c. Dextrose is used along with regular insulin to reduce the risk of developing hypoglycemia. It has no effect on the serum K+.

d. Sodium polystyrene sulfonate promotes K+ clearance across the bowel mucosa to be excreted, but it takes 6 hours to see the peak effect.

(Marino, 2014, pp. 682–684).

Clinical Pearl

Furosemide may not always convert oliguric to non-oliguric renal failure.

15 **The correct answer is C.**

Rationales:

a. Intermittent hemodialysis can remove life-threatening solutes in just a few hours.

b. There is no major trauma to red blood cells (RBC) during either intermittent hemodialysis or CRRT.

c. In patients who are already hemodynamically unstable, CRRT is less likely to increase the instability due to the slow gradual and continuous process.

d. Intermittent hemodialysis can remove 1–2 days' worth of excess fluid in just a few hours.

(Marino, 2014, p. 646).

16 **The correct answer is C.**

Rationales:

a. A serum sodium of 140 mEq/L is still within normal limits.

b. Urine osmolality is not used to diagnose hypernatremia, but it is used to assess for possible cause of hypernatremia.

c. Hypernatremia is defined as serum sodium greater than 145 mEq/L.

d. Serum osmolality greater than 300 mOsm/kg H$_2$O is not the definition of hypernatremia.

(Marino, 2014, p. 657; Papadakis & McPhee, 2019).

17 **The correct answer is A.**

Rationales:

a. Hypovolemic hypernatremia causes a decrease in plasma volume, which can lead to decreased tissue perfusion, so the first step in managing these patients is to fluid resuscitate them especially if they show signs of poor cardiac output state like hypotension or decreased urine output. After the patient is euvolemic, the free water deficit should be corrected at a rate of 0.5–1 mEq/L/hr.

b. Diuretics should not be used to correct Na+ in hypovolemia hypernatremia because they could cause hemodynamic instability in a person in low volume state.

c. When hypernatremia is corrected too rapidly, the patient may experience encephalopathy secondary to neuronal cell body shrinkage and osmotic demyelination.

d. The patient in the scenario is showing signs of low cardiac output secondary to hypovolemia; if he is not fluid resuscitated first, he may experience end-organ damage due to decreased tissue perfusion.

(Marino, 2014, pp. 658–661; Papadakis & McPhee, 2019).

18 **The correct answer is B.**

Rationales:

a. Nephrogenic DI is when the kidney's responsiveness to antidiuretic hormone (ADH) is impaired, and when compared to central DI, it is less severe. The use of corticosteroids in patients with DI will increase the renal free water loss.

b. Central DI is when ADH is not released from the pituitary and one of the common causes for central DI is traumatic brain injury. Administration of vasopressin in central DI is necessary because it will increase the urine osmolarity by 50% after the first dose.

Replacing the free water in central DI needs to be slowly done with close monitoring for water intoxication and hyponatremia, which can occur quickly when central DI starts to resolve.

c. Nephrogenic DI doesn't usually get so severe as to require aggressive fluid resuscitation.

d. Replacement of the free water deficit in central DI needs to be done slowly and monitored closely due to the high risk of water intoxication and hyponatremia whence central DI starts to resolve. Also, vasopressin administration should be started so that central DI can be reversed.

(Kasper et al., 2016; Marino, 2014, pp. 661–662; Papadakis & McPhee, 2019).

19 **The correct answer is D.**

Rationales:

a. DI is characterized as loss of urine that is dilute resulting in hypertonic plasma.

b. DI is caused by a defect in the release or response to ADH causing dilute urine and hypertonic plasma.

c. Patients with DI have hypertonic plasma secondary to hypernatremia from the inability to concentrate urine.

d. A hallmark finding for DI is dilute urine in the setting of hypertonic plasma.

(Marino, 2014, pp. 661–662).

20 **The correct answer is C.**

Rationales:

a. Ethanol level of 220 is likely normal for this patient and he drank his normal alcoholic intake on the day of admission, so he is not in withdrawal yet to have delirium tremens.

b. The patient's wife reported no change in drinking habits, so his ethanol level is likely his average and not an acute intoxication for him

c. Hyponatremia from beer potomania can occur with the consumption of a large amount of beer. Due to decreased solutes in the serum (from associated malnutrition), the free water excretion is decreased.

d. The patient has no history of psychiatric medication use that may cause polydipsia, and his wife denied any increase (or change) in his normal drinking habits.

(Papadakis & McPhee, 2019).

21 **The correct answer is A.**

Rationales:

a. Hyponatremia in the setting of hypovolemia is the result of Na+ loss with retention of excess free water, which commonly occurs with the use of hypotonic fluids in hospitalized patients.

b. Sodium-restrictive diets are not a common cause of hyponatremia in hospitalized patients.

c. Spironolactone use does not commonly cause hyponatremia in hospitalized patients.

d. Normal saline 0.9% is isotonic, and its use for fluid resuscitation does not cause hyponatremia in hospitalized patients.

(Marino, 2014, pp. 665–666; Papadakis & McPhee, 2019).

22 **The correct answer is B.**

Rationales:

a. Developing severe hypernatremia is not a common complication from hyponatremia treatment. Serum sodium levels are closely monitored, and for chronic hyponatremia, it is recommended to increase the serum sodium slowly with a max of 6 mEq/L increase in the first 24 hours.

b. Patients with chronic hyponatremia are at an increased risk of developing central pontine myelinolysis from treatment due to too rapid a correction in serum sodium.

c. Hyperchloremia is not a complication from hyponatremia treatment.

d. AKI is not a complication from hyponatremia treatment.

(Marino, 2014, p. 668; Papadakis & McPhee, 2019).

23 **The correct answer is C.**

Rationales:

a. This answer is a description of the pathophysiology of central pontine myelinolysis.

b. Acute cerebral atrophy is not a complication of hypotonic hyponatremia.

c. Cerebral edema with the risk of causing brain stem herniation is the life-threatening complication of hypotonic hyponatremia. Early symptoms include nausea, vomiting, and headaches.

d. This answer is a description of the pathophysiology of hepatic encephalopathy.

(Marino, 2014, p. 665; Shelat, 2018).

> **Clinical Pearl**
>
> Cardiac dysfunction can lead to renal failure due to low flow states.

24 **The correct answer is A.**

Rationales:

a. The hypokalemia and hypocalcemia associated with hypomagnesemia will be refractory to treatment until the hypomagnesemia is corrected.

b. Hypocalcemia associated with hypomagnesemia will be refractory to treatment until the hypomagnesemia is corrected.

c. This patient does not have hyperkalemia. Hyperkalemia is serum potassium greater than 4.5 mEq/L.

d. Hypokalemia associated with hypomagnesemia occurs in 40% of the time with hypomagnesemia. Treatment for hypokalemia will be refractory until the magnesium levels are corrected.

(Marino, 2014, pp. 690–692).

25 **The correct answer is D.**

Rationales:

a. Hypermagnesemia is not an electrolyte complication post massive blood transfusion. Hyperkalemia can occur post massive blood transfusion due to the steady leakage of potassium from the stored red blood cells in a unit of PRBC. One unit of PRBC can have 2–3 mEq/L of potassium in it.

b. Hypokalemia is not an electrolyte complication from massive blood transfusions. Hypocalcemia can occur due to calcium binding to the citrate anticoagulant in stored blood.

c. Hypercalcemia and hypomagnesemia are not an electrolyte complication from massive blood transfusions.

d. Hypocalcemia and hyperkalemia are two electrolyte abnormalities that can occur from massive blood transfusions for the reasons discussed above. With normal liver and renal function, a patient would likely be able to manage both without an intervention, but given that the patient in the question has an AKI, he will have a longer period of time clearing the extra potassium and citrate anticoagulant from his system.

(Marino, 2014, pp. 680–681, 704).

26 **The correct answer is B.**

Rationales:

a. Bradycardia is not a common problem from severe hypomagnesemia.

b. Torsades de pointes can occur in severe hypomagnesemia, and it is a ventricular tachycardia, which has a unique QRS that seems to twist around the baseline.

c. Supraventricular tachycardia is not a common problem from severe hypomagnesemia.

d. Atrial fibrillation is not a common problem from severe hypomagnesemia.

(Papadakis & McPhee, 2019).

27 **The correct answer is A.**

Rationales:

a. In the setting of hyperkalemia, the use of succinylcholine should be avoided because it promotes the movement of intracellular potassium out of the cells and can cause cardiac arrest secondary to severe hyperkalemia.

b. In the setting of hyperkalemia, there is no increased risk for life-threatening cardiac arrhythmias due to the use of rocuronium.

c. In the setting of hyperkalemia, there is no increased risk for life-threatening cardiac arrest due to the use of vecuronium.

d. In the setting of hyperkalemia, there is no increased risk for life-threatening cardiac arrest due to the use of cisatracurium.

(Marino, 2014, pp. 679–680).

28 **The correct answer is C.**

Rationales:

a. Inhaled B2-agonist bronchodilators at the normal therapeutic doses have mild effect on decreasing serum potassium levels by promoting an intracellular shift of the electrolyte.

b. Metabolic alkalosis can cause an intracellular shift of serum potassium, but the amount is variable and unpredictable.

c. In the setting of severe diarrhea, there can be serum potassium loss of 400 mEq a day.

d. Metabolic acidosis does not cause hypokalemia.

(Marino, 2014, pp. 673–684).

29 **The correct answer is B.**

Rationales:

a. Developing AKI does not mean that the patient will have CKD from then on.

b. TLS can occur after chemotherapy in any tumor but more often in hematologic malignances. TLS occurs due to a massive transcellular shift of electrolytes, and if coupled with impairment of excretion of electrolytes (e.g., AKI), it can cause life-threatening electrolyte imbalances.

c. DIC is not a complication postchemotherapy treatment, and the symptoms in the question are not specific to DIC.

d. Acute pancreatitis is not a complication postchemotherapy treatment, and the symptoms in the questions are not specific to pancreatitis.

(Marino, 2014, p. 679; Papadakis & McPhee, 2019).

 30 **The correct answer is D.**

Rationales:

a. AKI does not cause a discrepancy between the serum calcium assay level and ionized calcium level.

b. Hyponatremia does not cause a discrepancy between the serum calcium assay level and ionized calcium level.

c. Hypokalemia does not cause a discrepancy between the serum calcium assay level and ionized calcium level.

d. Hypoalbuminemia would cause the discrepancy between the calcium assay level and ionized calcium level. The calcium assay measures the total amount of calcium (biologically active and inactive) in the serum, while the ionized calcium measures the biologically active calcium level only. Eighty percent of calcium is bound to albumin, so in the setting of hypoalbuminemia, there will be a decrease in the total amount of calcium in the plasma, but ionized calcium is unbound and not affected by albumin levels.

(Marino, 2014, pp. 701–703).

References

Acute Kidney Injury Work Group. (2012). KDIGO clinical Practice guideline for acute kidney injury. *Kidney International Supplements, 2*(1), 1–141. doi:10.1038/kisup.2012.2

Kasper, D. L., Fauci, A. S., Hauser, S. L., Longo, D. L., Jameson, J. L., & Loscalzo, J. (Eds.). (2016). *Harrison's manual of medicine* (19th ed.). New York, NY: McGraw-Hill Education. Retrieved August 10, 2019, from http://accessmedicine.mhmedical.com.ezproxy2.library.drexel.edu/content.aspx?bookid=1820§ionid=127559610

Makris, K., & Spanou, L. (2016). Acute Kidney Injury: Definition, pathophysiology and clinical phenotypes. *The Clinical Biochemist Reviews, 37*(2), 85–98. Retrieved August 5, 2019, from https://www.ncbi.nlm.nih.gov/pmc/articles/PMC5198510/

Marino, P. L. (2014). *Marinos the ICU book* (4th ed.). Philadelphia, PA: Wolters Kluwer Health/Lippincott Williams & Wilkins.

Papadakis, M. A., & McPhee, S. J. (Eds.). (2019). *Current medical diagnosis and treatment 2019* (58th ed.). New York, NY: McGraw-Hill Education.

Shelat, A. M. (2018, April 30). *Osmotic demyelination syndrome: MedlinePlus Medical Encyclopedia.* Retrieved August 15, 2019, from https://medlineplus.gov/ency/article/000775.htm

CHAPTER 9

Endocrinology

Latesha Colbert-Mack, DNP, CRNP, AGACNP

Disease Questions

1 Which statement best describes diabetes?

a. Diabetes is a complex acute illness requiring intermittent medical care with multifactorial risk reduction strategies beyond glycemic control.

b. Diabetes is a complex chronic illness requiring intermittent medical care with multifactorial risk reduction strategies beyond glycemic control.

c. Diabetes is a simple chronic illness requiring intermittent medical care with multifactorial risk reduction strategies beyond glycemic control.

d. Diabetes is a simple acute illness requiring intermittent medical care with multifactorial risk reduction strategies beyond glycemic control.

2 A patient admitted to the medicine unit shares she was recently diagnosed with type 1 diabetes, but is not sure what this means. The best response from the AGACNP would be:

a. Type 1 diabetes is always diagnosed before the age of 20 secondary to pancreatic B-cell destruction that leads to insulin deficiency.

b. Type 1 diabetes can develop at any age but usually occurs before the age of 20. The lack of insulin as a hormone leads to the inability of the cells of the body to carry the glucose from the bloodstream, thus creating too much glucose in the bloodstream.

c. Type 1 diabetes is sometimes diagnosed before the age of 20 secondary to pancreatic B-cell destruction that leads to insulin deficiency.

d. Type 1 diabetes can develop at any age but usually occurs before the age of 20. The lack of glucose as a hormone leads to the inability of the cells of the body to carry the glucose from the bloodstream, thus creating too much glucose in the bloodstream.

3 A newly diagnosed patient with type 1 diabetes tells you that type 1 diabetes is always associated with pancreatic B-cell destruction. The adult-gerontology acute care nurse practitioner (AGACNP) knows this statement is false because:

a. A small minority of patients with type 1 diabetes will have permanent insulinopenia without any evidence of B-cell autoimmunity. These patients are prone to ketoacidosis and should be monitored closely.

b. A large majority of patients with type 1 diabetes will have permanent insulinopenia without any evidence of B-cell autoimmunity. These patients are prone to ketoacidosis and should be monitored closely.

c. A small minority of patients with type 1 diabetes will have intermittent insulinopenia without any evidence of B-cell autoimmunity. These patients are prone to ketoacidosis and should be monitored closely.

d. A large majority of patients with type 1 diabetes will have intermittent insulinopenia without any evidence of B-cell autoimmunity. These patients are prone to ketoacidosis and should be monitored closely.

Clinical Scenario:

Questions 4 through 14 refer to the following clinical scenario.

A.M. is a 52-year-old morbidly obese African American female with PMH significant for Prediabetes, HTN, COPD, and hypercholesteremia who presents to the emergency department with a blood sugar of 300 and complaints of polyuria, polydipsia polyphagia, and vaginitis over the last 2 weeks. HgbA1C in the ED is 17%. A.M. is surprised by her labs as symptoms as she was told she was on metformin to prevent diabetes. After gathering a focused H&P, the newly-hired AGACNP has expressed concerns that A.M. has a working diagnosis of diabetes that she would like to discuss with her preceptor.

4 On morning rounds, the resident states that A.M. is a patient with type 1 diabetes requiring immediate insulin therapy and treatment. Is the statement true or false?

a. False. A.M. has most likely developed type 2 diabetes secondary to a variety of factors—most likely insulin resistance and insulin deficiency. The lack of insulin production (type 1) most likely would have been identified in childhood. Many cases of type 2 diabetes are controlled without the use of insulin, but insulin may be used if necessary.

b. True. A.M. is a patient with type 1 diabetes with an A1C of 17%, which requires immediate insulin intervention that will continue at home.

c. True. A.M. is a patient with type 1 diabetes that will only improve if she has insulin initiated during this hospital visit.

d. False. A.M. has type 2 diabetes that will only respond to insulin.

5 Due to the presenting glucose and symptoms, the AGACNP has enough information to make the diagnosis of diabetes. Is this statement true or false?

a. False. Confirmation of diabetes may be made using one of the following diagnostic tests: plasma glucose criteria that include a fasting plasma glucose (FPG > 126 mg/dL after no caloric intake for 8 hours) or 2-hour plasma glucose (glucose >200 mg/dL after a 75 g oral glucose tolerance test) or A1C criteria ($\geq$6.5%) OR a patient who presents with random glucose greater than 200 mg/dL with classic symptoms of hyperglycemia/hyperglycemic crisis.

b. False. Confirmation of diabetes may be made using history of present illness (HPI), physical examination, and medication reconciliation.

c. True. Confirmation of diabetes may be made using only one of the following diagnostic tests: plasma glucose criteria that include an FPG (>126 mg/dL after no caloric intake for 8 hours) or 2-hour plasma glucose (glucose >200 mg/dL after a 75 g oral glucose tolerance test) or A1C criteria ($\geq$6.5%).

d. True. Confirmation of diabetes may be made using two diagnostic tests: plasma glucose criteria that include an FPG (>126 mg/dL after no caloric intake for 8 hours) or 2-hour plasma glucose (glucose >200 mg/dL after 75 g oral glucose tolerance test) or A1C criteria (≥6.5%) OR a patient who presents with random glucose greater than 200 mg/dL with classic symptoms of hyperglycemia/hyperglycemic crisis.

6 List all the factors that would steer the AGACNP to believe that A.M. is most likely a patient with type 2 versus type 1 diabetes.

a. Age, A1C, classic symptoms of hyperglycemia, and ethnicity

b. Age, A1C, classic symptoms of hyperglycemia, ethnicity, and morbid obesity

c. Age, A1C, classic symptoms of hyperglycemia, metformin, morbid obesity, and ethnicity

d. None of the above

7 The pathogenesis of type 2 diabetes is characterized by which of the following factors?

a. Impaired insulin secretion/insulin resistance

b. An excess of hepatic glucose production/abnormal fat metabolism

c. Both A and B

d. None of the above

8 First-line drugs in treating prediabetes and preventing diabetes include which of the following?

a. Metformin

b. Repaglinide

c. Sitagliptin

d. Combination therapy including insulin and oral agents

9 Social determinants of health, including access to health, low health literacy, lack of health insurance, and unreliable access to food, may impact a provider's decision on prescribing medications for a patient with type 2 diabetes. If you were caring for A.M. and she shared with you that she has food insecurity, which sulfonylurea would be the best choice due to its shorter half-life?

a. Metformin

b. Sitagliptin

c. Glipizide

d. Pioglitazone

10 Knowing that A.M. has a history of chronic kidney disease (CKD), which medication should NOT be advised?

a. Metformin

b. Sitagliptin

c. Glipizide

d. Both A and C

11 On rounds, the 2nd-year medical student suggests that A.M. is currently not at an increased risk of microvascular complications including retinopathy, diabetic kidney disease, and neuropathic complications. The AGACNP knows this statement is FALSE because:

a. Intensive glycemic control is associated with decreased rates of microvascular complications. An A1C of 17% is very concerning, and the goal is to reduce cardiovascular disease.

b. Intensive glycemic control is associated with increased rates of microvascular complications. An A1C of 17% is very concerning, and the goal is to reduce cardiovascular disease.

c. Intensive glycemic control is associated with variable rates of microvascular complications. An A1C of 17% is very concerning, and the goal is to reduce cardiovascular disease.

d. Intensive glycemic control is associated with no difference in rates of microvascular complications. An A1C of 17% is very concerning, and the goal is to reduce cardiovascular disease.

12 After presenting the patient, the AGACNP feels that A.M. should be admitted to the observation unit. Admission orders include a consult to the endocrine team. Prior to consulting the team, which parameters should be identified to distinguish between normal and abnormal glucose levels in a hospitalized patient?

a. Hyperglycemia is blood glucose level greater than 140 mg/dL.

b. Hypoglycemia is blood glucose level less than 70 mg/dL.

c. Severe hypoglycemia is blood glucose level less than 40 mg/dL.

d. All the above are true in classifying glucose abnormalities in the hospitalized setting.

13 A.M. is ready to be discharged, and the AGACNP is formulating a comprehensive discharge plan to promote optimal monitoring of glycemic control. Which factors MUST be included in this plan?

a. A follow-up with the primary provider to follow A1C levels

b. Self-monitoring of blood glucose (SMBG)

c. Patient education regarding food, nutrition, and glucose medications

d. B and C

e. A, B, and C

14 In addition, the endocrine team is considering initiating an oral agent for A.M. When discussing mechanism of action and contraindications, which medications would be contraindicated for A.M.?

a. Glibenclamide and metformin

b. Pioglitazone and metformin

c. Insulin and metformin

Clinical Scenario:

Questions 15 through 19 apply to the following scenario:

The AGACNP is en route to work at 2 p.m. when a family is encountered in the lobby. An adult male shares he feels shaky, clammy, confused and weak. On quick exam, the

NP notices that he is also sweating and with pallor. The family says to the AGACNP he is type 2 diabetic. They also shared that he took his insulin in hopes of eating after his colonoscopy. The patient is starting to look worse, but remains conscious. The NP calls for a rapid response team (RRT) and the team arrives asking for next steps. Of note, glucose level at time of arrival is 48 mg/dL.

15 The AGACNP instructs the team to administer 100 g of oral glucose immediately to increase blood sugar. Is this the appropriate action?

a. Yes, this is appropriate. The nurse practitioner (NP) should instruct the team to administer 100 g of oral glucose immediately to increase the blood sugar.

b. No, this is not appropriate. The appropriate dose of glucose is 15–20 g for a conscious patient. Oral medications should be avoided in the unconscious patient as the patient is not able to protect the airway.

16 In an emergency situation, glucagon should be only be administered by a health care professional. Is this statement true or false?

a. This statement is true because hypoglycemia prevention is critical for diabetes management. All caregivers should be educated on who should administer this lifesaving medication. This medication is limited to health care professionals.

b. This statement is false because hypoglycemia prevention is critical for diabetes management. All caregivers should be educated on how to administer this lifesaving medication. This medication is a medication that is not limited to health care professionals.

17 Glucagon kits are readily available to patients and families over-the-counter (OTC) and do not carry an expiration date. Is this statement true or false?

a. This statement is true. Allowing patients easy access to lifesaving medications was implemented by the Affordable Care Act in 2016.

b. This statement is false because glucagon must be prescribed and frequently reassessed for expired dates. Proper education to families is crucial to ensure that patients are not in possession of expired medications.

18 The family asks the AGACNP about the reason for the hypoglycemic incident. Which of the following is the best response from the NP?

a. Patients with type 1 diabetes are at increased risk of hypoglycemia.

b. Taking the a.m. insulin and fasting for a p.m. study increased the patient's risk of hypoglycemia.

c. I have to run to work; the RRT will be able to help you to the emergency department (ED) to explain further.

19 On repeat check, blood sugar is 120 and the patient is awake, talking, and feeling well. As the AGACNP, what should be recommended as next steps for the patient and family?

a. Nothing; allow the patient to proceed to colonoscopy.

b. Nothing, but reschedule colonoscopy for an earlier time on another day.

c. Encourage the patient to eat a meal or snack to prevent a repeat episode of hypoglycemia and reschedule the test.

20 An 18-year-old male is admitted to the medical intensive care unit (MICU) with resolving diabetic ketoacidosis (DKA) secondary to urosepsis. The patient has a past medical history (PMH) significant for type 1 diabetes and known to be noncompliant on medical therapy. The AGACNP recognizes that the patient's acidosis is resolving, but on rounds, the resident suggests the use of bicarbonate to facilitate resolution of acidosis. All of the statements below are FALSE except for which of the following?

a. The use of bicarbonate in DKA is proven to have no difference in resolution of acidosis.

b. The utilization of bicarbonate in DKA decreases overall length of stay for patients.

c. Bicarbonate is the preferred treatment in resolving metabolic acidosis in DKA in combination with treating the underlying cause.

Clinical Scenario:

Questions 21-26 relate to the scenario that follows:

A 40-year-old African American male with PMH significant for hypertension (HTN) for 20 years is currently being managed on amlodipine, metoprolol, and hydrochlorothiazide (HCTZ) to control his blood pressure. He presented to the ED in a hypertensive crisis, associated with acute onset of headache and palpitations after a workout in the gym.

21 The AGACNP develops a differential diagnosis list. Please check all that should be included:

a. Pheochromocytoma

b. Labile essential HTN

c. Cocaine and/or amphetamine use

d. Addison disease

e. A, C, and D

f. A, B, and C

22 After gathering an extensive history and physical (H&P), computed tomography of abdomen and pelvis (CT A/P) was performed and a right adrenal mass in the adrenal medulla was identified. How does this new information align with your working diagnosis above?

a. Pheochromocytomas arise in the adrenal cortex and secrete epinephrine and norepinephrine.

b. Pheochromocytomas arise in the adrenal cortex and secrete mineralocorticoids.

c. Pheochromocytomas arise in the adrenal medulla and secrete epinephrine and norepinephrine.

d. Pheochromocytomas arise in the adrenal medulla and secrete mineralocorticoids.

23 Once the retroperitoneal mass was identified, the new surgery resident suggests consulting radiology for a retroperitoneal biopsy to confirm the working diagnosis and rule out missing an adrenal cancer. What is the best response for the NP?

a. Agree with the plan and move forward with a biopsy as tissue diagnosis would be important in ruling out an adrenal cancer.

b. Agree with the plan as a biopsy is a pretty low-risk procedure and would assist with confirming diagnosis.

c. Disagree with the plan and suggest adding labs including serum metanephrines to rule out a functional tumor such as a pheochromocytoma.

24 Patients with pheochromocytomas are always symptomatic and complaining of palpitations and HTN. Is this statement true or false?

a. True

b. False

25 Paragangliomas are extra-adrenal pheochromocytomas that can be found anywhere throughout the body where sympathetic ganglia can be found. Is this statement true or false?

a. True

b. False

26 M.S. has a working diagnosis of a pheochromocytoma. Which part of the HPI would lead the NP to suspect this patient should have been worked up as an outpatient sooner for secondary causes of HTN?

a. Age in combination with multiple agents to treat HTN

b. Race/ethnicity in combination with multiple agents to treat HTN

c. Sex in combination with multiple agents to treat HTN

27 What test is most sensitive in confirming the diagnosis of a pheochromocytoma?

a. Serum metanephrines

b. Urine metanephrines

c. Clonidine suppression test

28 In gathering a comprehensive H&P, the AGACNP must include family history. All of the genetic syndromes that should be asked in the interview are associated with pheochromocytoma EXCEPT:

a. von Hippel–Lindau (VHL)

b. Multiple endocrine neoplasia type 1 (MEN 1) and MEN 1A

c. Multiple endocrine neoplasia type 2 (MEN 2) and MEN 2A

d. Neurofibromatosis 1 (NF1)

e. Succinate dehydrogenase (SDH)

29 The diagnosis of pheochromocytoma has been confirmed. As the AGACNP, which medications would be ordered for discharge to optimize the patient medically in preparation for a surgical resection that is planned in 2 weeks?

a. Alpha-blockers/calcium channel blockers (alone or in combination) with daily monitoring of blood pressure

b. Beta-blockers with daily monitoring of blood pressure

c. Beta-blockers/diuretics (alone or in combination) with daily monitoring of blood pressure

30 Post-surgical resection, which medication should NEVER be resumed on discharge even if the patient remains hypertensive postsurgery?

a. HCTZ 25 mg orally daily

b. Metoprolol 25 mg orally twice daily.

c. Phenoxybenzamine 10 mg orally twice daily.

31 Thyroid-stimulating hormone (TSH) deficiency causes the body's metabolism to slow down. Please select the endocrine disorder that best reflects this statement:

a. Cushing syndrome

b. Cushing disease

c. Hypothyroidism

d. Hyperthyroidism

32 What is the recommended screening for hypothyroidism or hyperthyroidism?

a. TSH and free T4

b. T3 and T4

c. Thyroid ultrasound

d. Fine needle aspiration

33 Which lab values are expected in confirming Hashimoto thyroiditis?

a. Elevated antithyroperoxidase and antithyroglobulin antibodies

b. Suppressed antithyroperoxidase and antithyroglobulin antibodies

34 Which lab values are more likely to be seen when confirming hyperthyroidism?

a. Suppressed TSH, elevated T3, increased iodine uptake; diffuse versus "cold" foci on scan

b. Suppressed TSH, elevated T3, increased iodine uptake; diffuse versus "hot" foci on scan

c. Elevated TSH, suppressed T3, increased iodine uptake; diffuse versus "cold" foci on scan

d. Elevated TSH, elevated T3, increased iodine uptake; diffuse versus "cold" foci on scan

35 Which diagnostic test is preferred when evaluating thyroid nodules?

a. MRI

b. CT

c. US

d. PET scan

36 A 40-year-old female presents to you with concerns for thyroid cancer. The patient has a PMH significant for MEN 2A. Which thyroid cancer is associated with MEN 2A?

a. Papillary thyroid cancer

b. Anaplastic thyroid cancer

c. Follicular thyroid cancer

d. Medullary thyroid cancer

37 The AGACNP is reviewing the differential diagnosis for a thyroid nodule with a patient on your unit, and the patient asks which nodule has a slight chance of not being cancer. Which disease would this refer to?

a. Follicular neoplasm

b. Anaplastic thyroid cancer

c. Medullary thyroid cancer

d. Papillary thyroid cancer

e. All of the options are cancer and should be clarified with the patient

38 A 42-year-old male with no PMH presents to the ED after his wife, who is a nurse, shared concerns that he was becoming more irritable, losing weight, getting thinning hair, and having frequent bowel movements with a rapid heart rate (HR). Vitals are notable for HR 112. In discussing differential diagnosis with the patient, the AGACNP shares that there is a possibility that he could have Graves disease. The patient asks for an explanation as to why this happens. Which is the best response below?

a. "Sometimes these things happen late in life."

b. "Graves disease is a disease of the thyroid gland. It is an autoimmune disorder characterized by an increase in synthesis and release of thyroid hormones."

c. "Graves disease is a disease of the thyroid gland. It is an autoimmune disorder characterized by a decrease in synthesis and release of thyroid hormones."

39 A patient being treated for Graves disease did not respond to radioactive iodine and wants to move forward to a total thyroidectomy. Which drug is most likely going to be lifelong for this patient?

a. Propranolol

b. Levothyroxine

c. Methimazole

d. SSKI

40 A newly married 35-year-old female is diagnosed with Graves disease and wants to discuss treatment options with the AGACNP. She shares that she and her husband are actively trying for pregnancy but she is not pregnant at this time. Which treatment plan would be best for this patient?

a. Propylthiouracil in the first trimester followed by methimazole

b. Radioactive iodine prior to conception and subtotal thyroidectomy in second trimester

c. Subtotal thyroidectomy followed by levothyroxine postoperatively

41 A 60-year-old female presents to the hospital with acute onset of sweating, chest palpitations, hyperreflexia, and hand tremors. Electrocardiogram (EKG) was performed and notable for HR 165 and atrial fibrillation with rapid ventricular response (RVR). The patient shares that she is surprised by this as she has been compliant with her medications, which include amiodarone and warfarin for the last 2 months. Labs were notable for high free T3 and T3 levels. What is the working diagnosis for this patient?

a. Acute thyroiditis

b. Graves disease

c. Uncontrolled atrial fibrillation

d. Amiodarone-induced thyrotoxicosis

42 A 50-year-old female has undergone radioactive iodine therapy for treatment of Graves disease. After a recent layoff, she lost her health insurance and was not able to follow up with the endocrinologist since treatment. While in the ED, the patient's husband reveals that over the last month, he has noticed she has become more fatigued and shared daily complaints of cold intolerance. He shared that this morning, she was hypothermic with a temperature of 95°F, having trouble breathing, and confused. Her husband says he called emergency medical service (EMS) because he was worried that she may have the same pneumonia that he had a week ago. Of note, labs were notable for Na 119. What would be the leading working admitting diagnosis?

a. Suspect community-acquired pneumonia and admit to observation status

b. Suspect myxedema crisis and admit to intensive care unit (ICU)

c. Suspect sepsis and admit to ICU

d. Suspect Graves disease exacerbation and admit to observation status

43 A 50-year-old male is currently being worked up for secondary causes of HTN refractory to medical management. The ED physician sent the patient for CT of the abdomen and pelvis prior to discharge from the observation unit. The radiologist called the AGACNP to share that there is a nodule noted in the adrenal cortex. Please select the most likely secondary cause for HTN in the list of differentials for this patient.

a. Pheochromocytoma

b. Renal stenosis

c. Aldosteronoma

44 A 43-year-old female is in the ED with physical examination findings concerning for Cushing syndrome. All of the following are examination findings of Cushing EXCEPT:

a. Moon face

b. Abdominal striae

c. Buffalo hump

d. Truncal weight loss

45 While diagnosing a patient with adrenal insufficiency, the following examination findings should be considered in differentiating primary and secondary adrenal insufficiency:

a. Hyperpigmentation: adrenocorticotropic hormone (ACTH) excess

b. Alabaster-colored pale skin: ACTH excess

c. Abdominal striae: ACTH neutral

46 The AGACNP is admitting a 35-year-old female who presents with disruption of her menstrual cycle, new-onset diabetes, and HTN. Which of the following diagnoses does the AGACNP know must be included in the differentials list?

a. Early menopause

b. Cushing disease

c. Polycystic ovary syndrome

d. Pheochromocytoma

47 Once Cushing disease is confirmed, the AGACNP should counsel the patient that the next steps for management would include which of the following?

a. Surgery

b. Supportive medical therapy

c. More frequent visits with the primary care physician (PCP)

d. Oral steroid taper

48 After gathering a comprehensive H&P, the AGACNP suspects a patient has Cushing syndrome. As the NP, it is essential to establish the correct diagnosis in identifying the appropriate management plan. Which lab will decide the approach to confirming the diagnosis?

a. Plasma ACTH

b. Urine ACTH

c. Urine metanephrines

d. Serum metanephrines

49 All of the following conditions are most likely associated with an excess of deficiency of steroids from the adrenal cortex EXCEPT:

a. Pheochromocytoma

b. Cushing syndrome

c. Aldosteronoma

d. Adrenal corticocarcinoma

50 A 65-year-old female is admitted to the observation unit after the PCP called EMS during a well visit. According to the family, the patient was in the office with complaints of worsening fatigue, postural HTN, hyponatremia, and decreased responsiveness. According to the family, the physician wanted the patient at the hospital to confirm a diagnosis of possible Addison disease. What is the next step in confirming a diagnosis of Addison disease?

a. Serum metanephrines

b. CT

c. MRI

d. Cosyntropin test

51 The loss of which two hormones can be used to characterize the clinical features of primary adrenal insufficiency (Addison disease)?

a. Glucocorticoid and mineralocorticoid

b. Mineralocorticoid ONLY

c. Epinephrine ONLY

52 A 35-year-old female presents to the floor with hyponatremia, hypotension, and a pituitary tumor. What diagnosis should be included in the differential diagnosis?

a. Primary adrenal insufficiency

b. Secondary adrenal insufficiency

c. Pheochromocytoma

d. Aldosteronoma

53 Secondary adrenal insufficiency can occur due to the dysfunction of which gland?

a. Thyroid gland

b. Pituitary gland

c. Pancreatic gland

54 Which of the following can be used to diagnose central diabetes insipidus from nephrotic diabetes insipidus and polydipsia?

a. Cosyntropin test

b. Vasopressin challenge test

c. Urine electrolytes

d. MRI

55 After administering the vasopressin challenge test in the ICU, it is suspected that the patient has nephrotic diabetes insipidus. What would the AGACNP expect to find in the test results?

a. No response in polydipsia or urine volume

b. Immediate improvement in polydipsia and urine volume

c. No response in polydipsia, improvement in urine volume

d. Improvement in polydipsia, but no response in urine volume

56 Another patient is post vasopressin challenge test in the ICU, and the AGACNP suspects the patient has central diabetes insipidus. What finding would be expected in the lab results?

a. No response in polydipsia, polyuria; serum sodium usually remains normal

b. Improvement in polydipsia and polyuria; serum sodium usually remains normal

c. No response in polydipsia; improvement in urine volume

d. Improvement in polydipsia, but no response in urine volume

57 Antidiuretic hormone (ADH) affects which two disorders directly?

a. Hypothyroidism and hyperthyroidism

b. Pheochromocytoma and aldosteronoma

c. Syndrome of inappropriate antidiuretic hormone secretion (SIADH) and diabetes insipidus (DI)

d. Type 1 and type 2 diabetes

58 The AGACNP is caring for a patient who was ruled in for central diabetes insipidus. Which of the following statements are true?

a. If it is a mild case of central diabetes insipidus, the patient may be controlled with regulating fluid intake; otherwise desmopressin acetate is the treatment of choice.

b. Mild, moderate, and severe cases of central diabetes insipidus must always be managed with desmopressin acetate.

c. Encouraging fluids is the gold standard for treating central diabetes insipidus.

d. Surgical resection of the pituitary gland is recommended to improve overall quality of life in these patients.

59 Which hormone is responsible for regulating plasma osmolality by controlling water excretion?

a. Thyroid-stimulating hormone (TSH)

b. Antidiuretic hormone (ADH)

c. Follicle-stimulating hormone (FSH)

d. Corticotropin-releasing hormone (CRH)

60 The AGACNP is caring for a patient in the surgical ICU (SICU) who is postop day (POD) no. 3 s/p Whipple. The lab calls with a critical sodium value of 118. On examination, the patient reports no surgical pain but a terrible headache. After examination, which labs would be crucial in the workup of acute severe symptomatic hyponatremia in this patient?

a. Basic metabolic panel (BMP), urine osmolality, serum osmolality, urine sodium

b. BMP, serum osmolality, urine sodium, urine creatinine

c. BMP, serum osmolality, urine creatinine, magnesium

d. BMP, urine osmolality, serum osmolality

61 A patient is euvolemic. Labs are as follows: serum osmolality 270, urine osmolality 150, and urine sodium 40. Which type of hyponatremia do you suspect?

a. Hypovolemic isotonic hyponatremia most likely due to SIADH in the setting of malignancy

b. Euvolemic hypotonic hyponatremia most likely due to SIADH in the setting of malignancy

c. Euvolemic hypertonic hyponatremia most likely due to SIADH in the setting of malignancy

62 During rounds, the team is discussing treatment plans for a patient with hypovolemic isotonic hyponatremia. All are treatment options for this condition EXCEPT:

a. Salt tablets

b. Tolvaptan (vasopressin receptor antagonist)

c. STAT renal consult

d. Encourage fluids

63 Osmotic demyelination syndrome (ODS) is a form of brain damage that occurs with:

a. Rapid correction of hyponatremia

b. Slow correction of hyponatremia

c. SIADH onset

d. DI onset

Disease Answers/Rationales

1 **The correct answer is B.**

Rationales:

a. Although diabetes is a complex condition, it is not characterized as an acute illness.

b. Diabetes is a complex chronic illness requiring intermittent medical care with multifactorial risk reduction strategies beyond glycemic control. Diabetes requires continuous medical care with multifactorial risk reduction strategies beyond glycemic control. Infrequent monitoring by a health profession may lead to increased morbidity and mortality.

c. This disease is not simple but very complex to manage as it has the potential to have multisystem impact if not managed properly.

d. Diabetes is not a simple acute illness requiring intermittent medical care with multifactorial risk reduction strategies beyond glycemic control.

(American Diabetes Association, 2016, p. 39; Kasper et al., 2015).

2 **The correct answer is B.**

Rationales:

a. Type 1 diabetes is not always diagnosed before the age of 20.

b. Type 1 diabetes can develop at any age but usually occurs before the age of 20. The lack of insulin as a hormone leads to the inability of the cells of the body to carry the glucose from the bloodstream, thus creating too much glucose in the bloodstream.

c. Type 1 diabetes is usually diagnosed before the age of 20 secondary to pancreatic B-cell destruction that leads to insulin deficiency.

d. This answer is incorrect because there is an overproduction of glucose but lack of the insulin hormone.

(American Diabetes Association, 2016, p. 39; Kasper et al., 2015).

3 **The correct answer is A**

Rationales:

a. A small minority of patients with type 1 diabetes will have permanent insulinopenia without any evidence of B-cell autoimmunity. These patients are prone to ketoacidosis and should be monitored closely.

b. This course of disease will impact a small minority of patients.

c. Patients with type 1 diabetes will not experience intermittent insulinopenia. This process is usually permanent.

d. This course of disease progress impacts a small minority of patients.

(American Diabetes Association, 2016, p. 39; Kasper et al., 2015).

4 **The correct answer is A.**

Rationales:

a. The resident's comment is false. A.M. has most likely developed type 2 diabetes secondary to a variety of factors, most likely insulin resistance and insulin deficiency. The lack of insulin production (type 1) most likely would have been identified in childhood. Many cases of type 2 diabetes are controlled without the use of insulin, but insulin may be used if necessary.

b. This answer is false because A.M. is most likely a patient with type 2 diabetes.

c. This answer is false because A.M. is most likely a patient with type 2 diabetes.

d. This answer is false. A.M. is a patient with type 2 diabetes; many patients with type 2 diabetes can be managed with oral medications alone or in combination with insulin.

(American Diabetes Association, 2016, p. 39; Kasper et al., 2015).

5 **The correct answer is D.**

Rationales:

a. False. The diagnosis is made by using two of the diagnostic tests. This statement is false because you would not only use one test to make the diagnosis.

b. False. Although the HPI, physical examination, and medication reconciliation are all important, they are not used to confirm the diagnosis.

c. False. The diagnosis is made by using two of the diagnostic tests. This statement is false because you would not only use one test to make the diagnosis.

d. True. Confirmation of diabetes may be made using two diagnostic tests: plasma glucose criteria that includes an FPG (>126 mg/dL after no caloric intake for 8 hours) or 2-hour plasma glucose (glucose >200 mg/dL after 75 g oral glucose tolerance test) or A1C criteria (≥6.5%) OR a patient who presents with random glucose greater than 200 mg/dL with classic symptoms of hyperglycemia/hyperglycemic crisis.

(American Diabetes Association, 2016, p. 39; Kasper et al., 2015).

6 **The correct answer is C.**

Rationales:

a. Age, HgbA1C, classic symptoms of hyperglycemia, and ethnicity would be associated with type 1 and type 2 diabetes.

b. Age, HgbA1C, classic symptoms of hyperglycemia, ethnicity, and morbid obesity may be associated with type 1 and type 2 diabetes.

c. Age, HgbA1C, classic symptoms of hyperglycemia, metformin, morbid obesity, and ethnicity as metformin is ONLY used in type 2 diabetes.

d. "None of the above" does not accurately reflect the classic symptoms associated with diabetes (type 1 or type 2).

(American Diabetes Association, 2016, p. 39; Kasper et al., 2015).

7 **The correct answer is C.**

Rationales:

a. Although impaired insulin secretion and insulin resistance are factors, this answer alone is not the most inclusive answer.

b. Although an excess of hepatic glucose production and abnormal fat metabolism are factors, this answer alone is not the most inclusive answer.

c. "A and B" is the best answer to the question.

d. This answer is incorrect as A and B explain the pathogenesis of type 2 diabetes.

(American Diabetes Association, 2016, p. 39; Kasper et al., 2015).

8 **The correct answer is A.**

Rationales:

a. Metformin has been used as the preferred agent in patients with prediabetes to reduce their risk of developing diabetes.

b. Repaglinide has NOT been used as the preferred agent in patients with prediabetes to reduce their risk of developing diabetes.

c. Sitagliptin has NOT been used as the preferred agent in patients with prediabetes to reduce their risk of developing diabetes.

d. Combination therapy including insulin and oral agents has NOT been used as the preferred agent in patients with prediabetes to reduce their risk of developing diabetes.

(American Diabetes Association, 2016, p. 39).

9 **The correct answer is C.**

Rationales:

a. Metformin is a biguanide.

b. Sitagliptin is a dipeptidyl peptidase 4 (DDP-4) inhibitor.

c. Glipizide is the only sulfonylurea listed in the list of medications.

d. Pioglitazone is a thiazolidinedione.

(American Diabetes Association, 2016, p. 39).

10 **The correct answer is D.**

Rationales:

a. Metformin is a biguanide that should be used in patients with renal insufficiency.

b. Sitagliptin is a DPP-4 inhibitor that may be administered to patients with renal insufficiency but in reduced doses.

c. Glipizide is a sulfonylurea. These medications are metabolized in the liver and cleared in the kidneys. Glipizide would not be advised for A.M. secondary to renal dysfunction.

d. This answer is correct because metformin and glipizide should be avoided in patients with renal dysfunction.

(Powers et al., 2018).

11 **The correct answer is A.**

Rationales:

a. The statement is false because intensive glycemic control is associated with decreased rates of microvascular complications. An A1C of 17% is very concerning, and the goal is to reduce cardiovascular disease.

b. This answer is incorrect because intensive glycemic control is associated with decreased rates of microvascular complications. An A1C of 17% is very concerning, and the goal is to reduce cardiovascular disease.

c. This answer is incorrect because intensive glycemic control is not associated with variable rates of microvascular complications. An A1C of 17% is very concerning, and the goal is to reduce cardiovascular disease.

d. This answer is incorrect because intensive glycemic control is associated with a difference in rates of microvascular complications. An A1C of 17% is very concerning, and the goal is to reduce cardiovascular disease.

(American Diabetes Association, 2016, p. 39).

12 **The correct answer is D.**

Rationales:

a. This answer is correct. Hyperglycemia is blood glucose level >140 mg/dL

b. This answer is correct. Hypoglycemia is blood glucose level <70 mg/dL

c. This answer is correct. Severe hypoglycemia is blood glucose level <40 mg/dL

d. This answer is the best answer to this question because all the above are true in classifying glucose abnormalities in the hospitalized setting

(American Diabetes Association, 2016, p. 39).

13 **The correct answer is E.**

Rationales:

a. This answer is correct. A follow-up with the primary provider to follow A1C levels.

b. This answer is correct. SMBG.

c. This answer is correct. Patient education regarding food, nutrition, and glucose medications ONLY.

d. This answer is correct as B and C is the first step in a comprehensive approach to achieve optimal glycemic control.

e. This is the best answer for this question because A, B, and C is the most comprehensive plan to achieve optimal glycemic control.

(American Diabetes Association, 2016, p. 39).

14 **The correct answer is A.**

Rationales:

a. This answer is correct because glyburide and metformin are contraindicated in patients with renal disease.

b. This answer is incorrect because Actos is a thiazolidinedione that is often associated with bladder cancer but can be used in patients with renal disease. Metformin is contraindicated.

c. This answer is incorrect because insulin is used in patients with renal insufficiency, while metformin is contraindicated.

(Powers et al., 2018).

15 **The correct answer is B.**

Rationales:

a. The dose of glucose is too high in this option. The appropriate dose of glucose is 15–20 g for a conscious patient.

b. The appropriate dose of glucose is 15–20 g for a conscious patient.

(American Diabetes Association, 2016, p. 39).

> **Clinical Pearl**
>
> HHNK is more lethal, with higher glucoses and greater volume loss than those with DKA.

16 **The correct answer is B.**

Rationales:

a. This statement is true because hypoglycemia prevention is critical for diabetes management. All caregivers should be educated on who should administer this lifesaving medication. This medication is one that is limited to health care professionals.

b. This statement is false because hypoglycemia prevention is critical for diabetes management. All caregivers should be educated on how to administer this lifesaving medication. This medication is one that is not limited to health care professionals.

(American Diabetes Association, 2016, p. 39).

c. Encouraging the patient to eat a meal or snack to prevent a repeat episode of hypoglycemia and rescheduling test are the next appropriate steps.

(American Diabetes Association, 2016, p. 39).

17 **The correct answer is B.**

Rationales:

a. This statement is true. Allowing patients easy access to lifesaving medications was implemented by the Affordable Care Act in 2016.

b. This statement is false because glucagon must be prescribed and frequently reassessed for expired dates. Proper education to families is crucial to ensure that patients are not in possession of expired medications.

(American Diabetes Association, 2016, p. 39).

18 **The correct answer is B.**

Rationales:

a. This answer is incorrect. Patients with type 1 diabetes are deficient in the insulin hormone and are most likely at increased risk of hyperglycemia.

b. This answer is correct. Taking the a.m. insulin and fasting for a p.m. study increased the patient's risk of hypoglycemia.

c. This answer is incorrect. The AGACNP should not dismiss the family's concerns.

(American Diabetes Association, 2016, p. 39).

19 **The correct answer is C.**

Rationales:

a. "Nothing; allow the patient to proceed to colonoscopy" is incorrect. Rebound hypoglycemia is possible if no additional steps are taken after the initial intervention.

b. "Nothing, but reschedule colonoscopy for an earlier time on another day" is incorrect for the reason above.

20 **The correct answer is A.**

Rationales:

a. This statement is true. The use of bicarbonate in DKA is proven to have no difference in resolution of acidosis.

b. This statement is false. "The utilization of bicarbonate in DKA decreases overall length of stay for patients" is not guided in evidence.

c. This statement is false. "Bicarbonate is preferred treatment in resolving metabolic acidosis in DKA in combination with treating the underlying cause" is not guided in evidence.

(American Diabetes Association, 2016, p. 39).

21 **The correct answer is D.**

Rationales:

a. Although correct, this is not the best answer. Pheochromocytoma should be included in the differential diagnosis.

b. Although correct, this is not the best answer. Labile essential HTN should be included in the differential diagnosis.

c. Although correct, this is not the best answer. Cocaine and/or amphetamine use should be included in the differential diagnosis.

d. This is the best answer in all of the responses. All of the differentials should be included except Addison disease as hypertensive crisis is not a part of the usual presentation

e. This answer is correct. A, C, and D should be included in the differential diagnosis.

f. A, B, and C should be included in the differential diagnosis.

(Kasper et al., 2015).

22 **The correct answer is C.**

Rationales:

a. This answer is incorrect. Pheochromocytomas arise in the adrenal medulla.

b. This answer is incorrect. Pheochromocytomas arise in the adrenal medulla and not in the cortex.

c. This is the correct answer. Pheochromocytomas arise in the adrenal medulla and secrete epinephrine and norepinephrine.

d. This answer is incorrect. Pheochromocytomas arise in the adrenal medulla and secrete epinephrine and norepinephrine.

(Kasper et al., 2015).

23 **The correct answer is C.**

Rationales:

a. This answer is incorrect. It is not recommended to biopsy retroperitoneal masses.

b. This answer is incorrect. A retroperitoneal biopsy is a high-risk procedure and should be avoided.

c. This is the correct answer. A provider should disagree with the plan and suggest adding labs including serum metanephrines to rule out a functional tumor such as a pheochromocytoma.

(Kasper et al., 2015).

24 **The correct answer is B.**

Rationales:

a. Patients are always symptomatic with complaints of palpitations and HTN, allowing for early intervention.

b. It is not uncommon (over 10% of cases) for patients to be asymptomatic and have tumor found on incidental imaging.

(Kasper et al., 2015).

25 **The correct answer is A.**

Rationales:

a. This is the basic definition of paragangliomas, which are extra-adrenal pheochromocytomas.

b. Pheochromocytomas are always found in the adrenal medulla and never found outside of the adrenal gland.

(Kasper et al., 2015).

26 **The correct answer is A.**

Rationales:

a. This answer is correct: age in combination with multiple agents to treat HTN. This patient was hypertensive since the age of 40 (20 years) and refractory to oral antihypertensives. Making the diagnosis is critical, and secondary causes for HTN should be explored to prevent fatalities.

b. This answer is incorrect. Although race/ethnicity in combination with multiple agents to treat HTN should be considered, it is not leading the nurse to suspect pheochromocytoma.

c. This answer is incorrect. Sex in combination with multiple agents to treat HTN would not lead the AGACNP to explore pheochromocytoma.

(Kasper et al., 2015).

27 **The correct answer is A.**

Rationales:

a. This is the correct answer. Serum metanephrines are the most sensitive test to confirm the diagnosis.

b. This is incorrect. Urine metanephrines are not the most sensitive test in confirming the diagnosis.

c. This is incorrect. Clonidine suppression test is not the most sensitive in confirming the diagnosis.

(Kasper et al., 2015).

28 **The correct answer is B.**

Rationales:

a. VHL is a genetic disorder that is associated with pheochromocytoma.

b. This is the correct answer. MEN 1 and MEN 1A are the genetic disorders that are associated with tumors seen in the pancreas, parathyroid, and pituitary gland.

c. MEN 2 and MEN 2A are genetic disorders associated with pheochromocytoma.

d. NF1 is a genetic disorder associated with pheochromocytoma.

e. SDH is a genetic disorder associated with pheochromocytoma.

(Kasper et al., 2015).

29 **The correct answer is A.**

Rationales:

a. Alpha-blockers/calcium channel blockers (alone or in combination) with daily monitoring of blood pressure is the first step in managing a pheochromocytoma.

b. "Beta-blockers with daily monitoring of blood pressure" is incorrect. Beta-blockers as initial therapy may lead to unopposed alpha causing paradoxical worsening of HTN. "A" is the only answer that does not start with beta-blockade prior to alpha-blocker initiation such as phenoxybenzamine or doxazosin.

c. "Beta-blockers/diuretics (alone or in combination) with daily monitoring of blood pressure" is incorrect as beta-blockers as initial therapy may lead to unopposed alpha causing paradoxical worsening of HTN. "A" is the only answer that does not start with beta-blockade prior to alpha-blocker initiation such as phenoxybenzamine or doxazosin.

(Kasper et al., 2015).

30 **The correct answer is C.**

Rationales:

a. HCTZ 25 mg orally daily may be used postoperatively.

b. Metoprolol 25 mg orally twice daily is often used postoperatively.

c. Phenoxybenzamine 10 mg orally twice daily: alpha-blockers are ONLY used preoperatively.

(Kasper et al., 2015).

> **Clinical Pearl**
>
> Myxedema coma is rare, but lethal if not identified early.

31 **The correct answer is C.**

Rationales:

a. This answer is incorrect. Cushing syndrome is not impacted by the TSH.

b. This answer is incorrect. Cushing disease is not impacted by the TSH.

c. This answer is correct. Hypothyroidism is caused by a TSH deficiency that leads to the slowing of the body's metabolism.

d. This answer is incorrect. Hyperthyroidism is not the result of TSH deficiency.

(Fitzgerald, 2018).

32 **The correct answer is A.**

Rationales:

a. TSH and free T4 are the screening tests for hypothyroidism and hyperthyroidism.

b. T3 and T4 are not the primary labs used to screen for hypothyroidism.

c. Thyroid ultrasound would not make the biochemical diagnosis.

d. Fine needle aspiration would not be used to determine the biochemical diagnosis.

(Fitzgerald, 2018).

33 **The correct answer is A.**

Rationales:

a. In Hashimoto thyroiditis, elevated antithyroperoxidase and antithyroglobulin antibodies are expected.

b. This answer is incorrect. Antithyroperoxidase and antithyroglobulin antibodies are not suppressed if Hashimoto thyroiditis is suspected.

(Fitzgerald, 2018).

34 **The correct answer is B.**

Rationales:

a. This answer is incorrect. In hyperthyroidism, the TSH is suppressed, but cancer is considered "cold" on the iodine uptake and scan.

b. Suppressed TSH, elevated T3, increased iodine uptake; diffuse versus "hot" foci on scan would be found with hyperthyroidism.

c. This answer is incorrect as the TSH is not elevated in hyperthyroidism.

d. This answer is incorrect as the TSH is not elevated in hyperthyroidism.

(Fitzgerald, 2018).

35 **The correct answer is C.**

Rationales:

a. MRI is not preferred as US is more sensitive in evaluating the thyroid and lymph nodes.

b. CT is not preferred as US is more sensitive in evaluating the thyroid and lymph nodes.

c. Ultrasound is preferred when evaluating thyroid nodules as it allows for a careful examination of the thyroid and is more sensitive for evaluating lymph node metastases than either CT or MRI scanning.

d. PET scan is not preferred as US is more sensitive in evaluating the thyroid and lymph nodes.

(Fitzgerald, 2018).

36 **The correct answer is D.**

Rationales:

a. Papillary thyroid cancer is not associated with MEN 2A.

b. Anaplastic thyroid cancer is not associated with MEN 2A.

c. Follicular thyroid cancer is not associated with MEN 2A.

d. Medullary thyroid cancer is the only thyroid cancer that is caused by an activating mutation of the ret protooncogene on chromosome 10. These patients will usually undergo a prophylactic thyroidectomy to prevent this type of cancer secondary to the genetic mutation.

(Fitzgerald, 2018).

37 **The correct answer is A.**

Rationales:

a. Follicular neoplasm is not always malignant. Almost 20% of the time, it is benign.

b. Anaplastic thyroid cancer is a malignancy.

c. Medullary thyroid cancer is a malignancy.

d. Papillary thyroid cancer is a malignancy.

e. This answer is incorrect as follicular neoplasm may not always be cancer.

(Fitzgerald, 2018).

38 **The correct answer is B.**

Rationales:

a. This answer is incorrect. "Sometimes these things happen late in life."

b. This is the correct response as Graves disease is an autoimmune disorder that is characterized by an increase in synthesis and release of thyroid hormones.

c. This answer is incorrect because Graves is characterized by an increase in synthesis and release of thyroid hormones.

(Fitzgerald, 2018).

39 **The correct answer is B.**

Rationales:

a. This is incorrect. Propranolol will not replace the loss of thyroid hormone post thyroidectomy.

b. Levothyroxine is the drug used as a synthetic hormone now that the patient does not have a thyroid. The other medications are used to treat hyperthyroidism, but in this clinical scenario, the patient does not have a thyroid now postsurgery.

c. Methimazole will not be resumed after surgery now that the thyroid has been completely removed.

d. SSKI will not be resumed after surgery now that the thyroid has been completely removed.

(Fitzgerald, 2018).

40 **The correct answer is C.**

Rationales:

a. Propylthiouracil in the first trimester followed by methimazole is not preferred as definitive treatment.

b. This answer is incorrect. Radioactive iodine (RAI) is toxic and should be avoided in patients who are actively trying to get pregnant. It is recommended that conception should be avoided for up to 1 year post-RAI.

c. Subtotal thyroidectomy followed by levothyroxine postoperatively is preferred as she requires a definitive treatment plan for her Graves disease as all the medications below may be dangerous to mom and baby.

(Fitzgerald, 2018).

41 **The correct answer is D.**

Rationales:

a. Acute thyroiditis is not the most likely cause for the labs.

b. Graves disease is not the most likely cause for the labs.

c. Although the patient is in atrial fibrillation, it does not provide a reason for the abnormal labs.

d. This is most likely amiodarone-induced thyrotoxicosis secondary to amiodarone's high iodine content.

(Fitzgerald, 2018).

42 **The correct answer is B.**

Rationales:

a. This is incorrect. The patient requires a workup for myxedema crisis in a critical care environment.

b. Suspect myxedema crisis and admit to ICU. The patient is most likely experiencing profound hypothyroidism secondary to RAI (destroys overactive thyroid tissue). Severe hypothyroidism secondary to RAI and lack of synthetic thyroid hormone replacement is the likely cause for the myxedema, hypothermia, hyponatremia, and profound hypothyroidism which must be managed in a critical care environment.

c. Although the patient should be evaluated and sent to the ICU, this patient is not presenting as a sepsis case.

d. This is incorrect. The patient is not presented as an appropriate observation status patient.

(Fitzgerald, 2018).

43 **The correct answer is C.**

Rationales:

a. Pheochromocytomas are not found in the adrenal cortex. They are found in the adrenal medulla.

b. Renal stenosis is not likely the secondary cause if the presumed source is from a nodule noted in the adrenal cortex.

c. Aldosteronoma is the correct answer. The adrenal cortex produces mineralocorticoids, glucocorticoids, and androgens. Aldosteronoma is an adrenal adenoma that produces excess aldosterone.

(Kasper et al., 2015).

44 **The correct answer is D.**

Rationales:

a. Moon face is often seen on physical examination.

b. Abdominal striae are often seen on physical examination.

c. Buffalo hump is often seen on physical examination.

d. Truncal weight loss is not a finding in Cushing syndrome. Truncal obesity is commonly seen as a physical examination finding.

(Kasper et al., 2015).

45 **The correct answer is A.**

Rationales:

a. Hyperpigmentation: ACTH excess is a distinguishing feature in primary adrenal insufficiency secondary to ACTH excess.

b. Alabaster-colored pale skin is not found in ACTH excess.

c. Abdominal striae are a physical examination finding in Cushing syndrome but do not distinguish primary and secondary adrenal insufficiency.

(Kasper et al., 2015).

46 **The correct answer is B.**

Rationales:

a. Early menopause may be included in the differential for disruption or menses, but the new onset of diabetes and HTN must be explored further for Cushing's.

b. Cushing syndrome should be included for any patient who experiences new-onset diabetes, HTN, and disruption of menses.

c. Polycystic ovary syndrome may be included in the differential for disruption or menses, but the new onset of diabetes and HTN must be explored further for Cushing's.

d. Pheochromocytoma may be included in the differential for HTN, but the new onset of diabetes and disruption of menses do not fit with this diagnosis.

(Kasper et al., 2015).

47 **The correct answer is A.**

Rationales:

a. Surgical intervention is recommended if the source of Cushing disease is most likely a pituitary tumor.

b. Supportive medical therapy is not curative, and surgical resection is recommended.

c. Cushing syndrome is life threatening, and more frequent visits with the PCP without intervention will negatively impact the patient's morbidity and mortality.

d. Oral steroid taper is an inappropriate plan.

(Kasper et al., 2015).

48 **The correct answer is A.**

Rationales:

a. Plasma ACTH will determine the differential diagnosis list. If ACTH is suppressed, it is ACTH-independent Cushing syndrome and an adrenal source should be explored further using unenhanced CT of adrenals. If ACTH is not suppressed, it is ACTH-dependent Cushing's, and Cushing disease should be explored further as a pituitary tumor may be the cause, and diagnosis may be made by using MRI, CPH, or high-dose DEX test.

b. Urine ACTH may be used, but this option did not specify if it was a 24-hour urine ACTH or random was being ordered.

c. Urine metanephrines are not the best option in the list above to make the diagnosis.

d. Serum metanephrines are not the best option in the list above to make the diagnosis.

(Kasper et al., 2015).

49 The correct answer is A.

Rationales:

a. Pheochromocytoma arises from the adrenal medulla where epinephrine and norepinephrine are produced.

b. Cushing syndrome may result from an excess of steroids from the adrenal cortex.

c. Aldosteronoma arises from the adrenal cortex.

d. Adrenal corticocarcinoma arises in the adrenal cortex.

(Kasper et al., 2015).

50 The correct answer is D.

Rationales:

a. Serum metanephrines are not the best test to aid in making the diagnosis of Addison disease.

b. CT scan is not the best test to aid in making the diagnosis of Addison disease.

c. MRI is not the best test to aid in making the diagnosis of Addison disease.

d. Cosyntropin test is a test that is used to confirm the diagnosis of Cushing syndrome.

(Kasper et al., 2015).

> **Clinical Pearl**
>
> In addition to BP control, liberal salt and fluid intake in the preceding 2 weeks before pheochromocytoma resection is an important aspect of preoperative care.

51 The correct answer is A.

Rationales:

a. This answer is correct; primary adrenal insufficiency is a loss of mineralocorticoids and glucocorticoids. Secondary adrenal insufficiency is the loss of glucocorticoid only (Addison disease).

b. Mineralocorticoid ONLY is an incomplete answer.

c. Epinephrine ONLY is an incomplete answer.

(Kasper et al., 2015).

52 The correct answer is B.

Rationales:

a. Primary adrenal insufficiency is the loss of both glucocorticoids and mineralocorticoids. The patient is not presenting with symptoms of both losses.

b. Secondary adrenal insufficiency is the correct answer.

c. Pheochromocytoma is incorrect. The symptoms are not aligned with the usual presentation of a pheochromocytoma.

d. Aldosteronoma is incorrect. The symptoms are not aligned with the usual presentation of a pheochromocytoma.

(Kasper et al., 2015).

53 The correct answer is B.

Rationales:

a. Thyroid gland is incorrect. A dysfunction of this gland does not cause secondary adrenal insufficiency.

b. Pituitary gland is correct. Dysfunction of this gland can lead to secondary adrenal insufficiency.

c. Pancreatic gland is incorrect. A dysfunction of this gland does not cause secondary adrenal insufficiency.

(Kasper et al., 2015).

54 The correct answer is B.

Rationales:

a. Cosyntropin test is not used to diagnose diabetes insipidus.

b. Vasopressin challenge test is a supervised test, in a controlled environment. Desmopressin acetate 0.05–0.1 ml (5–10 μg) intranasally (or 1 μg subcutaneously or intravenously) is given, with measurement of urine volume for 12 hours before and 12 hours after administration. A serum sodium is obtained at baseline, 12 hours after the desmopressin, and immediately if symptoms of hyponatremia develop.

c. Urine electrolytes are not used to diagnose diabetes insipidus.

d. MRI is not used to diagnose diabetes insipidus.

(Cho, 2018).

55 **The correct answer is A.**

Rationales:

a. No response in polydipsia or urine volume. Post vasopressin challenge test, the NP should suspect nephrotic DI if there is no response in symptoms of polydipsia or urine volume.

b. "Immediate improvement in polydipsia and urine volume" is incorrect.

c. "No response in polydipsia, improvement in urine volume" is incorrect.

d. "Improvement in polydipsia, but no response in urine volume" is incorrect.

(Cho, 2018).

56 **The correct answer is B.**

Rationales:

a. "No response in polydipsia, polyuria; serum sodium usually remains normal" is incorrect.

b. "Improvement in polydipsia and polyuria; serum sodium usually remains normal" is correct. Posttest, patients will report improvement in thirst and urine volume.

c. "No response in polydipsia, improvement in urine volume" is incorrect.

d. "Improvement in polydipsia, but no response in urine volume" is incorrect.

(Cho, 2018).

57 **The correct answer is C.**

Rationales:

a. "Hypothyroidism and hyperthyroidism" is incorrect as ADH has no impact.

b. "Pheochromocytoma and aldosteronoma" is incorrect as ADH has no impact.

c. SIADH and DI. The antidiuretic hormone affects DI and SIADH in opposing ways.

d. "Type 1 and type 2 diabetes" is incorrect as ADH has no impact.

(Cho, 2018).

58 **The correct answer is A.**

Rationales:

a. The goal of treatment is to improve symptoms of the disease. If it is a mild case of central diabetes insipidus, the patient may be controlled with regulating fluid intake; otherwise desmopressin acetate is the treatment of choice.

b. "Mild, moderate, and severe cases of central diabetes insipidus must always be managed with desmopressin acetate" is incorrect.

c. "Encouraging fluids is the gold standard for treating central diabetes insipidus" is incorrect.

d. "Surgical resection of the pituitary gland is recommended to improve overall quality of life in these patients" is incorrect.

(Cho, 2018).

59 **The correct answer is B.**

Rationales:

a. TSH is produced by the pituitary gland and stimulates the production of T4 from the thyroid gland and regulates conversion of T3 in the periphery.

b. ADH regulates the water concentration of the blood, which translates into osmolality.

c. FSH is essential to reproductive development of ovaries and testes.

d. CRH stimulates the pituitary, resulting in synthesis of ACTH.

(Cho, 2018).

60 **The correct answer is A.**

Rationales:

a. BMP, urine osmolality, serum osmolality, urine sodium are all the labs that are needed to distinguish between hypotonic hyponatremia, hypertonic hyponatremia, and isotonic hyponatremia.

b. "BMP, serum osmolality, urine sodium, urine creatinine" is not the complete list of labs that are needed to distinguish between hypotonic hyponatremia, hypertonic hyponatremia, and isotonic hyponatremia.

c. "BMP, serum osmolality, urine creatinine, magnesium" is not the list of labs needed in order to distinguish between hypotonic hyponatremia, hypertonic hyponatremia, and isotonic hyponatremia.

d. "BMP, urine osmolality, serum osmolality" is not the complete list of labs needed in order to distinguish between hypotonic hyponatremia, hypertonic hyponatremia, and isotonic hyponatremia.

(Cho, 2018).

61 **The correct answer is B.**

Rationales:

a. Hypovolemic isotonic hyponatremia most likely due to SIADH in the setting of malignancy is not the appropriate diagnosis based on the labs provided.

b. Euvolemic hypotonic hyponatremia most likely due to SIADH in the setting of malignancy. This patient is euvolemic with serum osmolality < 280 (hypotonic) and urine sodium > 20 in the setting of malignancy suggesting SIADH as the cause of hyponatremia

c. Euvolemic hypertonic hyponatremia most likely due to SIADH in the setting of malignancy is not the appropriate diagnosis based on the labs provided.

(Cho, 2018).

62 **The correct answer is D.**

Rationales:

a. Salt tablets are an appropriate intervention pending the severity of hyponatremia.

b. Tolvaptan (vasopressin receptor antagonist) is an appropriate intervention pending the severity of hyponatremia.

c. STAT nephrology consult is an appropriate option pending the severity of hyponatremia.

d. Encourage fluids is incorrect. Fluid restriction is encouraged and NOT encouraging fluids.

(Cho, 2018).

63 **The correct answer is A.**

Rationales:

a. Rapid correction of sodium beyond 0.5–1 mEq/L/h can lead to permanent brain damage.

b. Slow correction of sodium is preferred.

c. SIADH does not cause ODS.

d. DI onset does not cause ODS.

(Cho, 2018).

References

American Diabetes Association. (2016). Standards of medical care in diabetes. *Diabetes Care: The Journal of Clinical and Applied Research and Education, 39*(Suppl 1), S15–S35.

Cho, K. C. (2018). Electrolyte & acid-base disorders. In: M. A. Papadakis, S. J. McPhee, & M. W. Rabow, eds. *Current medical diagnosis & treatment 2019.* New York, NY: McGraw-Hill. Retrieved August 11, 2019, from http:// accessmedicine.mhmedical.com/content.aspx?bookid= 2449&sectionid=194574266.

Fitzgerald, P. A. (2018). Endocrine disorders. In: M. A. Papadakis, S. J. McPhee, & M. W. Rabow, eds. *Current medical diagnosis & treatment 2019.* New York, NY: McGraw-Hill. Retrieved Accessed July 9, 2019, from http://accessmedicine.mhmedical.com/content.aspx?bo okid=2449&sectionid=194577758.

Kasper, D. L., Fauci, A.S., et al., eds. (2015). *Harrison's principles of internal medicine* (19th ed.). New York, NY: McGraw-Hill.

Powers, A. C., et al. (2018). Diabetes mellitus: Management and therapies. In: J. Larry Jameson, et al., eds. *Harrison's principles of internal medicine* (20th ed.). New York, NY: McGraw-Hill. Retrieved from http://accessmedicine.mhmedical.com/content.aspx?bookid=2129&secti onid=192288412

CHAPTER 10

Vascular

Traci Stahl, MSN, FNP-BC, AGACNP-BC

Disease Questions

1 Which of the following patients is NOT at higher risk for developing deep vein thrombosis (DVT)?

a. A 74-year-old male who presents to the emergency department with fever, hypotension, and tachycardia

b. A 42-year-old female with BMI 38 who underwent gastric bypass surgery 6 months ago

c. A 21-year-old female who is 3 weeks post elective abortion

d. A 30-year-old female prescribed low dose birth control pills 2 weeks ago by her gynecologist

2 The AGACNP is called to the emergency room for evaluation of a 65-year-old male with PMH of hypertension, diabetes, and chronic systolic congestive heart failure, who is reporting pain of his right lower leg. The physical examination should include all of the following EXCEPT:

a. Dorsiflexion of the foot while the knee is fully extended

b. Palpation of distal pulses of BOTH lower extremities

c. Evaluation of capillary refill of the toes of the RIGHT foot

d. Passive movement and palpation of all joints

3 The AGACNP is called to the orthopedic floor to evaluate a patient who is postoperative day (POD) 2 from right total knee replacement surgery. On physical examination, bilateral lower leg varicosities are seen. The AGACNP is able to palpate a firm, tender erythematous fibrous cord in the right lower leg. The diagnosis is:

a. DVT

b. SVT (superficial venous thrombosis)

c. Unable to determine without further testing

d. None of the above

4 Which patient is at MOST risk to have a false-positive D-dimer result?

a. A 46-year-old male who underwent PTCA of LAD 2 days ago and is taking daily aspirin and clopidogrel

b. A 50-year-old male who is s/p CABG 2 weeks ago

c. A 57-year-old male with history of MI 6 months ago

d. A 64-year-old female with history of traumatic subdural hematoma 2 months ago

5 The AGACNP is being asked to admit a 65-year-old male with PMH of hypertension, diabetes mellitus II, and stage IV chronic kidney disease (creatinine clearance is less than 35 mL/min), who has acute VTE of the left lower extremity. The nurse practitioner orders:

a. Fondaparinux 5–10 mg subcutaneously every 24 hours

b. Enoxaparin 1 mg/kg subcutaneously every 12 hours

c. Apixaban 5 mg by mouth daily

d. Rivaroxaban 10 mg by mouth daily

6 The AGACNP is called to the emergency room to evaluate a patient with stage IIb acute limb ischemia of the right lower extremity. Physical examination findings will include:

a. Audible pedal pulse by arterial Doppler, no sensory loss, no muscle weakness

b. Inaudible pedal pulse by arterial Doppler, paralysis, numbness of entire RLE

c. Audible pedal pulse by arterial Doppler, numbness of the toes of the right foot, motor strength 5/5

d. Audible pedal pulse by arterial Doppler, numbness of the right foot AND pretibial leg, pain, and muscle weakness

7 The following are contraindications for thrombolysis EXCEPT:

a. A 76-year-old male with dementia

b. A 41-year-old male with cerebral aneurysm clipping 1 month ago

c. A 53-year-old female with blood pressure 195/110

d. A 34-year-old female with platelet count of 36,000

8 A 53-year-old female with history of tobacco abuse, HLD, HTN, and prior left superior mesenteric artery occlusion requiring small bowel resection is admitted for left inferior mesenteric artery occlusion. The patient undergoes endarterectomy of the left inferior mesenteric artery, and abdominal incision remains open with two drains in place. The nurse practitioner includes the following postoperative order:

a. Diazepam 5 mg IV every 6 hours

b. Warfarin 5 mg by mouth to start STAT

c. Streptokinase 1.5 million IU IV ×1 dose

d. Heparin infusion @ 40 units/kg/hr

9 The AGACNP is rounding in the ICU. He sees a 60-year-old male who is s/p successful distal embolization who is currently receiving rTPA treatment. When would the AGACNP initiate aspirin therapy?

a. Upon discharge from the hospital.

b. Immediately and concurrent with rTPA treatment.

c. Upon cessation of rTPA.

d. The AGACNP would change to LMWH and NOT start aspirin.

10 A 67-year-old male with history of nicotine addiction, diabetes mellitus type II, and BPH presents to the emergency room with progressive symptoms of cramping in his right lower leg. The nurse practitioner examines the patient and notes his lower leg to be cool to touch and dusky in color and a 1- × 0.5-in. stage 3 decubitus ulcer is present on the right heel. The diagnostic testing of choice is:

a. Duplex US

b. MRA

c. Digital angiography

d. None of the above

11 The AGACNP is called to evaluate a 72-year-old white male who is reporting that his feet are "cold." The bedside RN reports that dorsalis pedis pulse of the left foot is present only by doppler. Ankle brachial index (ABI) is conducted, and the result is 1. The AGACNP's next step is:

a. No further testing is indicated.

b. Perform toe–brachial index.

c. Consult vascular surgery team.

d. B and C.

12 A 46-year-old female presents to the emergency room with complaints of right arm numbness, coldness to touch, and pain when she was carrying groceries into the house. Initial vital signs are T 99.8, HR 90, RR 20, left arm BP 150/92, and right arm BP 110/84. Duplex US reveals reversal of flow in the right vertebral artery. The AGACNP suspects:

a. Acute CVA secondary to occlusion of vertebral artery

b. Livedo reticularis

c. DVT right arm

d. Subclavian steal syndrome

13 A 72-year-old female with history of polymyalgia rheumatica (PMR) presents to the ER with sudden onset of blurred vision in her right eye. She reports a 2-week history of low-grade fever, joint pains and headache, and jaw claudication. The most likely diagnosis is:

a. Acute ischemic stroke

b. Giant cell arteritis

c. Third nerve palsy

d. Lyme disease

14 A 78-year-old male who presents to the ER with unilateral blurred visions, fever, headaches, and jaw claudication would be expected to also have the following laboratory results EXCEPT:

a. Low serum albumin

b. Elevated alkaline phosphatase

c. Elevated leukocyte count

d. Elevated ESR and CRP

15 A 40-year-old male with no PMH presents to the ER with sudden onset of sharp abdominal pain that radiates to his back. Vital signs are as follows: T 99.9, p 92, RR 24, left arm BP 164/98, and right arm BP 190/105. On examination, the AGACNP notes absence of the right lower extremity popliteal and pedal pulse. The AGACNP immediately suspects:

a. Acute anterior wall MI (AWMI)

b. Acute aortic dissection

c. Acute embolic event to the RLE

d. None of the above

16 A patient with an acute aortic dissection would have CXR findings of which of the following?

a. Wide mediastinum

b. Pleural effusion of the right lower lobe of lung

c. Bilateral lung atelectasis

d. None of the above

17 The AGACNP evaluates a 40-year-old male with recent diagnosis of Marfan syndrome who is also a smoker and is presenting for elective cholecystectomy. A review of EMR includes CXR and lab work. Physical examination findings are normal. Vital signs are also within normal limits. Which diagnostic test must be completed prior to proceeding with surgery in this specific patient population?

a. EKG

b. PFT

c. CT scan of the chest

d. ABG

18 Which patient is at LEAST risk for developing abdominal aortic aneurysm (AAA)?

a. A 53-year-old African American female with uncontrolled diabetes mellitus type II on insulin

b. A 34-year-old white male who smokes 1 ppd for the past 14 years

c. A 40-year-old white male with well-controlled hypertension, on beta-blocker therapy

d. A 68-year-old white male with atherosclerotic heart disease

19 A 43-year-old white male with recent aortic dissection is in the ICU receiving a nitroprusside infusion. His current vital signs are as follows: T 99.4, HR 114, RR 22, and BP 136/86. The next appropriate intervention would be:

a. Diltiazem 30 mg by mouth every 6 hours

b. Metoprolol 2.5 mg IV every 6 hours

c. Enalapril 2.5 mg IV every 6 hours

d. None of the above

20 Ascending aortic dissections are more common than descending aortic dissections.

a. True

b. False

21 A 40-year-old white male presents to the emergency room for evaluation of chest pain after falling off his bicycle. He reports that his chest pain is relieved with morphine sulfate 2 mg IV. Vital signs are as follows: T 98.9, HR 84, RR 20, and BP 126/82. CT chest reveals 3 cm AAA. The AGACNP's NEXT intervention is:

a. Consult surgery.

b. Start metoprolol 12.5 mg by mouth twice daily.

c. Discharge to home and advise patient to follow up with surgery in 6 months.

d. Both A and B.

22 Which type of aortic dissection requires emergent surgical evaluation and treatment?

a. Ascending aorta

b. Descending aorta

c. Coarctation of the aorta

d. Both B and C

23 A 26-year-old white male with history of chronic pain syndrome presents to the emergency room with sudden onset of abdominal pain radiating to his back. CBC and CMP lab values were within normal limits. His heart rate is 102 and BP is 118/76. CT chest confirms diagnosis of 4.8 cm AAA. The AGACNP's next intervention is to order:

a. Surgery consult

b. Toxicology screen

c. Metoprolol 2.5 mg IV every 6 hours

d. All of the above

24 The AGACNP is conducting daily rounds on a 57-year-old white male with a history of ischemic heart disease, who is POD 31 from right femoral bypass surgery. The AGACNP knows that by starting cilostazol, this patient may be at increased risk for:

a. Angina pectoris.

b. Bradycardia.

c. Refractory hypertension.

d. All of the above are possible side effects.

25 Alteplase works in the body by:

a. Activating the production of plasmin

b. Deactivating the production of plasmin

c. Increasing fibrinogen

d. Decreasing prothrombin time

26 The AGACNP is performing discharge teaching for a 32-year-old female hospitalized for acute DVT of the right popliteal vein, s/p fracture of the right ankle NOT requiring surgical intervention. The AGACNP informs the patient of which of the following?

a. She will require anticoagulation therapy for 12 months.

b. She will require anticoagulation therapy for 3 months.

c. She will require anticoagulation therapy for 6 months.

d. She will require anticoagulation therapy for her lifetime.

27 Heparin is metabolized in the:

a. GI tract

b. Liver

c. Kidneys

d. Lung

28 The nurse practitioner is called to see a 44-year-old male who just returned to the ICU after undergoing a left carotid endarterectomy procedure. The patient is reporting difficulty swallowing, and the AGACNP notices a large expanding hematoma at the incision site. Vital signs are as follows: T 99, HR 84, RR 24, BP 100/70, and SaO_2 97% on nasal O_2. After briefly reviewing the operative record and noting that the patient did receive heparin 90 units/kg IV during the procedure, the AGACNP's next step is:

a. Protamine 50 mg IV ×1.

b. Obtain stat US.

c. Intubate the patient.

d. Give aminocaproic acid 5 g IV ×1.

29 The AGACNP is asked to admit a 72-year-old male diagnosed with thoracic abdominal aneurysm. On physical examination, the AGACNP notes edema of the right anterior cervical region extending upward to the jaw and laterally to the right arm. The AGACNP immediately suspects:

a. Compression of the tracheobronchial tree

b. Rupture of the aneurysm

c. SVC occlusion

d. Compression of a coronary artery

30 The most common aortic aneurysm is:

a. Thoracic.

b. Abdominal.

c. They are both equal in occurrence.

Disease Answers/Rationales

1 **The correct answer is B.**

Rationales:

a. A is incorrect because fever, hypotension, and tachycardia are symptoms of shock. Shock state will increase the risk for venous stasis.

b. B is the correct answer. BMI greater than 40 is obesity. Obesity is a risk factor for VTE. This patient has a BMI less than 40.

c. C is incorrect because all stages of pregnancy, including postabortion, are considered at risk.

d. D is incorrect because increased estrogen may cause hypercoagulability.

(McLendon & Attia, 2019).

2 **The correct answer is A.**

Rationales:

a. A is the correct answer. Dorsiflexion of the foot while the knee is fully extended, also known as Homans sign, is no longer used because it can potentially dislodge the DVT and then the blood clot may travel to the lung.

b. B is incorrect as the physical examination should always include both extremities.

c. C is incorrect as the capillary refill should be included in the examination.

d. D is incorrect as passive movement and palpation of all joints should be included in the physical examination to assess for arthritis and deformities.

(McLendon & Attia, 2019).

3 **The correct answer is B.**

Rationales:

a. A is incorrect because pain with DVT is usually more diffuse. Although both SVT and DVT can occur in lower extremities, DVT is most common in the lower extremities. The classic finding of SVT is a firm, tender, fibrous cord in the area of previous varicosity. A fibrous cord is rarely palpable with a DVT.

b. B is the correct answer. Pain with SVT is typically localized to the area of thrombosis.

c. C is incorrect because diagnosis CAN be made upon physical examination findings alone.

(McLendon & Attia, 2019).

4 **The correct answer is A.**

Rationales:

a. A is the correct answer.

b. B is incorrect as a false-positive D-Dimer can result from recent surgery.

c. C is incorrect as a false-positive D-Dimer can result from the inflammation related to recent cardiac events.

d. D is incorrect because false-positive D-dimer results can result from recent trauma.

(Binder et al., 2009, pp. 753–757).

5 **The correct answer is B.**

Rationales:

a. A is incorrect because fondaparinux should not be used in patients with CrCl less than 30 mL/min.

b. B is correct because enoxaparin is FDA approved at renal dosage of 1 mg/kg subcutaneously every 12 hr.

c. C is incorrect because subcutaneous medication is recommended for ACUTE treatment of DVT.

d. D is incorrect because subcutaneous medication is recommended for ACUTE treatment of DVT.

(Goldstein & Mishkel, 2011, pp. 381–389).

6 **The correct answer is D.**

Rationales:

The Rutherford ischemia staging:

    I. Limb is viable.

  IIA. Limb requires prompt intervention.

  IIB. Limb is salvageable with immediate revascularization.

   II. The limb has irreversible damage, major tissue loss, or permanent nerve damage.

a. A is an example of stage I.

b. B is an example of stage IIA.

c. C is an example of stage II.

d. D is an example of stage IIB.

(Goldstein & Mishkel, 2011, pp. 381–389).

7 **The correct answer is A.**

Rationales:

a. A is the correct answer. Dementia is associated with lower use of rTPA due to the FALSE perception that it raises the risk of hemorrhage.

b. B is incorrect because as per current AHA guidelines, AVM, aneurysm, or intracranial neoplasm are contraindications. Uncontrolled hypertension despite the use of antihypertensive medications to achieve adequate control of blood pressure is still associated with increased risk of poor outcomes.

c. C is incorrect because thrombolytic therapy is contraindicated in patients with SBP greater than 185 or DBP greater than 110.

d. D is incorrect because thrombolytic therapy is contraindicated in patients with platelet count less than 100,000.

(Fugate & Rabinstein, 2015, pp. 110–121).

8 **The correct answer is D.**

Rationales:

a. A is incorrect because it is a vasodilator.

b. B is incorrect because warfarin decreases blood clotting by blocking vitamin K, thus prolonging clotting. This patient will need to return to the OR for abdominal closure.

c. C is incorrect because streptokinase forms a complex with plasminogen that releases plasma. (It is derived from streptococci; therefore, patients with recent streptococcal infections can require much higher dosages.)

d. D is correct. Thromboplastin is a plasma protein aiding blood coagulation through catalyzing the conversion of prothrombin to thrombin. Heparin directly activates anticlotting factors. One of the inherent postoperative goals is to prevent reocclusion of the artery.

(Giammakakis et al., 2017, pp. 125–132).

9 **The correct answer is B.**

Rationales:

a. A is incorrect as patients with PAD have higher mortality due to cardiac disease, and aspirin therapy should be started immediately.

b. B is the correct answer. It is recommended to resume aspirin as soon as possible.

c. C is incorrect as aspirin therapy should be started immediately in these patients. Aspirin has also been shown to decrease the progression of atherosclerosis and occurrence of thrombotic complications.

d. D is incorrect because aspirin has been proven to reduce the possibility of suffering fatal or nonfatal vascular events by 25%. Low molecular weight heparin does not affect platelet function.

(Goldstein & Mishkel, 2011, pp. 381–389).

Clinical Pearl

Vasculitis is characterized by inflammation within the walls of arteries and is classified by the predominance of the size artery affected.

10 **The correct answer is C.**

Rationales:

Based upon the patient symptoms and physical examination findings, the nurse practitioner suspects the diagnosis of PAD.

a. A is incorrect because duplex US uses sound waves to create pictures of arteries. It can be lacking in quality.

b. B is incorrect because MRA is a noninvasive test, which eliminates exposure to ionizing radiation, but it has a higher cost and there is risk of contrast nephropathy.

c. C is the correct answer because digital angiography is the gold standard testing modality for PAD. This is a low-cost diagnostic test that provides additional information regarding luminal patency and presence of collaterals.

(Kollef, Bedient, Isakpw, & Witt, 2008).

11 **The correct answer is A.**

Rationales:

a. A is the correct answer. Normal ABI is 0.91–1.3.

b. B is incorrect because the patient has a normal ABI. If the ABI is greater than 1.3, obtain toe pressures.

c. C is incorrect because the patient has a normal ABI and does not require vascular surgery consultation. If ABI ≤ .90, then vascular surgery consult would be appropriate.

(Harvard Medical School, 2019).

12 **The correct answer is D.**

Rationales:

a. A is incorrect because US duplex does NOT confirm vertebral artery stroke. A CTA would be needed.

b. B is incorrect because livedo reticularis is a mottling pattern of the skin of the arms and legs.

c. C is incorrect because DVT of the right arm may have the same physical symptoms; however, the blood pressure would not be affected.

d. D is the correct answer. On examination, subclavian artery stenosis will exhibit a pressure difference between arms of greater than 40 mm Hg. US will show reversal of flow in the ipsilateral vertebral artery.

(Potter & Pinto, 2014, pp. 2320–2323).

13 **The correct answer is B.**

Rationales:

a. A is incorrect because acute ischemic stroke typically presents without joint pains and fever.

b. B is the correct answer. These are the classic symptoms of giant cell arteritis, and the patient's medical history suggests giant cell arteritis.

c. C is incorrect because symptoms of 3rd nerve palsy include diplopia, ptosis, paresis of eye adduction, and upward and downward gaze.

d. D is incorrect because although fever and joint pains can be symptoms of Lyme disease, the patient's PMH of PMR suggests that this is most likely not Lyme.

(Lazarewicz & Watson, 2019).

14 **The correct answer is C.**

Rationales:

a. A is incorrect because the serum albumin is moderately decreased initially until the initiation of glucocorticoids.

b. B is incorrect because 25%–35% of people will have elevation of alkaline phosphatase until glucocorticoid therapy is started.

c. C is the correct answer. The suspected diagnosis is giant cell arteritis. The leukocyte count is usually normal, despite inflammation.

d. D is an expected finding because the hallmark of GCA is elevation of ESR and CRP. ESR will increase naturally with age but also with inflammatory disease states. The same is true for CRP.

(Lazarewicz & Watson, 2019).

15 **The correct answer is B.**

Rationales:

a. A is incorrect because abdominal pain is an atypical location for pain with acute MI.

b. B is the correct answer. Pain is typically described as a sharp, tearing sensation. The patient may have a variance of blood pressure between each arm of ≥20 mm Hg.

c. C is incorrect because absence of pulse to the right lower extremity is present with acute limb ischemia; however, abdominal pain is not typical. Most often, pain is located in the area of the thrombus.

(Kuivaniemi, Ryer, Elmore, & Tromp, 2015, pp. 975–987).

16 **The correct answer is A.**

Rationales:

a. A is the correct answer. A widened mediastinum is a width of more than 6 cm on upright PA x-ray film.

b. B is incorrect because pleural effusion is not caused by aortic dissection.

c. C is incorrect because atelectasis is most commonly seen as a postoperative complication.

(Kuivaniemi et al., 2015, pp. 975–987).

17 **The correct answer is C.**

Rationales:

a. A is incorrect because baseline EKG is recommended for ALL patients undergoing surgery.

b. B is incorrect because PFT is not a NECESSARY test.

c. C is the correct answer. Per 2010 ACC/AHA/ AATS guidelines, patients with MFS should have cross-sectional imaging by CT every 3–5 years and prior to elective surgeries, due to the increased risk of aortic dissection.

d. D is incorrect because ABG would not be helpful in identifying aortic dimensions.

(Hiratzka et al., 2010, pp. 266–369).

18 **The correct answer is A.**

Rationales:

a. A is the correct answer. Female gender, diabetes, and non-white race are all associated with a decreased risk of AAA.

b. B is incorrect because this patient is a male, white, and a smoker, which are risk factors.

c. C is incorrect because this patient is male, is white, and has hypertension.

d. D is incorrect because risk factors associated with aneurysms include old age, male gender, hypertension, white race, family history, prior aneurysms, and smoking.

(Keisler & Carter, 2015, pp. 538–543).

19 **The correct answer is B.**

Rationales:

a. A is incorrect because diltiazem is acceptable IF the patient has no contraindications to beta-blockers but is not FIRST LINE.

b. B is the correct answer. Initial management of thoracic aortic dissection is aimed at decreasing aortic wall stress by controlling heart rate and blood pressure. Beta-blockers are recommended to decrease rate of ventricular contraction and maintain heart rate less than 60 bpm and SBP less than 120.

c. C is incorrect because ACE inhibitors cause vasodilation but do not decrease the rate of ventricular contraction.

(Gupta, Gupta, & Khoynezhad, 2009, pp. 66–76).

> **Clinical Pearl**
>
> Aortic dissections may be classified as type A or type B dissections. A type A dissection involves the aortic arch proximal to the subclavian artery and requires prompt surgical evaluation. Type B dissections typically occur in the proximal descending aorta beyond the left subclavian artery, and treatment (medical or surgical) depends on the presence of distal perfusion.

20 The correct answer is A.

Rationales:

a. A is the correct answer. Ascending aortic dissections are twice as common as descending aortic dissections.

(Kuivaniemi et al., 2015, pp. 975–987).

21 The correct answer is C.

Rationales:

a. A is incorrect because surgical treatment is recommended when aneurysms are ≥5 cm in diameter or are leaking.

b. B is incorrect because beta-blockers are recommended to control heart rate and blood pressure. This patient has stable vital signs with a heart rate less than 100 bpm and SBP less than 130 mm Hg.

c. C is the correct answer. This patient has stabilized and is pain free. It is safe to have him discharged to home with follow-up CT in 6 months.

(Kuivaniemi et al., 2015, pp. 975–987).

22 The correct answer is A.

Rationales:

a. A is the correct answer. Type A aortic dissection is a surgical emergency. Rupture of the dissected aorta is uncommon but will result in death without immediate intervention.

b. B is incorrect because descending aorta—type B—is treated initially by medical management. Surgery is reserved for patients with uncontrolled hypertension, persistent pain, dissection, or perfusion deficit compromising other organs.

c. C is incorrect because coarctation of the aorta is usually present at birth but not diagnosed until adulthood.

(Kuivaniemi et al., 2015, pp. 975–987).

23 The correct answer is B.

Rationales:

a. A is incorrect because the aneurysm is less than 5 cm and is not ruptured; therefore, surgery consult is not emergent.

b. B is the correct answer. A toxicology screen should be ordered on any patient presenting with acute aortic syndrome and no predisposing factors.

c. C is incorrect because beta-blockers are avoided in patients with cocaine toxicity. Current vital signs are stable. Obtain the toxicology screen PRIOR to starting beta-blocker therapy when vital signs are stable and the aneurysm is not ruptured.

(Kuivaniemi et al., 2015, pp. 975–987).

24 The correct answer is A.

Rationales:

a. A is the correct answer. This patient has a history of ischemic heart disease, and the vasodilatory effects of the medication may cause angina.

b. B is incorrect because cilostazol may induce tachycardia, NOT bradycardia.

c. C is incorrect because due to vasodilation, hypotension is a common side effect.

(Year-oldo, 2013, pp. 179–185).

25 The correct answer is A.

Rationales:

a. A is the correct answer. Altepase activates the production of plasmin.

b. B is incorrect because alteplase does not deactivate plasmin; it activates plasmin.

c. C is incorrect because alteplase decreases fibrinogen.

d. D is incorrect because plasmin breaks down fibrin and allows clots to disintegrate, and will increase prothrombin time.

(Fugate & Rabinstein, 2015, pp. 110–121).

26 **The correct answer is B.**

Rationales:

a. A is incorrect, as patients with provoked DVTs require anticoagulation for 3 months.

b. B is the correct answer. The correct answer is 3 months as the most likely source of the DVT was the patient's recent ankle fracture and the DVT is considered provoked.

c. C is incorrect, as her DVT is considered provoked, which requires 3 months of anticoagulation.

d. D is incorrect as patients with risk factors such as family history of DVT or clotting disorders, surgery, or recurrent DVT may require longer therapy if not an infinite duration of anticoagulation.

(Barnes, 2017).

27 **The correct answer is B.**

Rationales:

a. A is incorrect as heparin is not metabolized in the GI tract.

b. B is the correct answer. Heparin is metabolized in the liver.

c. C is incorrect, as heparin is not renally metabolized.

d. D is incorrect, as heparin is not metabolized in the lungs.

(Fugate & Rabinstein, 2015, pp. 110–121).

28 **The correct answer is A.**

Rationales:

a. A is the correct answer. Protamine is the antidote for heparin.

b. B is incorrect because the patient has an expanding hematoma. In order to stop the bleeding, the heparin antidote must be given.

c. C is incorrect because the patient is not hypoxic with airway compromise. The goal of care is to stop the bleeding.

d. D is incorrect because aminocaproic acid is used to reverse fibrinolytic therapy.

(Marino, 2007).

29 **The correct answer is C.**

Rationales:

a. A is incorrect because compression of the tracheobronchial tree would cause respiratory symptoms such as wheezing, cough, dyspnea, and hemoptysis.

b. B is incorrect because if an aneurysm has ruptured, symptoms would include chest pain and hypotension, leading to shock.

c. C is the correct answer. Compression of the central veins or SVC can cause thromboembolism or SVC syndrome.

d. D is incorrect because symptoms of MI would include chest pain and EKG changes.

(Janik, 2018).

Clinical Pearl

The goals of treatment for peripheral arterial disease center on cardiovascular risk reduction.

30 **The correct answer is B.**

Rationales:

a. A is incorrect, as abdominal aneurysms occur more frequently than do thoracic aneurysms. Both the thoracic aorta and the abdominal aorta have three layers (intimal, medial, and adventitial). The medial layer of the thoracic aorta is both avascular and vascular. The medial layer of the abdominal aorta is entirely avascular.

b. B is the correct answer. The majority of AAA are infrarenal and occur below the renal arteries.

c. C is incorrect, as thoracic and abdominal aneurysms do not occur with the same frequency.

(Kuivaniemi et al., 2015, pp. 975–987).

References

Barnes, G. (2017). Diagnosis and management of acute deep vein thrombosis. *American College of Cardiology.* Retrieved from https://www.acc.org/latest-in-cardiology/ten-points-to-remember/2017/09/28/14/14/diagnosis-and-management-of-acute-deep-vein-thrombosis (June 2019).

Binder, B., Lackner, H., Salmhofer, W., Kroemer, S., Custovic, J., & Hofmann-Wellenhof, R. (2009). Association between superficial vein thrombosis and deep vein thrombosis of the lower extremity. *Archives of Dermatology, 145*(7), 753–757. doi:10.1001/archdermatol.2009.12

Fugate, J., & Rabinstein, A. (2015). Absolute and relative contraindications to Iv rt-PA for acute ischemic stroke. *Neurohospitalist, 593,* 110–121.

Giammakakis, S., Galyfos, G., Sachmpazidis, I., Kapasas, K., Kerasidis, S., Stamatatos, I., et al. (2017). Thrombolysis in peripheral artery disease. *Therapeutic Advances in Cardiovascular Disease, 11*(4), 125–132.

Goldstein, J., & Mishkel, G. (2011). Choosing the correct therapeutic option for acute limb ischemia. *Interventional Cardiology, 3*(3), 381–389.

Gupta, P., Gupta, H., & Khoynezhad, A. (2009). Hypertensive emergency in aortic dissection and thoracic aortic aneurysm. *Pharmaceuticals, 2*(3), 66–76.

Harvard Medical School. (2019). Ankle brachial index. Retrieved from https://www.health.harvard.edu/newsletter_article/ankle-brachial-index (August 2019).

Hiratzka, L., Bakris, G., Beckman, J. A., Bersin, R. M., Carr, V. F., Casey, D. E., Jr., et al. (2010). 2010 ACC/AHA/AATS/ACR/ASA/SCA/SCAI/SIR/STS/SVM guidelines for the diagnosis and management of patients with thoracic aortic disease. *Circulation, 121*(13), 266–369.

Janik, L. (2018). *Cardiac diagnosis for acute care: The AGACNP and PA's guide to a comprehensive history and deciphering the differential.* New York, NY: Springer Publishing Company.

Keisler, B., & Carter, C. (2015). Abdominal aortic aneurysm. *American Family Physician, 91*(8), 538–543.

Kollef, M., Bedient, T., Isakpw, W., & Witt, C. (2008). *The washington manual of critical care.* Philadelphia, PA: Lippincott Williams & Wilkins.

Kuivaniemi, H., Ryer, E., Elmore, J., & Tromp, G. (2015). Understanding the pathogenesis of abdominal aortic aneurysms. *Expert Review of Cardiovascular Therapy, 13*(9), 975–987.

Lazarewicz, K., & Watson, P. (2019). Giant cell arteritis. *BMJ, 365,* l1964.

Marino, P. L. (2007). *The ICU book* (3rd ed.). Philadelphia, PA: Lippincott Williams & Wilkins.

McLendon, K., & Attia, M. (2019). *Deep vein thrombosis risk factors.* Treasure Island, FL: STAT Pearls Publishing, LLC.

Potter, B., & Pinto, D. (2014). Subclavian steal syndrome. *Circulation, 129*(22), 2320–2323.

Year-oldo, S. (2013). Efficacy of cilostazol on uncontrolled coronary vasospastic angina. *Cardiovascular Therapeutics, 31*(30), 179–185.

CHAPTER 11

Hematology and Oncology

Latesha Colbert-Mack, DNP, CRNP, AGACNP

Disease Questions

1 The cancer sites listed below are among the top five common new cancer cases in the United States EXCEPT:

a. Breast

b. Lung

c. Prostate

d. Colon and rectum

e. Leukemia

2 TNM is the most common classification system used in staging cancer. What does TNM stand for?

a. Tumor, Nodes, Metastasis

b. Timing, Nodes, Metastasis

c. Tissue Diagnosis, Nodes, Metastasis

d. Therapy, Nodes, Metastasis

3 A 74-year-old male is newly diagnosed with gastric cancer but unable to proceed to surgery secondary to decreased functional status. The medical oncologist and surgical oncologist agree that starting with chemotherapy with the intent for a curative surgery is the best oncologic approach. This approach is best described as:

a. Neoadjuvant chemotherapy prior to surgical resection

b. Adjuvant chemotherapy prior to surgical resection

4 A 52-year-old male underwent a computed tomography (CT) scan and was noted to have a colorectal cancer with liver lesion on diagnosis of disease. Which of the following clinical presentations best describes this patient?

a. Colorectal cancer with synchronous liver metastasis

b. Colorectal cancer with metachronous liver metastasis

5 The adult-gerontology acute care nurse practitioner (AGACNP) is rounding with the team on a patient with a pancreatic head mass. Differential diagnosis for a pancreatic mass includes pancreatic adenocarcinoma, pancreatic neuroendocrine tumor, or pancreatic pseudocyst. The nurse practitioner student asks what will be done to develop a thoughtful treatment plan. What is the best response?

a. Before we can develop a treatment plan, we will have to identify the tumor, stage the tumor using the TNM classification, and then treat the tumor with possibly chemotherapy, radiation therapy, surgical resection, or a combination of all three.

b. Pancreatic masses have terrible mortality rates, so we will most likely start with surgery.

c. In all solid tumors, surgery is the best chance for patient survival.

6 A 65-year-old male presents to the unit for new onset of nausea, bilious vomiting, and suspicion for a small bowel obstruction. Differential diagnosis for small bowel obstruction includes all of the following EXCEPT:

a. Malignancy

b. Intussusception

c. Adhesions

d. Gastritis

7 A CT confirms that a small bowel obstruction is most likely secondary to mass. It is not clear at this time if the mass is an adhesion or malignancy. The AGACNP suggests sending tumor markers to aid in developing the differential diagnosis list. Which tumor marker is associated with colon cancer?

a. Carcinoembryonic antigen (CEA)

b. CA19-9

c. BRAC1

d. Alpha-fetoprotein (AFP)

8 Tumor markers in solid tumors are often helpful with narrowing the differential diagnosis for a patient. Please select the appropriate tumor marker and oncologic disease association:

a. Prostate-specific antigen (PSA)—breast cancer

b. AFP—hepatocellular carcinoma

c. CEA—prostate cancer

d. BRAC1—thyroid cancer

9 A 52-year-old female presented to the hospital with a mass noted in the pancreas. Prior to making a surgical plan, the AGACNP orders tumor markers to assist diagnosis list. Which tumor marker is widely used in confirming pancreatic adenocarcinoma?

a. CEA

b. CA19-9

c. BRAC1

d. AFP

10 A patient presents with new onset of vocal hoarseness. Evaluation by otolaryngology identified vocal cord paralysis. Which solid tumor should be added to the differential for workup?

a. Breast cancer

b. Prostate cancer

c. Colorectal cancer

d. Non–small cell lung cancer (NSCLC)

11 A 49-year-old female presents to the unit with painless jaundice and concerns for hepatocellular carcinoma. Recent CT imaging reveals a mass in the biliary ducts as the possible cause for obstructive jaundice. The AGACNP suspects the final diagnosis postsurgery will be which of the following?

a. Hepatocellular carcinoma

b. Cholangiocarcinoma

c. Pancreatic cancer

d. Ovarian cancer

12 A 64-year-old male is diagnosed with cholangiocarcinoma. Which diagnostic test will be most useful in identifying the tumor in staging?

a. Endoscopic retrograde or percutaneous transhepatic cholangiography with biopsy

b. Endoscopic CT with fine needle aspiration of tumor

c. Electrocardiogram (EKG)

13 Treatment options for hepatocellular carcinoma include transarterial radioembolization (TACE), radiofrequency ablation (RFA), microwave ablation, and cryotherapy. Which treatment option is associated with curative outcome of disease?

a. TACE

b. RFA

c. Microwave ablation

d. None of the above

14 A patient is being admitted with distal gastric cancer. Which surgical procedure is most likely achieved rendered free of disease?

a. Total gastrectomy

b. Subtotal gastrectomy

c. Gastric enucleation

d. Gastrojejunostomy

15 Imatinib (Gleevec) is a chemotherapeutic targeted drug for which solid tumor?

a. Breast cancer

b. Lung cancer

c. Gastrointestinal stromal tumor (GIST)

d. Prostate cancer

16 The Philadelphia chromosome is specific to which type of cancer?

a. Chronic myelogenous leukemia (CML)

b. Acute lymphoblastic leukemia (ALL)

c. Acute myelogenous leukemia (AML)

d. Myelodysplastic syndrome (MDS)

17 The AGACNP is caring for a patient who reports that she was in her usual state of health until her last well visit when the primary care physician (PCP) stated that her labs were "abnormal." According to the office note, the patient has pancytopenia and is being admitted for a bone marrow biopsy. Results from the biopsy are consistent with a hypercellular bone marrow. Which diagnosis best fits this presentation?

a. AML

b. ALL

c. MDS

d. CML

18 The AGACNP is evaluating a patient in the oncology unit who is scared because he was told she may have leukemia. The patient shares that he was in usual state of health when, this a.m., celebrating his 47th birthday at breakfast with friends, he had a really bad nose bleed, which prompted him to seek medical attention in the ED. While examining the patient in the emergency department, the lab calls you with critical values: white blood cell (WBC) 76,000, hemoglobin (HGB) 8 g/dL, platelet count (PLT) 10,000, and absolute neutrophil count (ANC) 0.7. The patient was admitted for planned bone marrow biopsy. The AGACNP suspects that the patient has acute leukemia. What would you expect to find in the bone marrow biopsy?

a. Hypercellular bone marrow

b. Normal bone marrow

c. Hypercellular bone marrow that is dominated by blast cells

d. Fragmented marrow

19 A 19-year-old male who is home for college on Christmas break but needs a physical examination completed in order to play on the college soccer team. He reports being in his usual state of health but notices that he has had drenching night sweats over the last month but states his roommate was sick and it may have been a cold. At the time of the evaluation, vitals are normal, but on physical examination, painless lymphadenopathy is palpated in the neck and axilla as he is not showing any nonverbal cues of pain. Based on his presentation, which disease should be included in your differential diagnosis?

a. Mononucleosis

b. Lymphoma

c. Thyroglossal duct cyst

d. Upper respiratory infection

20 A 19-year-old male underwent a lymph node biopsy and is following up with you for the results. Prior to the appointment, the AGANCP reviews the pathology report, which notes the presence of Reed–Sternberg cells in an appropriate reactive cellular background. After reading the report, the AGACNP suspects he has which disease?

a. Non-Hodgkin lymphoma

b. Hodgkin lymphoma

c. Acute leukemia

d. MDS

21 At the time of diagnosis or initiation of chemotherapy, patients may develop life-threatening metabolic abnormalities that warrant immediate intervention. The AGACNP knows that which of the following are oncologic emergencies?

a. Tumor lysis syndrome (TLS), hypercalcemia, spinal cord compression, disseminated intravascular coagulopathy (DIC), and hyponatremia

b. TLS, hypercalcemia, spinal cord compression, DIC, and hypernatremia

c. TLS, hypocalcemia, spinal cord compression, DIC, and hyponatremia

d. TLS, hypocalcemia, spinal cord compression, DIC, and hypernatremia

22 Oncologic emergencies are never associated with the onset of chemotherapy or radiation therapy. Is the statement true or false?

a. False. Oncologic emergencies can occur at any time.

b. True. Oncologic emergencies are never associated with the onset of chemotherapy or radiation therapy.

c. True. Oncologic emergencies are never associated with the onset of chemotherapy, radiation therapy, or proton therapy.

23 The AGACNP is caring for a patient with ALL on the oncology unit who presented to the emergency department with seizures. Admission labs were drawn, and the lab calls with the following critical values: blood urea nitrogen (BUN) 30, creatinine level 2.1, phosphorus level 6, and calcium level 6.5. The AGACNP is most concerned that the patient is most likely experiencing which oncologic emergency?

a. Hypercalcemia

b. Spinal cord compression

c. TLS

d. DIC

24 Medical modalities to treat TLS may include all of the following EXCEPT:

a. Allopurinol

b. Rasburicase

c. Calcium gluconate

25 The AGACNP is caring for a patient on the oncology unit who is postoperative Day 1 from right breast radical mastectomy for recent diagnosis of metastatic breast cancer to bone. The nurse on rounds report that the patient has been more lethargic, confused, and persistently nauseated. The lab calls with a critical value: calcium 14, albumin 4, PTH 11 pg/mL, and creatinine level 1.8. All of the interventions below may treat severe hypercalcemia secondary to malignancy EXCEPT:

a. Zoledronic acid and pamidronate

b. Aggressive hydration with normal saline

c. Parathyroidectomy

d. Denosumab

26 The AGACNP is developing a management plan for the patient with severe hypercalemia with calcium 14, albumin 4, PTH 11 pg/mL, and creatinine level 1.8. Based on the labs available, which medication would be used cautiously?

a. Zoledronic acid and pamidronate

b. Aggressive hydration with normal saline

c. Parathyroidectomy

d. Denosumab

27 A patient presents to the unit with PMH significant for prostate cancer and new onset of bowel/bladder incontinence and left lower extremity weakness. The AGACNP suspects that the patient has a malignant cord compression and orders corticosteroids to reduce swelling. What change in clinical condition would warrant a stat neurosurgery consult for surgical intervention?

a. Known primary tumor

b. Positive response to radiation therapy

c. No compression of intraspinal bony fragments

d. Paraplegia less than 48 hours

28 A patient with which of the following tumors would be more predisposed to develop hyponatremia secondary to syndrome of inappropriate antidiuretic hormone secretion (SIADH)?

a. Lung cancer

b. Melanoma

c. Leukemia

d. Pancreatic cancer

29 Which drug is often used in the initial treatment of malignant cord compression?

a. Vasopressin

b. Ketorolac

c. Prednisone

d. Dexamethasone

30 The AGACNP is caring for a patient with acute promyelocytic leukemia who presented to the floor with severe bleeding. When examining the labs, the AGACNP suspects that the patient is developing DIC. If this was DIC, which statement below would be true?

a. High platelet, low fibrinogen level, decreased prothrombin time (PT), and activated partial thromboplastin time (aPTT)

b. Low platelet, low fibrinogen level, increased PT, and aPTT

c. Low platelet, low fibrinogen level, decreased PT, and aPTT

d. High platelet, high fibrinogen level, increased PT, and aPTT

Disease Answers/Rationales

1 The correct answer is E.

Rationales:

a. Breast—Listed as one of the top five cancer sites.

b. Lung—Listed as one of the top five cancer sites.

c. Prostate—Listed as one of the top five cancer sites.

d. Colon and rectum—Listed as one of the top five cancer sites.

e. Leukemia is correct. According to the SEER database, leukemia is not in the top five. Melanoma and skin cancers are the last in the top five group.

(Howlader et al., 2019).

2 The correct answer is A.

Rationales:

a. Tumor, Nodes, Metastasis—TNM stands for Tumor (name of primary tumor), Nodes (number of nearby lymph nodes that have cancer), and Metastasis (distant spread of disease). This staging system was created and is updated by the American Joint Committee on Cancer (AJCC) and the International Union Against Cancer (IUAC).

b. Timing, Nodes, Metastasis is incorrect.

c. Tissue Diagnosis, Nodes, Metastasis is incorrect.

d. Therapy, Nodes, Metastasis is incorrect.

(Edge & Compton, 2010, pp. 1471–1474).

3 The correct answer is A.

Rationales:

a. Neoadjuvant chemotherapy is administered prior to surgical resection.

b. This is an incorrect definition. Adjuvant chemotherapy is administered after surgical resection.

(Edge & Compton, 2010, pp. 1471–1474).

4 The correct answer is A.

Rationales:

a. Colorectal cancer with synchronous liver metastasis—the liver metastasis was diagnosed at the same time as the primary tumor, making it synchronous. If the liver metastasis were identified after surgery resection at interval follow-up visit, the metastasis would be metachronous.

b. Colorectal cancer with metachronous liver metastasis is incorrect.

(Edge & Compton, 2010, pp. 1471–1474).

5 **The correct answer is A.**

Rationales:

a. Before we can develop a treatment plan, we will have to identify the tumor, stage the tumor using the TNM classification, and then treat the tumor with possibly chemotherapy, radiation therapy, surgical resection, or a combination of all three. In order to develop a treatment plan, the steps would involve the ability to name the primary tumor, stage the primary tumor, and then develop a treatment plan that is appropriate.

b. "Pancreatic masses have terrible mortality rates, so we will most likely start with surgery" is incorrect. The medical and surgical oncologist will work together to develop the treatment plan as all pancreatic masses may not be cancerous.

c. "In all solid tumors, surgery is the best chance for patient survival" is not always true. This answer does not have enough information to be an accurate statement.

(Edge & Compton, 2010, pp. 1471–1474; Howlader et al., 2019).

6 **The correct answer is D.**

Rationales:

a. Malignancy may cause a small bowel obstruction.

b. Intussusception may cause a small bowel obstruction.

c. Adhesions may cause a small bowel obstruction.

d. Gastritis is inflammation in the stomach and does not cause a small bowel obstruction.

(Cornett et al., 2019).

7 **The correct answer is A.**

Rationales:

a. CEA is a tumor marker for colon cancers.

b. CA19-9 is a tumor marker for pancreatic cancers.

c. BRAC1 is a genetic mutation in breast cancers.

d. AFP is a tumor marker for hepatocellular cancers.

(Cornett et al., 2019).

Clinical Pearl

The most likely etiology of iron deficiency anemia is bleeding, unless proven otherwise.

8 **The correct answer is B.**

Rationales:

a. PSA—breast cancer is incorrect as PSA is used to aid in the diagnosis of prostate cancer.

b. AFP—hepatocellular carcinoma is correct.

c. CEA—prostate cancer is incorrect as CEA is used to aid in the diagnosis of colon cancer.

d. BRAC1—thyroid cancer is incorrect as BRAC1 is used to identify women who are high risk for breast cancer.

(Cornett et al., 2019).

9 **The correct answer is B.**

Rationales:

a. CEA is used to aid in the diagnosis of colon cancer.

b. CA19-9 is used to aid in the diagnosis of pancreatic cancer.

c. BRAC1 is used to identify women who are high risk for breast cancer.

d. AFP is used to aid in the diagnosis of hepatocellular carcinoma.

(Cornett et al., 2019).

10 **The correct answer is D.**

Rationales:

a. Breast cancer does not present as vocal paralysis.

b. Prostate cancer does not present as vocal cord paralysis.

c. Colorectal cancer does not present as vocal cord paralysis.

d. NSCLC can present with vocal cord paralysis.

(Seyed Toutounchi, Eydi, Golzari, Ghaffari, & Parvizian, 2014, pp. 47–50).

11 **The correct answer is B.**

Rationales:

a. Hepatocellular carcinoma is not the appropriate term to describe biliary cancer.

b. Cholangiocarcinoma is the term used to describe biliary cancer. In order to develop a treatment plan, the steps would involve the ability to name the primary tumor, stage the primary tumor, and then develop a treatment plan that is appropriate.

c. Pancreatic cancer is incorrect. Patient has cancer cells in the biliary ducts.

d. Ovarian cancer is incorrect. The patient does not have cancer in the ovaries.

(Cornett et al., 2019).

12 **The correct answer is A.**

Rationales:

a. Endoscopic retrograde or percutaneous transhepatic cholangiography with biopsy is the most appropriate diagnostic test.

b. Endoscopic CT with fine needle aspiration of tumor is incorrect. CT scans are not endoscopic.

c. EKG is not helpful with the diagnosis.

(Cornett et al., 2019).

13 **The correct answer is D.**

Rationales:

a. TACE is a palliative option.

b. RFA is a palliative option.

c. Microwave ablation is a palliative option.

d. "None of the above" is correct. All of the options listed are palliative options and NOT curative.

(Cornett et al., 2019).

14 **The correct answer is B.**

Rationales:

a. Total gastrectomy is not indicated as the patient has distal disease.

b. Subtotal gastrectomy is preferred in gastric tumors that are located in the distal two thirds of the stomach.

c. Gastric enucleation is not appropriate.

d. Gastrojejunostomy may be indicated if there is additional extensive disease, but the clinical case does not provide enough detail to suggest a bypass surgery is indicated.

(Cornett et al., 2019).

Clinical Pearl

Advanced vitamin B12 deficiency can lead to significant neurological symptoms, including paresthesias, gait dysfunction, and proprioception difficulties.

15 **The correct answer is C.**

Rationales:

a. Breast cancer is incorrect as imatinib is not targeted therapy for this disease.

b. Lung cancer is incorrect as imatinib is not targeted therapy for this disease.

c. Gastrointestinal stomal tumor is correct as imatinib is target therapy in the treatment of GISTs.

d. Prostate cancer is incorrect as imatinib is not targeted therapy for this disease.

(Cornett et al., 2019).

16 **The correct answer is A.**

Rationales:

a. CML—The Philadelphia chromosome is only seen in chronic myeloid leukemia.

b. ALL is not associated with the Philadelphia chromosome.

c. AML is not associated with the Philadelphia chromosome.

d. MDS is not associated with the Philadelphia chromosome.

(Damon & Babis Andreadis, 2019).

17 **The correct answer is C.**

Rationales:

a. AML typically presents with cytopenias but no hypercellular bone marrow.

b. ALL typically presents with cytopenias and hypercellular bone marrow that is dominated by blast cells.

c. MDS typically presents with cytopenias and hypercellular bone marrow.

d. CML typically presents with cytopenias but no hypercellular bone marrow.

(Damon & Babis Andreadis, 2019).

18 **The correct answer is C.**

Rationales:

a. Hypercellular bone marrow is not specific enough to answer the question.

b. Normal bone marrow is incorrect.

c. Hypercellular bone marrow that is dominated by blast cells.

d. Fragmented marrow is correct.

(Damon & Babis Andreadis, 2019).

19 **The correct answer is B.**

Rationales:

a. Mononucleosis is an infectious process that should be considered lower in the differential.

b. Lymphoma is a malignancy that should be suspected in an adult with painless lymphadenopathy and drenching night sweats. Answers A, C, and D are related to an infectious process but are least likely in this clinical scenario.

c. Thyroglossal duct cyst does not typically present as the clinical case above.

d. Upper respiratory infection does not present as the clinical case above.

(Damon & Babis Andreadis, 2019).

20 **The correct answer is B.**

Rationales:

a. Non-Hodgkin lymphoma will not have Reed-Sternberg cells on pathology.

b. Hodgkin lymphoma. The presence of Reed–Sternberg cells in an appropriate reactive cellular background distinguishes Hodgkin lymphoma from the other liquid tumors.

c. Acute leukemia will not have Reed–Sternberg cells noted on the pathology report.

d. MDS will not have Sternberg cells noted on the pathology report.

(Damon & Babis Andreadis, 2019).

21 **The correct answer is A.**

Rationales:

a. TLS, hypercalcemia, spinal cord compression, DIC, and hyponatremia are all life-threatening oncologic emergencies that require the practitioner to have knowledge of the disease process and treatments.

b. TLS, hypercalcemia, spinal cord compression, DIC, and hypernatremia are an incomplete list of all of the oncologic emergencies listed above. Hypernatremia is not usually present, but rather hyponatremia.

c. TLS, hypocalcemia, spinal cord compression, DIC, and hyponatremia are an incomplete list of the options. Patients will more likely have hypercalcemia.

d. TLS, hypocalcemia, spinal cord compression, DIC, and hypernatremia are an incomplete list of the options. Patients are more likely to have hyponatremia and hypercalcemia.

(Pi et al., 2016, pp. 625–638).

> ### Clinical Pearl
>
> von Willebrand disease is the most common inherited bleeding disorder, characterized by lack of von Willebrand factor (vWF), which is essential in clot formation. Most patients (75%–80%) have type 1, which is a quantitative lack of vWF, as opposed to type 2, which is characterized as a qualitative defect in the patient's vWF.

22 **The correct answer is A.**

Rationales:

False—Oncologic emergencies can occur at any time.

(Pi et al., 2016, pp. 625–638).

23 **The correct answer is C.**

Rationales:

a. Hypercalcemia can present with seizures, but the additional lab abnormalities and comorbidities would suggest the most likely diagnosis is TLS.

b. Spinal cord compression is not present with seizures and the abnormal labs above.

c. TLS—Patients with acute leukemia are at risk of developing TLS. In this case, the patient has the laboratory tumor lysis syndrome (LTLS), which is present when two or more metabolic values are present as well as clinical signs of TLS, such as renal insufficiency, seizures, or cardiac arrhythmias.

d. DIC does not present with seizures and the abnormal lab values noted in this clinical case.

(Pi et al., 2016, pp. 625–638).

24 **The correct answer is C.**

Rationales:

a. Allopurinol is used to prevent uric acid accumulation.

b. Rasburicase removes uric acid from the bloodstream.

c. Calcium gluconate is not used in the treatment of TLS.

(Pi et al., 2016, pp. 625–638).

25 **The correct answer is C.**

Rationales:

a. Zoledronic acid and pamidronate are an appropriate intervention.

b. Aggressive hydration with normal saline is an appropriate intervention.

c. Parathyroidectomy is not an appropriate medical intervention in treating hypercalcemia secondary to malignancy.

d. Denosumab is an appropriate intervention.

(Pi et al., 2016, pp. 625–638).

26 **The correct answer is A.**

Rationales:

a. Zoledronic acid and pamidronate are cleared renally and should be used cautiously in patients with renal dysfunction.

b. Aggressive hydration with normal saline is not an appropriate answer.

c. Parathyroidectomy is not an appropriate answer.

d. Denosumab is not an appropriate answer.

(Pi et al., 2016, pp. 625–638).

27 **The correct answer is D.**

Rationales:

a. Known primary tumor is not a necessary indication for surgery.

b. Positive response to radiation therapy is not an indication for surgery.

c. "No compression of intraspinal bony fragments" is not an indication for surgery.

d. Paraplegia less than 48 hours is an indication for surgery in a malignant spinal cord compression.

(Pi et al., 2016, pp. 625–638).

28 **The correct answer is A.**

Rationales:

a. Lung cancer is often associated with hyponatremia secondary to SIADH.

b. Melanoma is a skin cancer that is not associated with hyponatremia secondary to SIADH.

c. Leukemia is not associated with hyponatremia secondary to SIADH.

d. Pancreatic cancer is not associated with hyponatremia secondary to SIADH.

(Pi et al., 2016, pp. 625–638).

Clinical Pearl

The most common inherited thrombophilic disease is factor V Leiden, characterized as a resistance to activated protein C, and should be suspected in those with idiopathic thrombosis.

29 **The correct answer is D.**

Rationales:

a. Vasopressin is not used to treat malignant spinal cord compression.

b. Ketorolac may help with symptoms of a spinal cord compression, more specifically pain, but this is not a medication used in the treatment.

c. Prednisone is a steroid, but this is not the most common steroid used in the treatment of malignant spinal cord compression.

d. Steroids are often used to treat malignant spinal cord compression. Dexamethasone (16–100 mg/d) is used to delay the onset of neurologic deficits and decrease edema.

(Pi et al., 2016, pp. 625–638).

30 **The correct answer is B.**

Rationales:

a. High platelet, low fibrinogen level, decreased PT, and aPTT is incorrect. Low platelets are expected in DIC.

b. Low platelet, low fibrinogen level, increased PT, and aPTT are noted in DIC.

c. Low platelet, low fibrinogen level, decreased PT, and aPTT is incorrect. Increased PT is expected in DIC.

d. High platelet, high fibrinogen level, increased PT, and aPTT is incorrect. Low platelets are expected in DIC.

(Pi et al., 2016, pp. 625–638).

References

Cornett, P. A., Wang, S., Friedman, L. S., Cinar, P., Dea, T. O., McQuaid, K. R., ... Ryan, C. J. (2019). Cancer. In M. A. Papadakis, S. J. McPhee, & M. W. Rabow (Eds.), *Current medical diagnosis & treatment*. New York, NY: McGraw-Hill. Retrieved August 20, 2019, from http://accessmedicine.mhmedical.com/content.aspx?bookid=2449&sectionid=194858607

Damon, L. E., & Babis Andreadis, C. (2019). Blood disorders. In: M. A. Papadakis, S. J. McPhee, & M. W. Rabow (Eds.), *Current medical diagnosis & treatment*. New York, NY: McGraw-Hill. Retrieved August 26, 2019, from http://

accessmedicine.mhmedical.com/content.aspx?bookid=2449&sectionid=194437986

Edge, S. B., & Compton, C. C. (2010). The American Joint Committee on Cancer: The 7th edition of the AJCC cancer staging manual and the future of TNM. *Annals of Surgical Oncology, 17*(6), 1471–1474.

Howlader, N., Noone, A. M., Krapcho, M., Miller, D., Brest, A., Yu, M., ... Cronin, K. A. (Eds.) (2019). *SEER Cancer Statistics Review, 1975–2016*. Bethesda, MD: National Cancer Institute. Retrieved from https://seer.cancer.gov/

csr/1975_2016/. Based on November 2018 SEER data submission, posted to the SEER web site, April 2019.

Pi, J., Kang, Y., Smith, M., Earl, M., Norigian, Z., & McBride, A. (2016). A review in the treatment of oncologic emergencies. *Journal of Oncology Pharmacy Practice, 22*(4), 625–638.

Seyed Toutounchi, S. J., Eydi, M., Golzari, S. E., Ghaffari, M. R., & Parvizian, N. (2014). Vocal cord paralysis and its etiologies: A prospective study. *Journal of Cardiovascular and Thoracic Research, 6*(1), 47–50. doi:10.5681/jcvtr.2014.009

CHAPTER 12

Multisystem Trauma and Acute Care Surgery

Elizabeth Wirth-Tomaszewski, DNP, CRNP, CCRN, ACNP-BC, ACNPC

Disease Questions

1 Which of the following patients should be triaged as the priority of care in a mass casualty incident?

a. A 43-year-old female unrestrained driver with severe respiratory distress and severe facial trauma with BP 92/70 and heart rate 130.

b. A 37-year-old male unrestrained passenger with intact neurological status and obvious deformity of his right femur with BP 112/88 and heart rate 120.

c. A 34-year-old male restrained passenger confused with head laceration with BP 80/50 and heart rate 140.

d. An 18-year-old female restrained passenger with prolonged extrication with tender abdomen, BP 92/50, and heart rate 140.

2 A leading anatomical cause of liver laceration is:

a. Ligamentous arteriosum

b. Ligament of teres (round ligament)

c. Morison pouch

d. Hepatic vein

3 A 28-year-old male presents after sustaining a fall from a ladder. Emergency medical services (EMS) reported that he was awake and alert at the scene, but has rapidly deteriorated while en route to the hospital. He is immobilized with a cervical collar and long board. His Glasgow Coma Scale (GCS) on arrival is 7 (eyes open to pain, nonverbal, withdraws to pain). Given the above information, the AGACNP suspects:

a. Subdural hemorrhage

b. Intraventricular hemorrhage

c. Intracerebral hematoma

d. Epidural hemorrhage

4 A 65-year-old male restrained driver presents with evidence for traumatic brain injury. He opens his eyes to pain, makes incomprehensible verbal responses, and localizes only. The correct calculated GCS is:

a. 5

b. 7

c. 9

d. 11

5 Battle sign is suggestive of which of the following injuries?

a. Basilar skull fracture

b. Subdural hematoma

c. Intraperitoneal hemorrhage

d. Retroperitoneal hemorrhage

6 A 31-year-old male arrives with a gunshot wound to the chest. He is conscious and alert with the following vital signs: BP 78/40, heart rate 140, and respiratory rate 22. He has bilateral breath sounds, and his heart tones are muffled. There is venous jugular distention present. This presentation is most consistent with:

a. Virchow triad

b. Murphy triad

c. Cushing triad

d. Beck triad

7 A 30-year-old female arrives to the trauma bay after being stabbed in the central midback region. She is exhibiting sensory loss on the left side of her body, below the level of the injury, with motor loss on the right side below the level of the injury. This likely represents:

a. Anterior spinal cord injury

b. Posterior spinal cord injury

c. Brown-Séquard spinal cord injury

d. Central spinal cord injury

8 Spinal shock is best characterized as:

a. Hypotension and bradycardia associated with spinal injury, due to lack of vasomotor tone

b. Hypotension and tachycardia associated with spinal injury, due to lack of vasomotor tone

c. Loss of muscle tone and reflexes associated with spinal injury, without hemodynamic instability

d. Hypertension and bradycardia associated with traumatic brain injury

9 A 23-year-old female weighing 100 kg sustains full-thickness burns on her anterior torso. Large-bore intravenous access is achieved. According the Parkland formula, what is the correct volume of fluid to be administered over the first 8 hours postburn?

a. 4,550 mL of Ringer lactate

b. 3,900 mL of normal saline

c. 5,200 mL of normal saline

d. 2,250 mL of Ringer lactate

10 Pheochromocytoma is identified in a patient, who is scheduled for a surgical resection in 2 weeks. The most appropriate preoperative preparation is:

a. Beta-blockade and salt restriction

b. Fluid restriction and alpha-adrenergic antagonists

c. Liberal fluids and salt, adding phenoxybenzamine

d. Beta-blockade and liberal fluids

11 A 56-year-old male s/p motorcycle collision presents with complaints of severe pelvic pain and has an obvious deformity of the right lower extremity. He has crepitus across the right anterior chest wall and a distended abdomen. EMS have given a total of 2 L of normal saline for a BP of 80/50, with an increase of his BP to 100/60 prehospital. On arrival, his vital signs are BP 78/40, heart rate 140, respiratory rate 30, and SpO_2 of 94% on 100% FiO_2 via nonrebreather mask. This is an example of:

a. Rapid responder

b. Transient responder

c. Nonresponder

d. Minimal responder

12 A 19-year-old female unrestrained driver presents with unstable vital signs. Her airway was secured by prehospital medics. She has crepitus over her chest bilaterally, with diminished breath sounds on the right. Her trachea is deviated to the left, and her jugular veins are distended. Her BP is 70/38 with a heart rate of 146. The AGACNP suspects:

a. Right mainstem intubation

b. Left hemothorax

c. Diaphragmatic rupture

d. Right tension pneumothorax

13 A 32-year-old female presents status post GSW to the torso. Her abdomen is tense. Her BP is 82/56, with a heart rate of 136. Her respiratory rate is 32, and she is very anxious. The AGACNP recognizes this as which class of hypovolemic shock?

a. Class I

b. Class II

c. Class III

d. Class IV

14 A 70-kg male unrestrained driver presents with a severe head laceration with copious bleeding and a left femur fracture. He is confused and hypotensive, with a pulse of 146. He has received two liters of normal saline en route. What is the best course of action?

a. Hemorrhage control with direct pressure, splinting, and continue crystalloid infusion

b. Hemorrhage control with direct pressure, splinting, and begin balanced blood transfusion

c. Hemorrhage control with tourniquets, splinting, and administration of beta agonists to control his heart rate

d. Hemorrhage control with tourniquets and continue crystalloids

15 A 76-year-old male pedestrian presents after being struck by a motor vehicle. Witnesses state he was drinking alcohol prior to walking out in front of a pickup truck. He is currently belligerent, and has obvious severe facial and extremity trauma. He is refusing evaluation, and has pulled off his cervical collar. He is unwilling or unable to follow commands and is becoming drowsy. The best plan of care for this patient includes:

a. Allowing him to sign out against medical advice

b. Allowing him to sleep to allow his alcohol level to fall and reattempt evaluation

c. Establishing a secure airway utilizing rapid sequence intubation while maintaining inline cervical spine stabilization, and replacing his collar to better evaluate him

d. Sedating him to allow for further trauma and psychiatry evaluation

16 The AGACNP is screening a 65-year-old female for an elective hernia repair. Which of the following factors increases her intraoperative cardiac risk?

a. A personal history of insulin dependence and ischemic heart disease

b. A family history of ischemic heart disease and cerebrovascular disease

c. A moderate-risk surgery in the setting of acute kidney injury (AKI)

d. A personal history of diabetes type 2 and hypertension

17 A morbidly obese 46-year-old female is 36 hours postop from an uncomplicated, open cholecystectomy. Her vitals are as follows: BP 110/60, heart rate 106, respiratory rate 22, SpO$_2$ 92% on room air, and temperature 99.6°F. She has no indwelling devices, and her incision is open to air without exudate. The AGACNP suspects:

a. Sepsis and orders antibiotics

b. Surgical wound infection and orders a culture of the site

c. Bacteremia and orders blood cultures

d. Atelectasis and orders a chest x-ray and incentive spirometry

18 A 42-year-old obese female presents with an 8-hour history of abdominal pain and nausea. The nurse practitioner orders an abdominal ultrasound. When the sonographer positions the transducer in the right upper quadrant, the patient finds it difficult to breathe. This is known as:

a. Murphy sign as small

b. Virchow triad

c. Beck triad

d. Cullen sign

19 A 22-year-old male has been diagnosed with a subdural hematoma with mass effect. According to the Monro-Kellie doctrine, his intracranial pressure (ICP) will rise due to:

a. An increase in cerebrospinal fluid volume

b. An increase in intracranial blood volume

c. A decrease in parenchymal tissue

d. A decrease in cerebrospinal fluid volume

20 A 36-year-old female unrestrained driver presents to the emergency room with multisystem trauma. The correct order of evaluation according to primary survey in advanced trauma life support would be:

a. Vital signs, airway, hemorrhage control, neurological examination

b. Vital signs, neurological examination, airway, hemorrhage control

c. Airway, hemorrhage control, neurological examination, vital signs

d. Neurological examination, airway, hemorrhage control, vital signs

21 In which of the following cases might emergent cricothyrotomy be anticipated?

a. A 24-year-old male status post gunshot wound to the upper chest in cardiac arrest

b. A 36-year-old female unrestrained driver with obvious cribriform and mandibular fractures

c. A 28-year-old male status post assault with baseball bat with rib fractures and a pneumothorax

d. A 32-year-old female with a knife stab wound to the right chest and a tension pneumothorax

22 A 56-year-old male presented with traumatic brain injury and multiple rib fractures after falling 20 ft from a ladder yesterday. His neurologic examination is unchanged with a GCS of 3. His ICP is 28 as measured by a ventriculostomy device. Currently, his mean arterial pressure (MAP) is 65. The AGACNP:

a. Identifies the MAP as sufficient for this patient to prevent end organ damage

b. Calculates a cerebral perfusion pressure (CPP) that is too high, and orders vasodilators

c. Calculates a CPP that is too low, and orders pressors to increase the MAP

d. Identifies the ICP as too high and orders vasodilators

23 A 23-year-old female helmeted motorcyclist presents to the emergency room after having driven into a fence. She is having obvious signs of respiratory distress. Signs of laryngeal trauma include:

a. Palpable fracture, subcutaneous emphysema, and hoarseness

b. Shortness of breath and diminished breath sounds

c. Chest pain and difficulty swallowing

d. Crepitus in the anterior chest wall

24 A 62-year-old restrained male passenger presents in class III hemorrhagic shock status post motor vehicle collision. The most desirable site for intravenous access is:

a. Femoral

b. Jugular

c. Antecubital fossa

d. Subclavian

25 A 26-year-old pregnant female at 30 weeks' gestation is a restrained passenger involved in a motor vehicle crash with rollover. She presents with obvious head and chest injuries and is intubated by prehospital personnel for a GCS score of seven. On arrival, her blood pressure is 86/60 with a heart rate of 126. The AGACNP recognizes that:

a. She is compensating well hemodynamically.

b. She is experiencing significant hypovolemic shock with risk to the fetus.

c. These are normal variables in pregnancy.

d. Her tachycardia is likely due to anxiety related to the safety of her baby.

26 A 72-year-old female with a history significant for diastolic heart failure is admitted status post fall with traumatic brain injury and significant cerebral edema. Her family has decided to pursue do not resuscitate (DNR) status. Vital signs were stable overnight, with no acute changes in her mental status. GCS is calculated at 3. The nurse now calls the AGACNP with an acute change in vital signs. Her blood pressure is 212/102, heart rate is 42 and sinus bradycardia, and her respirations have become irregular on a ventilator. The AGACNP recognizes this as:

a. Cushing triad and impending herniation

b. Beck triad and pericardial tamponade

c. Neurogenic shock with acute deterioration

d. Cardiogenic shock with acute decompensation

27 A pregnant 24-year-old at 28 weeks' gestation presents after a physical assault. She is complaining of abdominal pain, cramping, and vaginal bleeding. Vital signs are 126/72, heart rate 94, respiratory rate of 24, and oxygen saturation of 96% on room air. Of the following, which is the most appropriate course of treatment after physical assessment?

a. Complete blood count (CBC), basic metabolic profile (BMP), urinalysis (UA), fetal heart tones

b. CBC, BMP, urine toxicology screen, alcohol level, fetal heart tones

c. CBC, BMP, UA, coagulation studies, type and screen, fetal heart tones

d. CBC, BMP, UA, coagulation studies, fetal heart tones

28 Rovsing sign is best described as:

a. Right lower quadrant pain elicited from palpation of the left lower quadrant

b. Hypogastric pain upon internal and external rotation of the hip while supine

c. Right lower quadrant pain when the right hip is hyperextended while the knee is flexed

d. Pain elicited when the right upper quadrant is palpated

29 A 57-year-old male with history of chronic pancreatitis presents for acute abdominal pain, with nausea and vomiting. Lab data are consistent with acute on chronic pancreatitis. His physical examination is significant for ecchymosis on his left flank. This finding is most consistent with:

a. Cullen sign indicating retroperitoneal hemorrhage

b. Battle sign indicating intra-abdominal hemorrhage

c. Kehr sign indicating intra-abdominal hemorrhage

d. Grey Turner sign indicating retroperitoneal hemorrhage

30 A 54-year-old female with past medical history significant for atrial fibrillation and a mechanical aortic valve replacement on warfarin has sustained a fall. A CT scan of the brain reveals a large subdural hematoma with intraparenchymal hematoma, and her mental status has begun to deteriorate. Her family wishes full code status. The best course of action regarding the patient's anticoagulation is:

a. Continue the anticoagulation due to the patient's mechanical aortic valve.

b. Discontinue the anticoagulation and allow the INR to drift down.

c. Discontinue the anticoagulation and actively reverse with vitamin K.

d. Discontinue the anticoagulation and actively reverse with prothrombin complex concentrate or fresh frozen plasma.

Disease Answers/Rationales

1 The correct answer is A.

Rationales:

a. This patient has a high potential for airway obstruction and is exhibiting signs of shock.

b. Although this patient is tachycardic, he is compensating with a stable blood pressure.

c. The airway issue exhibited in A is a higher priority than the shock state in this patient.

d. The airway issue exhibited in A is a higher priority than the shock state in this patient.

(American College of Surgeons Committee on Trauma, 2012, pp. 339–340).

2 The correct answer is B.

Rationales:

a. The ligamentous arteriosum is the remainder of fetal structures in the heart, sometimes responsible for aortic tears.

b. The ligament of teres is often referred to as the cheese slicer of the liver, arising from a component of fetal circulation.

c. Morison pouch is an anatomical location near the liver that is assessed on FAST examination (Focused Assessment with Sonography for Trauma), which fills with blood in the setting of hemoperitoneum or liver laceration.

d. The hepatic vein can be injured but is not a major cause of injury to the liver itself.

(National Association of Emergency Medical Technicians (NAEMT), 2016, p. 69).

3 **The correct answer is D.**

Rationales:

a. A subdural hemorrhage has a predictable (if any) deterioration in mental status, depending on its chronicity.

b. Intraventricular hemorrhages are largely hypertensive in nature, and present with headaches and photophobia.

c. Intracerebral contusions tend to develop over time (hours to days) as opposed to rapid presentation.

d. The classic presentation of an epidural hemorrhage is characterized by a period of lucidity after the insult, with rapidly deteriorating or complete loss of consciousness shortly thereafter.

(American College of Surgeons Committee on Trauma, 2012, p. 156).

4 **The correct answer is C.**

Rationales:

a. This answer is incorrect based on the GCS.

b. This answer is incorrect based on the GCS.

c. Eye opening to pain is scored 2, incomprehensible sounds are scored 2, and localizing is scored 5.

d. This answer is incorrect based on the GCS.

(American College of Surgeons Committee on Trauma, 2012, p. 156).

5 **The correct answer is A.**

Rationales:

a. Battle sign is an ecchymosis behind the ear, suggesting basilar skull fracture.

b. Subdural hematomas often have no external signs, although a patient with a skull fracture may have a subdural hematoma.

c. Intraperitoneal hemorrhage may result in Cullen sign (periumbilical ecchymosis).

d. Retroperitoneal hemorrhage may result in Grey Turner sign (flank ecchymosis).

(American College of Surgeons Committee on Trauma, 2012, p. 155).

Clinical Pearl

Decreased levels of consciousness can lead to loss of airway control. If GCS less than 8 = intubate.

6 **The correct answer is D.**

Rationales:

a. Virchow triad consists of stasis, vessel injury, and hypercoagulability and relates to vascular thrombosis formation.

b. Murphy triad consists of pain, vomiting, and fever related to appendicitis.

c. Cushing triad is described as bradycardia, bradypnea, and hypertension and is a late sign associated with impending brain herniation.

d. Beck triad consists of venous distention, muffled heart tones, and hypotension and indicates pericardial tamponade, which can occur with penetrating trauma to the chest.

(American College of Surgeons Committee on Trauma, 2012, p. 101).

7 **The correct answer is C.**

Rationales:

a. Presentation of anterior cord injury is characterized by paraplegia, sensory loss, and loss of temperature and pain sensations bilaterally distal to the injury (with dorsal functions remaining intact).

b. Presentation of posterior cord injury is characterized by loss of proprioception, vibration, and deep pressure sensation bilaterally and distal to the injury.

c. Brown-Séquard spinal cord injury (SCI). Brown-Séquard is a rare phenomenon that results from hemisection of the spinal cord, resulting in sensory loss on one side of the body distal to the injury, with contralateral motor loss below the level of the injury.

d. Central cord injury presents as a greater loss of motor function in the upper extremities than that of the lower extremities, with varying degrees of sensory loss.

(American College of Surgeons Committee on Trauma, 2012, p. 181).

8 **The correct answer is C.**

Rationales:

a. This answer refers to neurogenic shock associated with cervical or upper thoracic spinal cord injuries (as opposed to intracranial injuries, which do not cause neurogenic shock).

b. This answer describes hemorrhagic shock associated with additional injuries in the setting of a SCI. Loss of vasomotor tone would not cause tachycardia.

c. Spinal shock is defined as loss of motor and sensory function after SCI.

d. Hypertension and bradycardia are associated with increased ICP and impending herniation in the setting of traumatic brain injury.

(American College of Surgeons Committee on Trauma, 2012, pp. 179–180).

9 **The correct answer is D.**

Rationales:

a. Total fluids for 24 hours based on 3.5 mL/kg with 13% BSA.

b. Total fluids for 24 hours based on 3 mL/kg with 13% BSA.

c. Total fluids for 24 hours based on 4 mL/kg with 13% BSA.

d. Fluids for first 8 hours based on 3.5 mL/kg with 13% BSA, half of which is infused in the first 8 hours.

(Doherty, 2015, pp. 230–231).

10 **The correct answer is C.**

Rationales:

a. Beta-blockade will provide some symptom mitigation, but not the alpha stimulation. Salt restriction will make fluid retention more difficult.

b. Hypovolemia occurs as a result of increased catecholamines, and fluid restriction would worsen the deficit.

c. Pheochromocytomas cause excessive catecholamine release, which depletes fluid volumes and can cause cardiomyopathies. This must be mitigated by using alpha-adrenergic antagonists (phenoxybenzamine preferred) and fluid volumes restoration preoperatively, as manipulation of the tumor can cause hypertensive crisis intraoperatively.

d. Beta antagonists will not mitigate the catecholamine release.

(Doherty, 2015, p. 789).

Clinical Pearl

If cervical spine injury is a possibility, maintaining immobilization is paramount during intubation, which requires inline traction by a team member whose only responsibility is ensuring that immobilization.

11 **The correct answer is B.**

Rationales:

a. A rapid responder is one who maintains hemodynamic stability after a fluid bolus.

b. A transient responder initially responds but then becomes hypotensive once again.

c. A nonresponder does not respond to fluid resuscitation and likely requires damage control/exploratory laparotomy.

d. A minimal responder responds only minimally to fluids, and is treated like a nonresponder.

(American College of Surgeons Committee on Trauma, 2012, pp. 73–74).

d. Class IV shock is characterized by hypotension, heart rate greater than 140, respiratory rate greater than 35, and confusion or lethargy.

(American College of Surgeons Committee on Trauma, 2012, pp. 69–70).

12 **The correct answer is D.**

Rationales:

a. A right mainstem intubation would yield diminished breath sounds on the left, and unlikely would cause tracheal deviation or jugular vein distention.

b. Left hemothorax would produce diminished breath sounds on the left and dull percussion. Due to hypovolemia, jugular vein distention would not likely occur.

c. Diaphragmatic rupture would not cause tracheal deviation.

d. Tension pneumothorax is characterized by absent or hyperresonance on the affected side, with tracheal deviation to the contralateral side. Due to increased intrathoracic pressure and decreased venous return, tension pneumothorax will produce jugular venous distention and signs of shock.

(Klingensmith, Aziz, Bharat, Fox, & Porembka, 2012, p. 499).

13 **The correct answer is C.**

Rationales:

a. Class I shock is characterized by a normal blood pressure, heart rate less than 100, and respiratory rate 14–20. Patients may be slightly anxious.

b. Class II shock is characterized by compensated BP, pulse rate 100–120, and respiratory rate 20–30. Patients will be mildly anxious.

c. Class III shock is characterized by hypotension, heart rate 120–140, respiratory rate 30–40, and anxiousness or confusion.

14 **The correct answer is B.**

Rationales:

a. While hemorrhage control is indicated, he has received adequate crystalloid. Balanced blood transfusions should be considered for class IV hemorrhagic shock.

b. He is exhibiting class IV hemorrhagic shock. Hemorrhage control and balanced blood transfusion are indicated, as he has received an adequate fluid bolus prehospital.

c. Tourniquets are not indicated for hemorrhage control in this patient, and beta-blockers will worsen his shock state.

d. Tourniquets are not indicated for hemorrhage control in this patient, and his femur fracture should be splinted for control. He has had adequate crystalloid resuscitation. Balanced blood transfusions should be considered.

(American College of Surgeons Committee on Trauma, 2012, pp. 69–70).

15 **The correct answer is C.**

Rationales:

a. This patient has an obvious head injury and is likely intoxicated. He lacks capacity to sign out against medical advice due to his declining mental status.

b. This patient requires immediate evaluation for possible closed head injuries, hypoxia, or cervical spine injuries. His mental status limits his ability to protect himself or sense injuries, and is declining.

c. This patient may have life-threatening injuries that require immediate evaluation. His mental status may be declining due to intoxicants or hypoxia, and his examination may be rendered unreliable. By intubating the patient, his airway is secured and a thorough assessment can be performed safely.

d. This patient is exhibiting signs of intoxicants and/or hypoxia in the setting of a head injury with declining mental status. Sedation should be avoided.

(American College of Surgeons Committee on Trauma, 2012, p. 33).

Clinical Pearl

The primary survey is composed of Airway, Breathing, Circulation, Disability, and Environment. Life-threatening injuries and conditions should be identified during the primary survey.

---

16 **The correct answer is A.**

Rationales:

a. Risk factors associated with increased cardiac risk according to the Revised Cardiac Risk Index (RCRI) include insulin therapy for diabetes and ischemic heart disease. These two factors increase her risk by 0.9%.

b. Family history does not factor into RCRI.

c. Although a serum creatinine will increase her risk, a moderate surgery does not. Her risk would be calculated at 0.4%.

d. Diabetes without insulin use and hypertension do not factor into RCRI.

(Klingensmith et al., 2012, pp. 5–6).

17 **The correct answer is D.**

Rationales:

a. There is no indication that the patient has a urinary tract infection. Antibiotics would not be recommended without culture data.

b. Surgical wound infection is not likely at 36 hours. There is no indication that there is an issue with the site.

c. Bacteremia would be unlikely at 36 hours.

d. Atelectasis is a common complication in the first 48 hours, and is especially prevalent in those who are obese and those who have had abdominal surgery.

(Klingensmith et al., 2012, pp. 53–54).

18 **The correct answer is A.**

Rationales:

a. Murphy sign is elicited by palpation of the right upper quadrant and arrests breathing. This is an example of a radiographic Murphy sign.

b. Virchow triad describes stasis, vascular injury, and hypercoagulability that are related to deep vein thrombosis.

c. Beck triad describes jugular venous distention, muffled alternatives, and hypertension related to pericardial tamponade.

d. Cullen sign is periumbilical ecchymosis related to intraperitoneal hemorrhage.

(Doherty, 2015, p. 490).

19 **The correct answer is B.**

Rationales:

a. Cerebrospinal fluid volume is expected to decrease to compensate for the increased volume occupied by the hematoma.

b. The Monro-Kellie doctrine dictates that the intracranial space is fixed, and the three components (brain parenchyma, cerebrospinal fluid volume, blood volume) within it must compensate for one another, or increased ICP will result. In this case, the increase is occupied by blood volume in the form of a subdural hematoma.

c. There is no decrease in parenchymal brain tissue.

d. Although the volume of cerebrospinal fluid may decrease to compensate for increased pressure, this will not result in increased ICP.

(Doherty, 2015, p. 871).

20 **The correct answer is C.**

Rationales:

a. Although important, vital signs are to be performed between the primary and secondary surveys. The order of evaluation in the primary survey should be airway, followed by breathing, circulation and hemorrhage control, neurologic disability, and exposure/environment.

b. Although important, vital signs are to be performed between the primary and secondary surveys. The order of evaluation in the primary survey should be airway, followed by breathing, circulation and hemorrhage control, neurologic disability, and exposure/environment.

c. The order of evaluation in the primary survey should be airway, followed by breathing, circulation and hemorrhage control, neurologic disability, and exposure/environment.

d. Although some elements of the neurological examination might be observed upon arrival, detailed neurological evaluation should be performed later in the primary survey. The order of evaluation in the primary survey should be airway, followed by breathing, circulation and hemorrhage control, neurologic disability, and exposure/environment.

(Doherty, 2015, pp. 194–198).

Clinical Pearl

The secondary survey involved a head-to-toe assessment for injuries not identified on the primary survey. This is followed by a tertiary survey conducted once the evaluation is complete, to identify any injuries missed due to distraction or alteration in mental status.

---

21 **The correct answer is B.**

Rationales:

a. This patient would likely require an emergency thoracotomy.

b. Given the extent of facial injuries, this patient may require emergency cricothyrotomy due to inaccessibility or obstruction of the upper airway.

c. This patient would likely require a tube thoracostomy.

d. This patient would require a needle decompression or emergent tube thoracostomy.

(Doherty, 2015, pp. 194–198).

22 **The correct answer is C.**

Rationales:

a. Although the MAP is sufficient for other organs, we have a direct measurement of the ICP. When calculating the CPP by subtracting the ICP from the MAP, the CPP is low at 37 mm Hg. Either the ICP must be lowered or the MAP must be increased to elevate the CPP to at least 70 mm Hg.

b. Vasodilators would further decrease the blood pressure, and possibly increase the ICP by vasodilator vessels within the intracranial compartment.

c. Vasopressors would increase the MAP, allowing for higher ICPs to prevail without sacrificing this cerebral perfusion pressure. Conversely, one could utilize measures to attempt to decrease the ICP such as using sedation, opening the ventriculostomy to relieve cerebrospinal fluid, or osmotic measures to reduce cerebral swelling.

d. Although the ICP is too high, vasodilators may increase the ICP by dilating vessels within the intracranial compartment and dropping systemic blood pressure.

(Doherty, 2015, p. 871).

23 **The correct answer is A.**

Rationales:

a. The presence of a palpable fracture, subcutaneous emphysema, and hoarseness are all signs of possible laryngeal trauma.

b. Shortness of breath and diminished breath sounds are nonspecific, and could be attributed to multiple conditions.

c. Chest pain and difficulty swallowing may indicate esophageal obstruction or caustic ingestion, however not typical of laryngeal trauma.

d. Crepitus in the anterior chest wall is likely related to a pneumothorax, as opposed to an upper airway injury.

(American College of Surgeons Committee on Trauma, 2012, p. 33).

24 **The correct answer is C.**

Rationales:

a. The femoral vein is acceptable but is not favored.

b. The jugular vein is relatively inaccessible in most trauma patients to cervical spine immobilization.

c. Short, large, or peripheral lines in the antecubital fossa are favored strongly in trauma patients. This is due to Poiseuille law, which states the rate of flow is proportional to the fourth power the radius of the cannula and inversely related to the length.

d. Subclavian lines carry a significant risk of pneumothorax and arterial cannulation.

(American College of Surgeons Committee on Trauma, 2012, p. 71).

25 **The correct answer is B.**

Rationales:

a. Although she is maintaining what appears to be a sufficient MAP, her vital signs are significant due to increased intravascular volume present in pregnant patients.

b. Pregnant patients will lose significant amounts of blood before heart rate and blood pressure are affected due to the increased intravascular volume associated with pregnancy. Once hypotension and tachycardia are present, the fetus has likely experienced distress due to lack of perfusion. Fetal distress or demise can occur despite absence of catastrophic maternal injury.

c. Although blood pressure tends to fall 5–15 mm Hg in the second trimester, and heart rate increases gradually by 10–15 beats/min, the patient's vital signs exceed these normal parameters.

d. Tachycardia is likely related to hypovolemia. Her prevailing head injury and altered mental status require intubation.

(American College of Surgeons Committee on Trauma, 2012, pp. 290–292).

Clinical Pearl

If a patient deteriorates during a trauma evaluation, the provider should begin again with a primary survey to ascertain if there has been a change in the patient's condition (e.g., a tension pneumothorax).

26 **The correct answer is A.**

Rationales:

a. Cushing triad is characterized by bradycardia, hypertension, and irregular respirations. It is a sign of impending herniation, which would be consistent in this patient's clinical presentation.

b. Beck triad is characterized by muffled heart tones, hypotension, and tachycardia related to pericardial tamponade. This patient's clinical presentation is not consistent with pericardial tamponade.

c. Neurogenic shock is characterized by hypotension and bradycardia. This patient's clinical presentation is not consistent with neurogenic shock.

d. Cardiogenic shock is characterized by hypotension. This patient's clinical presentation is not consistent with cardiogenic shock.

(Doherty, 2015, p. 867).

27 **The correct answer is C.**

Rationales:

a. Although all of these are important, the type and screen is essential in a pregnant patient with vaginal bleeding.

b. The alcohol level and toxicology screen are standard in most trauma patients. Although the others are important, the type and screen is essential in a pregnant patient with vaginal bleeding.

c. This answer provides the most comprehensive evaluation for a pregnant trauma patient experiencing vaginal bleeding, including hemoglobin, platelets, and coagulation profile. The type and screen is essential to determine if the mother is Rh negative. Immunoglobulin should be administered in cases where the mother is Rh negative.

d. Although all of these are important, the type and screen is essential in a pregnant patient with vaginal bleeding.

(American College of Surgeons Committee on Trauma, 2012, p. 294).

28 **The correct answer is A.**

Rationales:

a. This best describes the Rovsing sign, a sign of appendicitis.

b. This best describes the obturator sign, a sign of appendicitis.

c. This best describes the iliopsoas sign, a sign of appendicitis.

d. This best describes the Murphy sign, a sign of cholecystitis.

(Klingensmith et al., 2012, pp. 283–284).

29 **The correct answer is D.**

Rationales:

a. Cullen sign is characterized by periumbilical ecchymosis, and is associated with severe pancreatitis.

b. Battle sign is characterized by retroauricular ecchymosis, and is associated with basilar skull fractures.

c. Kehr sign is left upper quadrant pain referred to the left shoulder. This is largely associated with splenic ruptures.

d. Grey Turner is flank ecchymosis, and is associated with severe pancreatitis with hemorrhage.

(Klingensmith et al., 2012, p. 325).

30 **The correct answer is D.**

Rationales:

a. Continuing her anticoagulation will likely worsen her bleeding, and could likely be life threatening. The risk of bleeding must be mitigated with the risk of thrombosis related to her atrial fibrillation mechanical valve, requiring an honest conversation with the family and the patient.

b. Discontinuing the anticoagulation is necessary to prevent further bleeding; however, her coagulopathy may actively contribute to the deterioration of her mental status related to her intracranial hemorrhage if active reversal is not employed.

c. Discontinuing the anticoagulation is necessary to prevent further bleeding; however, vitamin K takes 1–2 days to reverse anticoagulation related to warfarin. This may not mitigate her deterioration in status quickly enough, and her intracranial hemorrhage may continue to worsen.

d. Discontinuing the anticoagulation is necessary to prevent further bleeding, and active reversal of her anticoagulation is necessary to prevent further worsening of her intracranial hemorrhage.

(Klingensmith et al., 2012, p. 141).

References

American College of Surgeons Committee on Trauma. (2012). *ATLS student course manual* (9th ed.). Chicago, IL: American College of Surgeons.

Doherty, G. M. (2015). *Current diagnosis and treatment: Surgery* (14th ed.). New York, NY: McGraw Hill.

Klingensmith, M. E., Aziz, A., Bharat, A., Fox, A. C., & Porembka, M. R. (2012). *Washington manual of surgery* (6th ed.). Philadelphia, PA: Wolters Kluwer.

National Association of Emergency Medical Technicians (NAEMT). (2016). *PHTLS: Prehospital trauma life support* (8th ed.). Burlington, MA: Jones and Bartlett.

CHAPTER 13

Critical Care

Anne Dabrow Woods, DNP, RN, CRNP, ANP-BC, AGACNP-BC, FAAN and
Elizabeth Wirth-Tomaszewski, DNP, CRNP, CCRN, ACNP-BC, ACNPC

Disease Questions

1 In hypovolemic shock, which hemodynamic parameter is correct?

   a. Central venous pressure (CVP) is low.

   b. Systemic vascular resistance (SVR) is low.

   c. Cardiac output is high.

   d. Mixed venous oxygen saturation (SvO_2) is high.

2 In cardiogenic shock, which hemodynamic parameter is correct?

   a. CVP is low.

   b. SVR is low.

   c. Cardiac output is low.

   d. SvO_2 is high.

3 In distributive shock, which hemodynamic parameter is correct?

   a. CVP is high.

   b. SVR is low.

   c. Cardiac output is low.

   d. SvO_2 is low.

4 In obstructive shock due to pulmonary embolism, which hemodynamic parameter is correct?

   a. CVP is high.

   b. SVR is low.

   c. Cardiac output is high.

   d. SvO_2 is high.

5 The pressure the left ventricle has to overcome to eject its contents is the definition of which hemodynamic parameter?

a. Preload

b. Stroke volume

c. Afterload

d. Pulmonary capillary wedge pressure

6 The venous return to the heart or stretch of the right ventricle is the definition of which hemodynamic parameter?

a. Pulmonary capillary wedge pressure

b. Stroke volume

c. Afterload

d. Preload

7 A patient is in shock and presents with these hemodynamic parameters: CO 8.6, CI 4.8, SVR 400, and CVP 0 mm Hg. What type of shock is the patient experiencing?

a. Cardiogenic

b. Obstructive

c. Distributive

d. Hypovolemic

8 A patient is in shock and presents with these hemodynamic parameters: CO 3.8 L/min, CI 1.9 L/min/m^2, SVR 2,000 dynes/seconds/cm^{-5}, CVP 0 mm Hg. What type of shock is the patient experiencing?

a. Cardiogenic

b. Obstructive

c. Distributive

d. Hypovolemic

9 A patient is in shock and needs to be placed on vasopressor support. Which vasopressor is an alpha agonist only and does not affect heart rate?

a. Norepinephrine

b. Epinephrine

c. Nicardipine

d. Phenylephrine

10 A 78-year-old patient presents with a 2-day history of fever of 102°F, chills, and nausea. This morning the patient is confused and oriented only to his name. The patient was brought to the emergency department and was found to have the following vital signs: BP 70/42 mm Hg, heart rate 110 bpm, respiratory rate 24/min, and SpO$_2$ 92%. Blood cultures, urine culture, complete blood count (CBC), chemistry, and lactate were ordered. What is the next best intervention for this patient?

a. Start norepinephrine at 4 µg/min.

b. Start dobutamine at 2 µg/min.

c. Start 30 mL/kg of crystalloid fluid resuscitation bolus.

d. Administer 500 mL of 5% albumin.

11 A patient has cardiomyopathy and an ejection fraction of 10% and requires an inotropic agent. His vital signs are BP 98/54 mm Hg, heart rate of 70 bpm, and respiratory rate of 20/min. Which inotropic agent would be best suited for the patient?

a. Dopamine

b. Dobutamine

c. Milrinone

d. Epinephrine

12 A patient is in cardiogenic shock, and his blood pressure is now 110/72 mm Hg and his CVP is 18 mm Hg. Which medication would work best to decrease the CVP pressure?

a. Phenylephrine

b. Nitroglycerin

c. Metoprolol

d. Diltiazem

13 In distributive shock secondary to sepsis, what hemodynamic effect does the inflammatory mediator release cause to occur?

a. Massive vasoconstriction of the vascular bed and decrease in cardiac output

b. Massive anticoagulation with increased risk of bleeding

c. Massive increase in the SVR and preload

d. Vasodilation of the vascular bed causing a decrease in SVR

14 A patient is being treated for septic shock and remains hypotensive despite 30 mL/kg of crystalloids. What would be the next best course of action for this patient?

a. Administer a vasopressin infusion.

b. Administer a norepinephrine infusion.

c. Administer a milrinone infusion.

d. Start stress-dose steroids.

15 A patient is in septic shock secondary to community-acquired pneumonia. He was intubated and placed on the ventilator for airway and breathing support 4 days ago. He is on propofol and fentanyl for sedation and comfort. He has developed oliguria, a creatinine of 5.6 mg/dL (from 2 mg/dL), CPK of 10,000, elevated liver function tests, triglyceride level of 1,500, and

a metabolic acidosis. What is the best immediate intervention?

a. Start a furosemide infusion.

b. Administer 5% dextrose with 150 mEq of sodium bicarbonate.

c. Stop the propofol, start an isotonic crystalloid, and consult nephrology.

d. Start fenofibrate.

16 A patient exhibits multiple Kerley B lines on his chest x-ray. The adult-gerontology acute care nurse practitioner (AGACNP) knows that this finding is indicative of which diagnosis?

a. Pneumonia

b. Pneumothorax

c. Pulmonary edema

d. Pleural effusion

17 A patient is admitted with anaphylactic shock and has a blood pressure of 70/50 mm Hg and continues to have severe wheezing. Which vasopressor is preferred in this situation?

a. Norepinephrine

b. Epinephrine

c. Dobutamine

d. Dopamine

18 A patient is experiencing a blood pressure of 82/60 mm Hg and a heart rate of 50 bpm despite receiving 30 mL/kg of crystalloids. Which vasopressor would be most appropriate in this situation to increase both the blood pressure and the heart rate?

a. Dopamine at 5 µg/kg/min

b. Dobutamine at 10 µg/kg/min

c. Milrinone at 0.375 µg/kg/min

d. Nitroglycerin at 20 µg/min

19 A patient is admitted with septic shock and has received 30 mL/kg of crystalloids and is on 15 µg/min of norepinephrine and vasopressin at 0.03 units/min and was hemodynamically stable. You are called to his room because suddenly his blood pressure dropped from 100/68 to 68/40 mm Hg and his CVP has now dropped from 10 to 2 mm Hg. He is now complaining of abdominal pain and nausea. What would be the next best intervention?

a. Stat CBC, type and screen, and give the patient a crystalloid fluid bolus.

b. Stat chemistry and give the patient a crystalloid fluid bolus.

c. Stat troponin and give the patient a crystalloid fluid bolus.

d. Stat lactate and give the patient a crystalloid fluid bolus.

20 A patient with a history of UGI bleed received 1 unit of packed red blood cells (PRBCs) yesterday, and his hemoglobin increased from 7 to 7.9 mg/dL. This morning his hemoglobin is 7.6 mg/dL. The patient shows no active signs of bleeding, and he is hemodynamically stable. What is the next best intervention?

a. Transfuse 2 units of PRBCs.

b. Transfuse 2 units of fresh frozen plasma (FFP).

c. Check the hemoglobin and hematocrit in the a.m.

d. Check the hemoglobin and hematocrit in 72 hours.

21 A patient is in septic shock and has received 30 mL/kg of crystalloids as a bolus and has been started on a norepinephrine infusion, and it is now at 20 µg/min. His hemodynamics are CO 8.2, CI 4.2, CVP 8, and SVR 500. What would be the next best course of action?

a. Administer 500 mL of 5% albumin.

b. Start a vasopressin infusion.

c. Start a dobutamine infusion.

d. Start a milrinone infusion.

22 The AGACNP is called to the room of a 56-year-old patient who was admitted 8 hours ago after vomiting 500 mL of dark red blood at home. The patient was placed on a pantoprazole infusion and is scheduled for an endoscopy tomorrow. The patient vomited 1,000 mL of bright red blood twice in the past 15 minutes and is diaphoretic, and his blood pressure is 70/50 mm Hg. He is ordered a 1,000-mL bolus of LR, a stat CBC and a transfusion of 2 units of PRBCs. What would be the next best course of action?

a. Give him another bolus of pantoprazole.

b. Give him a bolus of octreotide and start him on an infusion.

c. Give him 4 units of FFP.

d. Start him on a norepinephrine infusion.

23 What is vasopressin's mechanism of action?

a. Stimulates the alpha receptors

b. Stimulates the beta 1 and beta 2 receptors

c. Stimulates the release of nitric oxide in the endothelium

d. Regulates the kidney reabsorption of water, regulates smooth muscle vascular tone, and modulates brainstem autonomic function

24 The AGACNP is admitting a patient who has a C-spine fracture after a diving accident. What type of shock describes the hemodynamic changes of hypotension, bradycardia, low CVP, and low SVR due to the disruption of autonomic pathways?

a. Hypovolemic shock

b. Neurogenic shock

c. Spinal shock

d. Cardiogenic shock

25 A 62-year-old man describes having sudden chest pain with a tearing and ripping sensation and pain in his chest and back. He becomes hypertensive with a blood pressure of 200/120 mm Hg. What would the most likely diagnosis be for this patient?

a. Acute myocardial infarction

b. Acute peptic ulcer perforation

c. Acute aortic dissection

d. Acute pancreatitis

26 A patient presents after a syncopal episode and has a blood pressure of 72/48 mm Hg. He describes having symptoms of anorexia, nausea, vomiting, weight loss, weakness, fatigue, and orthostatic hypotension for the past month, and his admission labs reveal him to have hyponatremia and a low cortisol level. Which is the most likely diagnosis?

a. Hypovolemic shock

b. Multiple sclerosis

c. Cushing syndrome

d. Adrenal crisis

27 A patient is diagnosed with hyponatremia; his plasma osmolality is 250 mOsm/L, urine osmolality is 110 mOsm/L, and urine sodium level is 22 mEq/L, and he is euvolemic. What is the most likely cause of the hyponatremia?

a. Syndrome of inappropriate diuretic hormone (SIADH)

b. Heart failure

c. Hyperaldosteronism

d. Vomiting

28 A patient has hyponatremia and is being corrected with 3% saline. What can occur if the sodium is corrected too quickly?

a. Central pontine myelinolysis

b. Seizures

c. SIADH

d. Nephrotic syndrome

29 A patient has a sodium level of 155 mEq/L, and the urine volume for the past 24 hours is less than 800 mL, the urine osmolality is greater than 800 mOsm/L, and the urine sodium is less than 10 mEq/L. What is the most likely cause of the hypernatremia?

a. Osmotic diuresis glucosuria

b. SIADH

c. Diuretic use

d. Lithium

30 In patients experiencing anaphylactic shock, what is the first medication that should be given?

a. Intramuscular epinephrine .3–.5 mg of a 1:1,000 solution

b. Intramuscular epinephrine .3–.5 mg of a 1:10,000 solution

c. Epinephrine infusion

d. Methylprednisolone 1–2 mg/kg daily for 1–2 days

31 The AGACNP has been called to see a patient admitted with intractable vomiting, who is now lethargic and confused. He has been NPO since yesterday. Vital signs are blood pressure 106/60, HR 102, RR 8, and temperature 97.9°F. The most appropriate first step would be:

a. Order a fingerstick glucose.

b. Order a stat CT brain.

c. Order NS 1 L bolus.

d. Order neuro checks every hour until resolved.

32 A 23-year-old female is admitted this morning with viral pneumonia. Her respiratory effort is becoming labored, and her oxygen saturations are falling despite being placed on 100% nonrebreather mask. She is unable to reposition herself in bed without significant distress. Her breath sounds are diminished bilaterally. Chest x-ray reveals bilateral fluffy infiltrates, and ABG reveals PaO_2 of 70. The AGACNP suspects the patient has developed:

a. Pulmonary emboli

b. Diastolic congestive heart failure (CHF)

c. Pneumothorax

d. Acute respiratory distress syndrome (ARDS)

33 Which of the following are modalities utilized in the patient with ARDS?

a. Lung-protective ventilation strategies, airway pressure release ventilation

b. Proning, sedation, and neuromuscular blockade

c. Venous–venous extracorporeal oxygenation and pulmonary vasodilators

d. All of the above

34 A 35-year-old male with an ideal body weight of 70 kg is admitted with a polypharmacy overdose, resulting in acute hypoxemic and hypercapneic respiratory failure. He was intubated in the emergency room (ER), and was placed on the ventilator with the following settings: AC rate 10, tidal volume 560, FiO_2 40%, and PEEP +5. His new ABG results are pH 7.23, PaO_2 160 mm Hg, $PaCO_2$ 65 mm Hg, HCO_3 31 mEq/L, and SpO_2 98%. What ventilator changes would the AGACNP make?

a. Decrease the tidal volume to 480.

b. Increase the PEEP to +10.

c. Increase the respiratory rate to 14.

d. Make no changes.

35 A 32-year-old pregnant female presents with pleuritic chest pain and shortness of breath. She smokes 1 pack of cigarettes per day. Her vital signs are BP 124/60, HR 134 sinus tachycardia, respiratory rate of 24, and SpO_2 94% on 6 L oxygen via nasal cannula. The AGACNP suspects pulmonary embolism and orders:

a. D-dimer

b. CTA of the chest to rule out PE

c. Thrombolytics

d. Warfarin

36 A 64-year-old male with past medical history of DM2, hypertension, and hyperlipidemia presents to the emergency department with a 2-hour history of crushing substernal chest pain. EKG reveals ST-segment elevation in leads II, III, and AVF. Which of the following is the most appropriate intervention, given the cited situation?

a. Nitroglycerin, aspirin, and heparin drip with admission to the step down unit

b. Full dose anticoagulation as primary percutaneous coronary intervention (PCI) is not available for 3 hours

c. Fibrinolytics as PCI is not available for 30 minutes

d. Emergent catheterization with PCI as this is available within 90 minutes of arrival

37 A 45-year-old male was admitted to the ICU for acute hypoxemic respiratory failure requiring intubation 6 days ago. He was extubated this morning. The nurse calls the AGACNP at 9 p.m. to report that the patient is actively hallucinating, cannot follow directions, and is becoming agitated. The most likely cause for this set of symptoms is:

a. Recreational drugs

b. Early-onset dementia

c. ICU delirium

d. Alcohol withdrawal

38 A 57-year-old female with past medical history of recreational drug use (heroin and cocaine) and bacterial endocarditis presents to the ER with complaints of anxiety and constant chest pressure for the last hour. She is hypertensive and tachycardic. Which set of orders is the most appropriate for the AGACNP to order first?

a. CBC, BMP, troponin, urine metanephrines

b. CBC, BMP, urine drug screen, troponins, metoprolol 5 mg IV

c. EKG, CBC, BMP, UA, urine drug screen, troponin

d. EKG, metoprolol 5 mg IV, CBC, urine drug screen, troponins

39 A 28-year-old female presents with a recreational overindulgence of MDMA and cocaine. The AGACNP knows the priorities of care are:

a. Lorazepam, control of seizures, monitoring for cardiac ischemia, supportive care

b. Naloxone, intubation, and mechanical ventilation

c. Vasopressor support, intubation, and mechanical ventilation

d. Naloxone, beta blockade, neuro checks

40 A 46-year-old female presents with an intentional overdose of acetaminophen. She isn't sure how much she took but advises the AGACNP that it occurred 10 hours ago. Which of the following is correct regarding this patient's clinical presentation?

a. Jaundice and transaminitis would be present.

b. Her AST would be elevated by twice normal levels.

c. No signs or symptoms may be present.

d. Fulminant hepatic failure would be present.

41 The antidote for acetaminophen is *N*-acetylcysteine (NAC). Based on the Rumack–Matthew nomogram, under which condition would this be administered?

a. The timing of the overdose is unknown.

b. The timing of the overdose is unknown, and the level falls below the treatment line.

c. The dose of the ingestion is known, and the level falls above the treatment line.

d. The timing of the overdose is known, and the level falls above the treatment line.

42 A 52-year-old male with past medical history of hypertension, diabetes type II, and CAD presents to the emergency room with a chief complaint of headache and blurred vision. Vital signs are BP 210/120, HR 89, RR 16, temperature 98.6°F, and SpO$_2$ 98% on room air. The most appropriate diagnosis for this patient is:

a. Hypertension

b. Hypertensive urgency

c. Hypertensive emergency

d. Stroke

43 A 66-year-old female with past medical history of hypertension has presented to the emergency department with new-onset right-sided weakness and expressive aphasia for the past hour. Her vital signs are BP 212/126, HR 88, RR 18, temperature 98.2°F, and SpO$_2$ 97% on room air. Her initial CT of the brain is negative. The AGACNP recommends the following treatment regimen:

a. Labetalol 10 mg IVP once, followed by thrombolytic administration.

b. Labetalol 10 mg IVP bolus, followed by a labetalol drip titrated to SBP less than 185 and DBP less than 110. If parameters are met, thrombolytics may be given within 3 hours of symptom onset.

c. Nicardipine infusion at 5 mg/hr, titrated to DBP less than 90, up to 15 mg/hr with thrombolytic administration if BP parameters are met and within 3 hours of symptom onset.

d. Nicardipine infusion to start at 15 mg/hr, with thrombolytics to follow.

44 A 43-year-old male is status post alteplase administration for stroke. Upon arrival to the ICU, staff reports that the patient is complaining of a severe headache. The alteplase is discontinued. Stat CT of the brain reveals intracranial hemorrhage. To stop this life-threatening bleeding, the AGACNP orders which of the following to reverse the alteplase?

a. PRBCs, fresh frozen plasma, and cryoprecipitate

b. Fresh frozen plasma and platelets

c. PRBCs and fresh frozen plasma

d. Cryoprecipitate and fresh frozen plasma

45 A 67-year-old female with past medical history of diabetes type II, atrial fibrillation on warfarin, and hypercholesterolemia presents to the emergency department with palpitations, pallor, and hypotension. Vital signs are BP 86/48, HR 122, RR 22, and SpO$_2$ 93% on room air. The patient's daughter has concerns that the patient has been forgetful lately and some of her medication bottles are empty. Her labs begin to result while she is in radiology, with an INR of greater than 9 and hematocrit of 17.8%. Her CT reveals a large psoas muscle hemorrhage. Which of the following would the AGACNP order to reverse this patient's warfarin?

a. Vitamin K and prothrombin complex concentrate (PCC)

b. PRBCs

c. Platelets and PCC

d. PRBCs and platelets

46 A 22-year-old male status post motor vehicle collision is admitted to the trauma ICU with multiple injuries and severe blood loss anemia. As a result he has received 22 units of packed red blood cells, 10 units of fresh frozen plasma, and 4 units of platelets. His hemoglobin and blood pressure have stabilized. Nursing calls to report that he is now anuric with high peak pressures on the ventilator. His abdomen is distended and firm. A measured bladder pressure is 28 mm Hg. Based on this clinical picture, the AGACNP suspects:

a. Ileus

b. Abdominal compartment syndrome (ACS)

c. Constipation

d. Acute kidney injury related to hypovolemia

47 A 32-year-old female with no past medical history presents to the ICU status post cholecystectomy, unable to be extubated due to extreme agitation upon emergence from anesthesia. She was sedated with propofol prior to departure from the suite. Upon arrival to the ICU, her vital signs are BP 180/100, HR 112, RR 22, SpO$_2$ 98% on 40% FiO$_2$ via the ventilator, and temperature 105.6°F. The AGACNP notes that her extremities are rigid and suspects which of the following is most likely the cause?

a. Neuroleptic malignant syndrome

b. Infection from intestinal spillage

c. Seizures

d. Malignant hyperthermia

48 Alveolar hypoventilation can occur with which of the following conditions?

a. Opiates, opioids, benzodiazepines

b. Opiates in the setting of obesity

c. Hypophosphatemia

d. All of the above

49 A 22-year-old female presents to the emergency department with intense thirst, polyuria, and dysuria. She is diagnosed with a urinary tract infection. Her routine lab work also reveals a serum glucose of 369 and 3+ urinary ketones. Her CO_2 on her BMP is 12. This presentation is suspicious for:

a. Diabetic ketoacidosis (DKA)

b. Hyperosmolar nonketotic state (HHNK)

c. Incidental hyperglycemia

d. Nothing, as this is normal with a urinary tract infection

50 A 59-year-old male is hospitalized with CHF, and has been on furosemide for several days. His latest BMP reveals a sodium of 130, chloride of 98, and CO_2 of 10. The AGACNP orders an arterial blood gas, which reveals a metabolic alkalosis (pH 7.55) despite a $PaCO_2$ of 55 mm Hg. Which of the following is the most appropriate treatment?

a. Bumetanide 2 mg IVP

b. Sodium bicarbonate 50 mEq IVP

c. Acetazolamide 250 mg IVP

d. Furosemide 60 mg IVP

51 The AGACNP is responding to a rapid response call for a 38-year-old male on the floor admitted for intractable headaches. Upon arrival, the patient does not follow commands, withdrawing to pain only. He does not open his eyes to pain, and is completely nonverbal. His fingerstick glucose is 98. Which is the most appropriate next step?

a. Stat CT of the brain

b. Neurological consultation

c. Intubation and mechanical ventilation

d. Administration of mannitol in anticipation of surgery

52 Prolonged neuromuscular blockade can lead to which of the following complications?

a. Critical illness myopathy, pressure ulcers, venous thromboembolism

b. Hyperglycemia, hypotension, parasthesias

c. Hypoglycemia, hypotension, anxiety

d. Hyponatremia, hypertension, clonus

53 A 54-year-old male with past medical history of diabetes type II presents with hyperglycemia and polyuria. His serum glucose is 1,023 mg/dL and serum osmolality 334 mOsm/kg. Of note, his pH is 7.39 on a venous blood gas. His urinalysis is remarkable only for a high glucose level. Vital signs are BP 96/48, HR 122, RR 16, and SpO_2 98% on room air. This clinical presentation is most consistent with:

a. DKA

b. Addison disease

c. Hyperglycemic hyperosmolar nonketotic state

d. Cushing disease

54 A 21-year-old male is hospital day 5, transferred to the ICU status post isolated traumatic brain injury with evacuation of a subdural hematoma. Nursing reports that his urine output has increased over the course of the evening to 400 mL/hr during the past 4 hours. His vital signs have remained stable. The AGACNP orders a urinalysis, BMP, and serum osmolality, suspecting which of the following?

a. SIADH

b. Mobilization of resuscitation fluids

c. Hypoalbuminemia

d. Central diabetes insipidus (DI)

55 A 45-year-old female with a past medical history of dilated cardiomyopathy is admitted to the ICU status post cardiac arrest. Targeted temperature management is being considered. All of the following are potential complications of therapeutic hypothermia during cooling, EXCEPT:

a. Osborne waves on EKG

b. Bradycardia

c. Peripheral vasodilatation

d. Hypotension

Disease Answers/Rationales

1 **The correct answer is A.**

Rationales:

a. In hypovolemic shock, the volume returning to the heart, also called preload, is low.

b. In hypovolemic shock, the body compensates by vasoconstricting the arteries, thus causing the SVR to be elevated.

c. In hypovolemic shock, the cardiac output is low due to insufficient circulating volume and stroke volume.

d. In hypovolemic shock, the SvO_2 is low due to the reuptake of oxygen in the cells in the periphery on remaining hemoglobin.

(Bhat et al., 2016, pp. 239–248).

2 **The correct answer is C.**

Rationales:

a. In cardiogenic shock, the CVP is elevated due to increased preload or venous return to the heart.

b. In cardiogenic shock, the SVR is elevated due to elevated afterload or vasoconstriction in the arteries the left ventricle has to overcome to eject its contents.

c. In cardiogenic shock, the cardiac output is low due to the inability of the myocardium to pump effectively.

d. In cardiogenic shock, the SvO_2 is low due to the update of oxygen in the periphery.

(Bhat et al., 2016, pp. 239–248).

3 **The correct answer is B.**

Rationales:

a. The CVP is low in distributive shock due to the immune response that causes massive vasodilation. This vasodilation also affects the venous system leading to a decrease in preload.

b. The SVR is low in distributive shock due to the immune response that causes massive vasodilation.

c. The cardiac output is elevated in distributive shock due to the heart trying to compensate for the low preload and afterload states.

d. The SvO_2 is high in distributive shock due to the inability of the capillary bed to uptake oxygen due to sluggish blood flow and microemboli.

(Bhat et al., 2016, pp. 239–248).

4 **The correct answer is A.**

Rationales:

a. The CVP is elevated in obstructive shock due to pulmonary embolism due to inability of the blood to flow forward into the pulmonary vasculature.

b. The SVR is normal to elevated in obstructive shock due to pulmonary embolism due to compensatory mechanisms.

c. The cardiac output is low in obstructive shock due to pulmonary embolism due to lack of stroke volume.

d. The SvO_2 is low in obstructive shock due to pulmonary embolism due to lack of oxygenated blood leaving the lungs.

(Bhat et al., 2016, pp. 239–248).

Clinical Pearl

Preload is reflected in the right atrium pressure or CVP. Volume overload will increase preload, and dehydration or hemorrhage will decrease preload.

---

5 **The correct answer is C.**

Rationales:

a. Preload is the venous return to the heart and the stretch of the right ventricle.

b. Stroke volume is the amount of blood pumped out of the heart every minute.

c. Afterload is the pressure the left ventricle has to overcome to eject its contents into the aorta and is also called SVR, and reflects the vasoconstriction or vasodilation in the arterial system.

d. Pulmonary capillary wedge pressure is the pressure in the pulmonary capillary bed when a pulmonary artery catheter balloon is inflated; it reflects what is occurring in the left atrium.

(Bhat et al., 2016, pp. 239–248).

---

6 **The correct answer is D.**

Rationales:

a. Pulmonary capillary wedge pressure is the pressure in the pulmonary capillary bed when a pulmonary artery catheter balloon is inflated; it reflects what is occurring in the left atrium.

b. Stroke volume is the amount of blood pumped out of the heart every minute.

c. Afterload is the pressure the left ventricle has to overcome to eject its contents into the aorta and is also called system vascular resistance or the vasoconstriction or vasodilation in the arterial system.

d. Preload is the venous return to the heart and the stretch of the right ventricle.

(Bhat et al., 2016, pp. 239–248).

---

7 **The correct answer is C.**

Rationales:

a. In cardiogenic shock, the CVP and SVR are elevated and the CO/CI and SvO_2 are decreased.

b. In obstructive shock, the CVP is elevated and the SVR is normal to high, the CO/CI is low, and the SvO_2 is normal to low.

c. In distributive shock, the CVP and SVR are low, the CO/CI is elevated, and the SvO_2 is elevated.

d. In hypovolemic shock, the CVP is low, the SVR is elevated, the CO/CI is low, and the SvO_2 is low.

(Bhat et al., 2016, pp. 239–248).

---

8 **The correct answer is D.**

Rationales:

a. In cardiogenic shock, the CVP and SVR are elevated and the CO/CI and SvO_2 are decreased.

b. In obstructive shock, the CVP is elevated and the SVR is normal to high, the CO/CI is low, and the SvO_2 is normal to low.

c. In distributive shock, the CVP and SVR are low, the CO/CI is elevated, and the SvO_2 is elevated.

d. In hypovolemic shock, the CVP is low, the SVR is elevated, the CO/CI is low, and the SvO_2 is low.

(Bhat et al., 2016, pp. 239–248).

---

9 **The correct answer is D.**

Rationales:

a. Norepinephrine is both an alpha and beta agonist.

b. Epinephrine is both an alpha and beta agonist.

c. Nicardipine is a dihydropyridine calcium channel blocker that is used to decrease blood pressure.

d. Phenylephrine is an alpha agonist only.

(Bhat et al., 2016, pp. 239–248).

10 **The correct answer is C.**

Rationales:

a. Norepinephrine is a vasopressor agent that is started after the patient is adequately volume resuscitated.

b. Dobutamine is an inotropic agent that is used to increase cardiac output. This patient requires volume resuscitation because he is in septic shock.

c. In septic shock, the goal is to achieve and maintain an MAP greater than 65 mm Hg; therefore, administering volume resuscitation at 30 mL/kg over the first 3 hours is the recommended intervention.

d. In septic shock, administration of crystalloids, either Ringer lactate or normal saline, at 30 mL/kg over the first 3 hours is recommended.

(Rhodes et al., 2017, pp. 486–552).

11 **The correct answer is C.**

Rationales:

a. In a patient with an adequate blood pressure, milrinone is recommended. Dopamine is recommended with hypotension and with bradycardia.

b. Dobutamine is a good inotropic agent; however, because this patient has an adequate blood pressure, milrinone is recommended.

c. Milrinone is recommended to increase contractility and cardiac output when the patient has an adequate blood pressure.

d. Epinephrine is both an alpha and beta agonist and it strengths contraction; however, it is reserved for patients who are hypotensive and bradycardic when other medications do not work.

(Manaker, 2019).

12 **The correct answer is B.**

Rationales:

a. Phenylephrine is an alpha agonist and increases SVR; it does not decrease the preload.

b. Nitroglycerin is a vasodilator that decreases preload because it predominantly works on the venous side of the vascular system.

c. Metoprolol is a beta-blocker and will not decrease the preload.

d. Diltiazem is a nondihydropyridine calcium channel blocker that decreases heart rate; it does not affect the preload.

(Manaker, 2019).

13 **The correct answer is D.**

Rationales:

a. In distributive shock, the inflammatory response causes vasodilation of the vascular bed and an increase in cardiac output.

b. In distributive shock, the inflammatory response causes microembolization.

c. In distributive shock, the SVR and the preload are both decreased.

d. The inflammatory response in septic shock causes vasodilation of the vascular bed and a decrease in SVR and preload.

(Bhat et al., 2016, pp. 239–248).

Clinical Pearl

Mixed venous oxygen saturation is only elevated in distributive shock; it is decreased with all of the other shock states.

14 **The correct answer is B.**

Rationales:

a. Vasopressin is a second-line vasopressor in septic shock.

b. If a patient remains hypotensive despite adequate volume resuscitation, a norepinephrine infusion is the first-line vasopressor to use to increase the mean arterial pressure to a goal of 65 mm Hg or greater.

c. Milrinone is an inotropic agent used to increase myocardial function and cardiac output; however, it can cause vasodilation and hypotension.

d. Stress-dose steroids are only started in septic shock if the patient has a known cortisol deficiency or the patient remains hypotensive despite vasopressor therapy.

(Rhodes et al., 2017, pp. 486–552).

15 **The correct answer is C.**

Rationales:

a. The patient is exhibiting propofol infusion syndrome, and furosemide is not indicated.

b. The patient is exhibiting propofol infusion syndrome, and an IV with bicarbonate is not indicated unless the patient's pH is less than 6.19.

c. Stopping the propofol infusion, starting isotonic crystalloid to flush the kidneys of myoglobin, and consulting nephrology are recommended.

d. Although the patient's triglycerides are elevated, they are elevated due to the propofol and the level should decrease once the infusion is stopped. In addition, fenofibrate cannot be administered through an oral or nasogastric tube.

(Bhat et al., 2016, pp. 239–248).

16 **The correct answer is C.**

Rationales:

a. Kerley B lines are associated with fluid in the fissures, not pneumonia. Pneumonia is seen as an infiltrate on chest x-ray.

b. Pneumothorax is seen as a lack of lung markings on chest x-ray, not Kerley B lines.

c. Kerley B lines are associated with fluid overload and pulmonary edema.

d. Pleural effusions are viewed as opacities on a chest x-ray, not Kerley B lines.

(Bhat et al., 2016, pp. 239–248).

17 **The correct answer is B.**

Rationales:

a. Norepinephrine is an alpha and beta 1 agonist and not a beta 2 agonist; therefore, it would not help in this situation.

b. Epinephrine would increase the blood pressure and relax the bronchial smooth muscle, relieving the wheezing. This occurs due to its alpha and beta 1 and beta 2 effects.

c. Dobutamine is a beta 1 agonist and increases the strength of myocardial contraction; it does not affect the bronchial smooth muscle.

d. Dopamine has beta 1 effects at lower doses and alpha effects at higher doses; it does not affect bronchial smooth muscle.

(Manaker, 2019).

18 **The correct answer is A.**

Rationales:

a. Dopamine has beta 1 effects at doses of 5–10 µg/kg/min and has alpha effects at doses of 10–20 µg/kg/min and therefore, would be the best drug in this situation.

b. Dobutamine increases the cardiac output but will not increase the blood pressure or heart rate and in fact can cause vasodilation.

c. Milrinone increases cardiac output; however, it can cause hypotension, and it does not affect heart rate.

d. Nitroglycerin is a vasodilator that decreases preload and blood pressure, and it does not increase the heart rate.

(Manaker, 2019).

Clinical Pearl

Nitroglycerin works predominantly to decrease preload while nitroprusside works predominantly to decrease afterload.

19 **The correct answer is A.**

Rationales:

a. This patient's sudden decline in blood pressure and CVP along with his symptoms of abdominal pain and nausea point to a gastrointestinal issue, and GI bleed needs to be ruled out. Ordering a stat CBC to assess Hgb change, type and screen so you are able to transfuse packed red blood cells as needed, and giving the patient a crystalloid fluid bolus to increase his CVP is warranted.

b. A stat chemistry will not give you information about whether the patient is actively bleeding.

c. A stat troponin level will not give you information about whether the patient is actively bleeding.

d. A stat lactate level will not give you information about whether the patient is actively bleeding.

(Bhat et al., 2016, pp. 239–248).

20 **The correct answer is C.**

Rationales:

a. The patient's hemoglobin and hematocrit are only slightly lower and the patient is not actively bleeding; no packed red blood cell transfusion is warranted.

b. The patient's hemoglobin and hematocrit are only slightly lower and the patient is not actively bleeding; no fresh frozen plasma is warranted.

c. The hemoglobin and hematocrit can be evaluated in the morning as long as the patient remains hemodynamically stable and is not actively bleeding.

d. Waiting 72 hours is too long for a patient who had a recent GI bleed.

(Carson et al., 2016, pp. 2025–2035).

21 **The correct answer is B.**

Rationales:

a. The CVP is within normal limits; no albumin is warranted.

b. The SVR is still low; therefore, adding vasopressin as a second-line agent would be appropriate.

c. The patient's cardiac output is high; no dobutamine is warranted.

d. The patient's cardiac output is elevated; no milrinone is warranted.

(Bhat et al., 2016, pp. 239–248).

22 **The correct answer is B.**

Rationales:

a. The patient is actively GI bleeding on a pantoprazole infusion; giving an additional bolus is not recommended.

b. The patient is actively vomiting bright red blood while on a pantoprazole infusion. You must consider that he has esophageal varices; therefore, an octreotide bolus and infusion are recommended to decrease the bleeding from esophageal varices.

c. Fresh frozen plasma will decrease an elevated INR; it will not stop the active bleeding.

d. Norepinephrine is a potent vasopressor that will increase his blood pressure; however, the patient is actively bleeding and the cause needs to be treated. Norepinephrine will not treat the cause of the bleed.

(Bhat et al., 2016, pp. 239–248).

Clinical Pearl

If a patient remains hypotensive despite adequate fluid resuscitation and pressors, consider adding stress-dose steroids for possible adrenal insufficiency. Also assess for profound acidosis, which will render pressors ineffective.

23 **The correct answer is D.**

Rationales:

a. Vasopressin stimulates the V2 receptors, not the alpha receptors.

b. Vasopressin does not stimulate the beta 1 or beta 2 receptors.

c. Vasopressin does not stimulate the release of nitric oxide from the vascular endothelium.

d. Vasopressin stimulates the V2 receptors, regulates the kidney reabsorption of water, regulates smooth muscle vascular tone, and modulates brainstem autonomic function.

(Manaker, 2019).

24 **The correct answer is B.**

Rationales:

a. Hypovolemic shock causes a low CVP, high SVR, and tachycardia.

b. Neurogenic shock characterizes the hemodynamic response of the body to a spinal cord injury. These responses include bradycardia, hypotension, low CVP, and low SVR due to disruption of autonomic pathways.

c. Spinal shock characterizes the loss of movement or sensation below the level of spinal injury.

d. Cardiogenic shock causes a high CVP and SVR and a low cardiac output.

(Bhat et al., 2016, pp. 239–248).

Clinical Pearl

Neurogenic shock and spinal shock are not the same. Neurogenic shock is a type of distributive shock that characterizes the hemodynamic response of the body to a spinal cord injury. Spinal shock is characterized by the loss of movement below the level of injury.

25 **The correct answer is C.**

Rationales:

a. Acute myocardial infarction is characterized by chest heaviness, diaphoresis, nausea, shortness of breath, and pain radiating to the neck, teeth, or left arm.

b. Acute peptic ulcer perforation is characterized by severe epigastric pain and nausea; it does not cause a tearing or ripping sensation in the chest or back.

c. Acute aortic dissection is characterized by sudden chest pain that is characterized by a tearing or ripping sensation in the chest or back, and it is often accompanied by hypertension.

d. Acute pancreatitis is characterized by abdominal and back pain, not a tearing or ripping sensation.

(Bhat et al., 2016, pp. 239–248).

26 **The correct answer is D.**

Rationales:

a. The symptoms described by the patient occurred over the past month; hypovolemic shock occurs suddenly.

b. Multiple sclerosis is characterized by weakness and fatigue, visual disturbance in one eye, foot dragging, bowel dysfunction, and imbalance.

c. Cushing syndrome is characterized by weakness, facial rounding, and hirsutism.

d. Adrenal crisis is characterized by symptoms of anorexia, nausea, vomiting, weight loss, weakness, fatigue, orthostatic hypotension, hyponatremia, and a low cortisol level.

(Bhat et al., 2016, p. 767).

27 **The correct answer is A.**

Rationales:

a. SIADH is a cause of euvolemic hyponatremia.

b. Heart failure can cause hypervolemic hyponatremia.

c. Hyperaldosteronism may cause hypovolemic hyponatremia.

d. Vomiting may cause hypovolemic hyponatremia.

(Bhat et al., 2016, p. 361).

28 **The correct answer is A.**

Rationales:

a. Central pontine myelinolysis results from damage to the neurons due to rapid osmotic shifts that occur with sodium correction that is too rapid.

b. Seizures are an effect of hyponatremia.

c. SIADH can be a cause of euvolemic hyponatremia.

d. Nephrotic syndrome can be a cause of hypervolemic hyponatremia.

(Bhat et al., 2016, p. 361).

29 **The correct answer is C.**

Rationales:

a. Osmotic diuresis glucosuria can be a cause of hypovolemic/euvolemic hypernatremia.

b. SIADH can cause euvolemic hyponatremia.

c. Diuretic use can cause hypovolemic hypernatremia, and the patient would have a urine sodium less than 10 mEq/L and the urine volume would be less than 800 mL in 24 hours.

d. Lithium can cause hypovolemic/euvolemic hypernatremia.

(Bhat et al., 2016, p. 365).

30 **The correct answer is A.**

Rationales:

a. Intramuscular epinephrine 1:1,000 concentration, .3–.5 mg is the recommended first-line drug for anaphylactic shock.

b. The 1:10,000 epinephrine solution is given IV, not IM.

c. An epinephrine infusion would be given if the patient continues to have severe symptoms of anaphylaxis after receiving IM epinephrine.

d. Methylprednisolone is used in anaphylactic shock; however, it prevents recurrence of symptoms but does not stop the initial reaction.

(Bhat et al., 2016, pp. 239–248).

31 **The correct answer is A.**

Rationales:

a. A fingerstick glucose can be performed quickly at the bedside, and failure to identify and treat life-threatening hypoglycemia can lead to rapid deterioration.

b. A CT brain may be considered after ensuring adequate glucose levels.

c. This patient's MAP is greater than 65, and hypotension is not present.

d. Ordering neuro checks will not alter this patient's course. Repeat assessment is necessary, but the cause must be discovered.

(Marino, 2014, p. 800).

32 **The correct answer is D.**

Rationales:

a. Given the clinical picture and fluffy infiltrates on CXR, pulmonary emboli are not the likely culprit.

b. There is no evidence for fluid overload or CHF on CXR.

c. Pneumothorax is not reported on the CXR, and breath sounds are present.

d. ARDS is defined by an acute onset of hypoxia, with P/F ratio less than or equal to 300 mm Hg, and bilateral fluffy infiltrates developing within 24 hours in the absence of left heart failure or fluid overload.

(Marino, 2014, p. 449).

33 **The correct answer is D.**

Rationales:

a. Lung-protective ventilation strategies and airway pressure release ventilation assist in limiting pressures exerted by the ventilators and increase recruitment, respectively.

b. Proning, sedation, and neuromuscular blockade are considered supportive treatments that allow for increased surface area on the posterior aspect of the lungs to participate in gas exchange. The sedation and neuromuscular blockade are used to assist in the tolerance of higher intrathoracic pressures that translate into higher peak and plateau pressures.

c. Venous–venous extracorporeal oxygenation and pulmonary vasodilators are considered rescue modalities, when refractory hypoxemia is present.

d. All of the above are modalities of treatment in ARDS.

(Fish & Talmor, 2019).

34 **The correct answer is C.**

Rationales:

a. Decreasing the tidal volume would increase the acidosis due to further accumulation of carbon dioxide.

b. Increasing the PEEP is not necessary, as the patient is not hypoxemic.

c. Increasing the respiratory rate to 14 will allow for more minute volume, which would decrease the $PaCO_2$.

d. Making no changes will not improve the patient's status, and he may decompensate further.

(Marino, 2014, pp. 516–517).

35 **The correct answer is B.**

Rationales:

a. A D-dimer should only be ordered in those with low suspicion for PE. Also, pregnancy gestations over 16 weeks will have an elevated D-dimer, rendering the test nondiagnostic for negative PEs.

b. Benefits outweigh risks to mother and fetus when CTA of the chest is used to rule out PE.

c. Thrombolytics should only be used in those who are hemodynamically unstable. Treatment is not deferred due to pregnancy.

d. Warfarin should not be administered to pregnant patients (particularly in the first trimester) due to teratogenic effects.

(Dries, 2012).

36 **The correct answer is D.**

Rationales:

a. These interventions are appropriate for hemodynamically stable, unstable angina. They are not sufficient for STEMI.

b. If PCI intervention door-to-device time is not expected within 90 minutes, fibrinolytics should be employed.

c. Fibrinolytics should be used when PCI intervention door-to-device time is not expected within 90 minutes.

d. PCI intervention has a 90-minute door-to-device window.

(Tomey & Gidwani, 2019).

37 **The correct answer is C.**

Rationales:

a. Recreational drugs are unlikely given his length of stay, unless brought into the ICU by visitors. Although this is possible, it is not as likely as ICU delirium.

b. Early-onset dementia is a gradual, and sometimes insidious, process whereas delirium is an acute mental status change.

c. ICU delirium is characterized by an acute mental status change or inattentiveness, with disorganized thinking or altered level of consciousness.

d. Alcohol withdrawal would typically be noted in the first 48–72 hours of admission. These symptoms started later in the course of his hospitalization.

(Hsieh, 2019).

38 **The correct answer is C.**

Rationales:

a. Urine metanephrines are increased in pheochromocytoma, which has an intermittent pattern of symptoms that include sweating, headaches, palpitations, and hypertension. Her symptoms are constant in nature.

b. Beta-blockers should be avoided in patients at risk for cocaine ingestion, due to unopposed alpha activity that may worsen hypertension.

c. EKG and troponins are central to chest pain evaluation, but this patient presents with a concern for continued drug use. Drug screening is imperative, as beta-blockers are a mainstay in cardiac ischemia. If given concurrently with cocaine, unopposed alpha activity may worsen a hypertensive emergency.

d. Beta-blockers should be avoided in patients with cocaine ingestion, due to unopposed alpha activity that may worsen hypertension into crisis.

(Mossop & DiBlasio, 2019).

39 **The correct answer is A.**

Rationales:

a. Lorazepam, control of seizures, monitoring for cardiac ischemia, and supportive care are mainstays of treatment for sympathomimetic ingestion. Hyperthermia, arrhythmias, and rhabdomyolysis are also common, and patients should be monitored closely for these complications.

b. Naloxone, intubation, and mechanical ventilation are supportive care for depressants, such as opiates, opioids, and benzodiazepines.

c. Vasopressor support, intubation, and mechanical ventilation are supportive care for depressant toxidromes with hemodynamic instability.

d. Naloxone is not indicated for sympathomimetic overdose, and beta blockade could be harmful (as alpha stimulation is unopposed, leading to hypertensive emergency).

(Mossop & DiBlasio, 2019).

> **Clinical Pearl**
>
> Lorazepam is the agent of choice for sympathomimetic toxidromes, by suppressing seizures, and is also effective treating arrhythmias due to stimulant ingestions.

40 **The correct answer is C.**

Rationales:

a. Hepatotoxicity in acetaminophen overdose does not manifest in the first 24 hours.

b. Hepatotoxicity does not manifest in the first 24 hours.

c. Signs of hepatotoxicity do not manifest in the first 24 hours.

d. Hepatotoxicity does not manifest in the first 24 hours.

(Marino, 2014, pp. 966–967).

41 **The correct answer is D.**

Rationales:

a. The Rumack–Matthew nomogram cannot be used when the timing of the ingestion is unknown.

b. The Rumack–Matthew nomogram cannot be used when the timing of the ingestion is unknown.

c. The Rumack–Matthew nomogram denotes risk of hepatotoxicity based on timing and corresponding levels. Dosage of ingestion does not factor into the decision to give NAC.

d. The Rumack–Matthew nomogram utilizes the timing and corresponding levels to determine risk of hepatotoxicity. Any patient with a level above the treatment line should be initiated on NAC.

(Marino, 2014, pp. 966–967).

42 **The correct answer is C.**

Rationales:

a. This patient has been diagnosed with hypertension but has symptoms concerning for end-organ damage, which elevates the diagnosis to hypertensive emergency.

b. Hypertensive urgency is defined as accelerated hypertension, without signs of end-organ damage.

c. This patient has neurological symptoms in the setting of extreme hypertension, concerning for end-organ damage. This defines hypertensive emergency and must be treated with caution to prevent hypoperfusion to end organs.

d. The symptoms and vital signs in this scenario do not confirm a diagnosis of stroke.

(Papadakis & McPhee, 2018, p. 479).

43 **The correct answer is B.**

Rationales:

a. Blood pressure must be reevaluated with SBP less than 185 and DBP less than 110 before thrombolytics can be administered. In order to qualify for thrombolytic therapy, the patient's symptoms must be within 3 hours.

b. Blood pressure must be reevaluated with SBP less than 185 and DBP less than 110 before thrombolytics can be administered. In order to qualify for thrombolytic therapy, the patient's symptoms must be within 3 hours.

c. Blood pressure must be reevaluated with SBP less than 185 and DBP less than 110 before thrombolytics can be administered. A DBP of 90 is too low, and may result in hypoperfusion. In order to qualify for thrombolytic therapy, the patient's symptoms must be within 3 hours.

d. The starting dose of nicardipine is 5 mg/hr, titratable to a maximum of 15 mg/hr. In order to qualify for thrombolytic therapy, the patient's symptoms must be within 3 hours.

(Marino, 2014, pp. 838–839).

> **Clinical Pearl**
>
> Nicardipine and labetalol are the antihypertensives of choice to reduce BP in the setting of stroke. Care must be taken to ensure that end organs are not hypoperfused due to rapid reduction of arterial pressure. Mean arterial pressures should not be reduced less than 25% within hours to prevent hypoperfusion.

44 **The correct answer is D.**

Rationales:

a. The fresh frozen plasma and cryoprecipitate will assist in reversal of alteplase, which acts on plasminogen bound to fibrin (which creates the clot). There is not enough volume loss with an intracranial hemorrhage to warrant packed red blood cell transfusion.

b. Fresh frozen plasma should be given after cryoprecipitate, and platelets will not affect the bleeding unless the patient is known to be thrombocytopenic.

c. Fresh frozen plasma may be given after cryoprecipitate; however, packed red blood cells will not reverse alteplase.

d. Cryoprecipitate should be given, followed by fresh frozen plasma until the serum fibrinogen level reaches greater than 1mg/mL to reverse the effects of alteplase.

(Marino, 2014, p. 310).

45 **The correct answer is A.**

Rationales:

a. Vitamin K and PCC are used together to reverse the effects of warfarin.

b. PRBCs may be required for her hemorrhage but will not alter the effects of warfarin.

c. Although PCC may assist in the reversal of warfarin, platelets will not.

d. PRBCs and platelets do not counter the effects of warfarin.

(Marino, 2014, p. 382).

46 The correct answer is B.

Rationales:

a. Although this patient is at risk for ileus, this would not cause anuria in a euvolemic patient. Ileus would be unlikely to cause increased peak pressures on the ventilator or elevated bladder pressures.

b. ACS is characterized by elevated bladder pressures (which translate to increased intrathoracic pressures) and new end-organ dysfunction due to hypoperfusion. Bladder pressures are consistently greater than 20 mm Hg.

c. Constipation is unlikely to result in anuria and increased intrathoracic pressures, unless extreme.

d. This patient's volume appears to have been restored with stabilized BPs. He may be developing acute kidney injury related to compression of the renal arteries due to increased intra-abdominal pressures secondary to ACS.

(Marino, 2014, p. 643).

47 The correct answer is D.

Rationales:

a. Although this is possible, it is unlikely that her symptoms are related to drugs that inhibit dopaminergic transmission (CNS stimulants, for example) or withdrawal from those that facilitate dopaminergic transmission (levodopa, as an example).

b. Systemic inflammatory responses from infection would not likely produce a fever this high, and would not lead to muscle rigidity.

c. Seizures would be unlikely in a patient who has not had a history of epilepsy, and would not likely occur while on propofol (which can be used in status epilepticus). Her muscle rigidity is not likely related to seizure activity, which would be more tonic–clonic in nature.

d. Malignant hyperthermia (MH) can result from the inhalation of halogenated anesthetic gases or succinylcholine administration. It is characterized by fever, muscle rigidity, and myonecrosis leading to rhabdomyolysis from the muscle rigidity. MH is an autosomal dominant disorder.

(Marino, 2014, pp. 764–766).

 Clinical Pearl

Malignant hyperthermia is a medical emergency and requires a team effort. Early recognition and treatment can reduce mortality from over 70% to less than 10%. The treatment for MH is dantrolene sodium, a muscle relaxant that blocks release of calcium from the sarcoplasmic reticulum in the muscles.

48 The correct answer is D.

Rationales:

a. Opiates, opioids, and benzodiazepines can cause hypoventilation.

b. Obesity can cause hypoventilation.

c. Hypophosphatemia can cause hypoventilation.

d. All of these can cause alveolar hypoventilation.

(Marino, 2014, p. 399).

 Clinical Pearl

Hypophosphatemia can be caused by refeeding syndrome and can lead to failure to wean from ventilatory support.

49 The correct answer is A.

Rationales:

a. DKA is characterized by exaggerated diabetic symptomatology, with ketone production and acidosis.

b. Hyperosmolar nonketotic state is characterized by severely elevated serum glucose and hypovolemia. There is little to no production of ketones due to the pancreas' ability to manufacture enough insulin to prevent ketosis.

c. The symptoms are characteristic of diabetes, and specifically DKA.

d. Urinary tract infections in type I diabetics may cause DKA, but this clinical picture is not normal.

(Marino, 2014, p. 610).

50 **The correct answer is C.**

Rationales:

a. Further diuresis with a loop diuretic will increase sodium and chloride losses and further promote alkalosis.

b. Sodium bicarbonate will not fix the issue, and will potentially make the alkalosis worse.

c. Acetazolamide inhibits the reabsorption of bicarbonate, which will increase urinary excretion and resolve the metabolic derangement. The $PaCO_2$ will normalize with treatment.

d. Further diuresis with a loop diuretic will increase sodium and chloride losses and further promote alkalosis.

(Marino, 2014, p. 627).

51 **The correct answer is C.**

Rationales:

a. Given this patient's clinical picture, he should be intubated to secure his airway prior to any travel for imaging.

b. Although neurological consultation is important, this patient's GCS is less than 8 and requires immediate intervention to protect his airway.

c. His GCS is 6. Airway reflexes are typically impaired with GCS scores less than 8, which warrant securing his airway.

d. There is no current indication for surgery or mannitol.

(Marino, 2014, pp. 808–809).

52 **The correct answer is A.**

Rationales:

a. All of these are potential complications of neuromuscular blockade.

b. Use of NMB does not typically cause this constellation of symptoms.

c. Use of NMB does not typically cause this constellation of symptoms, although anxiety can result from too little sedation if the patient becomes aware.

d. Use of NMB does not typically cause this constellation of symptoms, and clonus should not occur with drug-induced paralysis.

(Marino, 2014, pp. 826–827).

> **Clinical Pearl**
>
> When utilizing neuromuscular blockers, patients should always be sedated adequately. Failure to do so can result in long-term psychological damage.

53 **The correct answer is C.**

Rationales:

a. This patient exhibits severe hyperglycemia and is not acidotic. DKA characteristically has glucoses 250–600 mg/dL, acidosis, in the setting of ketonuria.

b. Addison disease does not exhibit these symptoms.

c. Hyperglycemic hyperosmotic nonketotic state is characterized by severe hyperglycemia, serum osmolality greater than 310 mOsm/kg, and profound fluid losses due to osmotic diuresis.

d. Cushing disease does not exhibit these symptoms.

(Papadakis & McPhee, 2018, p. 1258).

> ### Clinical Pearl
>
> HHNK is more common in type II diabetics who make enough insulin to prevent ketosis, whereas DKA occurs in those with very little to no insulin production. HHNK is associated with higher glucoses and more severe hypovolemia, sometimes requiring 6–10 L of volume resuscitation.

d. Central DI is most consistent with this clinical picture in the setting of head trauma. The AGACNP should expect serum hyperosmolality, low urine specific gravity, and possibly hypernatremia from significant losses.

(Papadakis & McPhee, 2018, pp. 901–902).

54 **The correct answer is D.**

Rationales:

a. SIADH will result in reduced urine output and hyponatremia. Although associated occasionally with head trauma, this patient has increased urine output that is inconsistent with SIADH.

b. The timing of the increased urine production is more suspicious for a recent event, as opposed to fluids given 5 days previously. High-volume resuscitation would not be indicated in an isolated head trauma.

c. There is no indication that this patient is hypoalbuminemic. In cases of low albumin levels, patients tend to have third space sequestering and hypervolemic hyponatremia.

55 **The correct answer is C.**

Rationales:

a. Osborne waves appear as global J waves at the QRS-T wave junction, and are not specific to hypothermia (both induced and unintentional environmental).

b. Bradycardia may be observed due to drop in metabolic rate.

c. Vasodilatation is observed during the warming phase, as opposed to the cooling phase when vasoconstriction may be problematic.

d. Hypotension may occur due to cold diuresis and cardiac depression.

(Marino, 2014, pp. 336–339).

References

Bhat, P., et al. (2016). *The Washington manual of medical therapeutics* (35th ed.). Philadelphia, PA: Wolters Kluwer.

Carson, J. L., et al. (2016). Red blood cell transfusion: A clinical practice guideline for AABB. *JAMA, 316*(19), 2025–2035.

Dries, D. J. (2012). *Fundamentals of critical care support* (5th ed., pp. 14–20). Mount Prospect, IL: Society of Critical Care Medicine.

Fish, E., & Talmor, D. (2019). The acute respiratory distress syndrome. In J. M Oropello, S. M. Pastores, V. Kvetan (Eds.), *Critical care*. New York, NY: McGraw-Hill. Retrieved from http://accessmedicine.mhmedical.com.ezproxy2.library.drexel.edu/content.aspx?bookid=1944&sectionid=143516870. Accessed October 16, 2019.

Hsieh, S. (2019). Delirium in the intensive care unit. In J. M Oropello, S. M. Pastores, V. Kvetan (Eds.), *Critical care*. New York, NY: McGraw-Hill. Retrieved from http://accessmedicine.mhmedical.com.ezproxy2.library.drexel.edu/content.aspx?bookid=1944&sectionid=143519348. Accessed October 17, 2019.

Manaker, S. (2019). Use of vasopressors and inotropes. *UpToDate.*

Marino, P. L. (2014). *The ICU book* (4th ed.). Philadelphia, PA: Wolters Kluwer.

Mossop, E., & DiBlasio, F. (2019). Overdose, poisoning, and withdrawal. In J. M Oropello, S. M. Pastores, V. Kvetan (Eds.), *Critical care*. New York, NY: McGraw-Hill. Retrieved from http://accessmedicine.mhmedical.com.ezproxy2.library.drexel.edu/content.aspx?bookid=1944&sectionid=143520164. Accessed October 17, 2019.

Papadakis, M. A., & McPhee, S. J. (2018). *Current medical diagnosis and treatment* (58th ed.). New York, NY: McGraw Hill Publishing.

Rhodes, A., et al. (2017). Surviving sepsis campaign guidelines. *Critical Care Medicine, 45*(3), 486–552.

Tomey, M. I., & Gidwani, U. K. (2019). Acute cardiac ischemia. In J. M Oropello, S. M. Pastores, V. Kvetan (Eds.), *Critical care*. New York, NY: McGraw-Hill. Retrieved from http://accessmedicine.mhmedical.com.ezproxy2.library.drexel.edu/content.aspx?bookid=1944&sectionid=143517163. Accessed October 17, 2019.

CHAPTER 14

Palliative Care and Pain Management

Kristy I. Dawe, MSN, AGACNP-BC, NP-C

Disease Questions

1 Informed consent can be defined as:

a. The health care provider making decisions on the patient's behalf

b. A patient's family making decisions for the patient, even if the patient has capacity and is willing to make his or her own decisions

c. Decision making that involves the patient and fosters a culture of mutual respect between the patient and provider

d. Deferring decision making to insurance companies

2 Which of the following is NOT a key element of informed consent?

a. The patient must have the ability to understand the information being presented to him or her.

b. The patient must exhibit competency.

c. The patient must have the capacity to make a decision.

d. The patient must be able to make the decision voluntarily.

3 A patient admitted to the intensive care unit (ICU) has just received a diagnosis of a terminal illness. While having a goals-of-care discussion with a patient and the patient's family members, the nurse practitioner witnesses the patient's son telling him, "Dad, you need to continue treatment. You can't stop now and leave us. I won't forgive you if you stop treatment." The nurse practitioner has disclosed all relevant information to the patient and family, and it is clear that the patient understands the information and has the capacity to make his own decisions. After further discussion, the patient elects to continue his full code status and to continue aggressive treatment. Which key element of informed consent has been violated in this example?

a. Voluntary choice

b. Ability to understand information

c. Disclosure of information

d. Decision-making capacity

4 Which of the following are elements of decision-making capacity?

a. The ability to communicate a choice

b. The ability to understand relevant information

c. The ability to understand the situation and its consequences

d. All of the above

5 Which one of the following scenarios violates an element of decisional capacity?

a. When explaining a diagnosis and treatment options, the patient easily communicates his or her understanding and decisions regarding his or her care.

b. When the nurse practitioner asks the patient to explain back the information he or she has been given, the patient is unable to fully explain it, mixes up details, and seems generally confused about his or her diagnosis and options.

c. The patient can verbalize the effects of the disease and his or her treatment choices on both self and family.

d. The patient verbalizes his or her decision-making rationale when explaining his or her treatment choices.

6 What is advanced care planning?

a. The process in which patients delineate their health care state, goals, and objectives with the help of trained professionals

b. Decision making performed by the health care team for the patient

c. End-of-life plans discussed and carried out by the patient's family

d. Legal documents that deal with the patient's financial concerns

7 POLST (Physician Orders for Life-Sustaining Treatment) and MOLST (Medical Orders for Life-Sustaining Treatment) are examples of which of the following?

a. Strict orders that must be followed when a patient is admitted to the hospital

b. Orders that are written to keep patients alive as long as possible for their families

c. A guide that helps patients with advanced illness and their families discuss care options in the event of exacerbations and end-of-life scenarios

d. Orders that will always involve comfort care measures

8 A living will can be described as which of the following?

a. A guideline created by the patient for a specific set of medical circumstances. It can list acceptable and unacceptable types of treatment for these medical circumstances.

b. A list of orders to be followed for terminal diagnoses.

c. Guidelines for a patient's family listing the patient's funeral arrangements.

d. Guidelines for a patient's family listing the patient's financial concerns upon his or her death.

9 What is a durable power of attorney for health care?

a. A surrogate named by the patient to make financial decisions for the patient if the patient is incapacitated

b. A surrogate named by the patient to make medical decision for the patient if the patient is incapacitated and unable to make decisions for self

c. A form that allows the hospital or health care provider to make decisions for the patient if the patient is incapacitated

d. A form that allows an attorney to make medical decisions for a patient

10 The nurse practitioner is caring for a patient in the ICU with a terminal diagnosis. He sets ups meetings with the family and whole clinical care team to help present information and clarify the patient's goals of care to help the patient and family make decisions regarding the patient's care. This is an example of:

a. A living will

b. A health care proxy

c. A POLST

d. Shared decision making

11 What is the focus of palliative care?

a. Treatment of symptoms

b. Providing psychological and spiritual support to patients and families

c. Ensuring communication between patients and the health care teams to help align treatment modalities with the patients' goals of care

d. All of the above

12 Analgesics and techniques used to reduce pain work in which of the following ways?

a. Interruption of neural impulses in the spinal cord

b. Inhibiting the production of pain mediators

c. Central nervous system (CNS) alteration of pain perception

d. All of the above

13 Which of the following is NOT a goal of pain control for patients suffering from acute pain?

a. To keep the patient quiet and not complaining

b. To provide optimum patient comfort

c. To help control anxiety and agitation

d. To prevent the development of chronic pain syndromes

14 When prescribing opioid medications to a patient with chronic pain, the nurse practitioner knows which of the following practices is important to help minimize the risk of noncompliance with regulatory agencies?

a. The nurse practitioner knows it is necessary to be aware of national standards for prescribing opioids.

b. The nurse practitioner knows that he/she will need to adequately evaluate patients at regular intervals.

c. The nurse practitioner knows it is NOT necessary to consistently document compliance and pain assessment tools.

d. The nurse practitioner knows it is necessary to engage interventions that have safeguards in place for both the patient and the nurse practitioner when prescribing opioids.

15 Which of the following chart entries is adequate when documenting the prescribing of opioids to a patient with chronic pain?

a. The patient presents for routine follow-up for prescription of chronic oxycodone therapy for chronic neck pain. The patient rates his pain as a "2" on 1–10 scale and describes it as intermittent, sharp, and tingling. The oxycodone keeps the pain at a "2," and he reports it is an "8" without it. He reports no side effects from the oxycodone. He has not seen any other providers for his pain issues, and there have not been other prescriptions filled upon the nurse practitioner's review of the database. His medication list includes oxycodone 10 mg every 12 hours, acetaminophen 650 mg every 6 hours as needed, and lisinopril 10 mg daily for hypertension. Today he will be prescribed oxycodone 10 mg every 12 hours, 60 pills dispensed, no refills. The patient will return in 30 days for a follow-up.

b. The patient presents for routine follow-up for prescription of chronic oxycodone therapy for chronic neck pain. The patient rates his pain as a "2" on 1–10 scale and describes it as intermittent, sharp, and tingling. The oxycodone keeps the pain at a "2," and he reports it is an "8" without it. He reports no side effects from the oxycodone. He has not seen any other providers for his pain issues, and there have not been other prescriptions filled upon the nurse practitioner's review of the database.

c. The patient presents for routine follow-up for prescription of chronic oxycodone therapy for chronic neck pain. He reports no side effects

from the oxycodone. He has not seen any other providers for his pain issues, and there have not been other prescriptions filled upon the nurse practitioner's review of the database. His medication list includes oxycodone 10 mg every 12 hours, acetaminophen 650 mg every 6 hours as needed, and lisinopril 10 mg daily for hypertension. Today he will be prescribed oxycodone 10 mg every 12 hours, 60 pills dispensed, no refills. The patient will return in 30 days for a follow-up.

d. The patient presents for routine follow-up for prescription of chronic oxycodone therapy for chronic neck pain. The patient rates his pain as a "2" on 1–10 scale and describes it as intermittent, sharp, and tingling. The oxycodone keeps the pain at a "2," and he reports it is an "8" without it. He reports no side effects from the oxycodone. His medication list includes oxycodone 10 mg every 12 hours, acetaminophen 650 mg every 6 hours as needed, and lisinopril 10 mg daily for hypertension. Today he will be prescribed oxycodone 10 mg every 12 hours, 60 pills dispensed, no refills. The patient will return in 30 days for a follow-up.

Disease Answers/Rationales

1 **The correct answer is C.**

Rationales:

a. Heteronomy is the term describing a provider using his or her will to make decisions for the patient.

b. A patient's family cannot make decisions on behalf of the patient if the patient has capacity and is willing to make his or her own decisions.

c. The definition of informed consent is decision making that involves the patient and fosters a culture of mutual respect between the patient and provider.

d. Deferring decision making to insurance companies is not informed consent.

(Oropella, Pastores, & Kvetan, 2016, Chapter 81).

2 **The correct answer is B.**

Rationales:

a. Being able to understand the information presented is a key element of informed consent.

b. Competency is the patient's ability to perform the actions that are needed to put a decision he or she made into effect and is not a key element of informed consent.

c. The patient must have the capacity to make a decision as an element of informed consent.

d. The patient must have the ability to make a decision voluntarily, that is, without external forces or coercion.

(Oropella et al., 2016, Chapter 81).

3 **The correct answer is A.**

Rationales:

a. In this instance, the patient's voluntary choice has been violated, as he was not free to make his decision without external influences and coercion from his family.

b. The patient had the ability to understand, so this element was not violated.

c. The nurse practitioner disclosed all relevant information to the patient and family, so this element was not violated.

d. The patient had decision-making capacity.

(Oropella et al., 2016, Chapter 81).

4 **The correct answer is D.**

Rationales:

a. The ability to communicate a choice is an element of capacity.

b. The ability to understand relevant information is an element of capacity.

c. The ability to understand the situation and its consequences is an element of capacity.

d. The fourth element of capacity is the ability to deliberate and make judgments regarding the treatment options being given.

(Oropella et al., 2016, Chapter 81).

Clinical Pearl

Double effect is defined as an intervention that is meant to alleviate suffering but also can harm or hasten the moment of death. The intent of the action defines the ethical construct of the intervention.

5 **The correct answer is B.**

Rationales:

a. The ability to communicate a choice is an element of capacity.

b. The ability to understand relevant information is an element of capacity. In this instance, it does not appear that the patient understands the information the patient has been given.

c. The ability to understand the situation and its consequences is an element of capacity.

d. The fourth element of capacity is the ability to deliberate and make judgments regarding the treatment options being given.

(Oropella et al., 2016, Chapter 81).

6 **The correct answer is A.**

Rationales:

a. Advanced care planning is the process in which patients delineate their health care state, goals, and objectives with the help of trained professionals.

b. Decision making performed by the health care team for the patient is not advanced care planning.

c. End-of-life plans discussed and carried out by the patient's family are not advanced care planning.

d. Legal documents that deal with the patient's financial concerns are not advanced care planning.

(Oropella et al., 2016, Chapter 81).

7 **The correct answer is C.**

Rationales:

a. POLST and MOLST are not strict orders that must be followed when a patient is admitted to the hospital. They are guidelines already set forth by the patient or the patient's proxy.

b. POLST and MOLST are not orders that are written to keep patients alive as long as possible for their families.

c. POLST and MOLST are a guide that helps patients with advanced illness and their families discuss care options in the event of exacerbations and end of life scenarios.

d. POLST and MOLST are not orders that will always involve comfort care measures.

(Oropella et al., 2016, Chapter 81).

8 **The correct answer is A.**

Rationales:

a. A living will is a guideline created by a patient for a specific set of medical circumstances that lists acceptable and unacceptable types of treatments for those medical circumstances.

b. A living will is not a list of orders to be followed for terminal diagnoses.

c. A living will is not a guideline for a patient's family listing the patient's funeral arrangements.

d. A living will is not a guideline for a patient's family listing the patient's financial concerns upon his or her death.

(Oropella et al., 2016, Chapter 81).

9 **The correct answer is B.**

Rationales:

a. A durable power of attorney for health care is not a surrogate named by the patient to make financial decisions for the patient if the patient is incapacitated.

b. A durable power of attorney for health care is a surrogate named by the patient to make medical decision for the patient if the patient is incapacitated and unable to make decisions for self.

c. A durable power of attorney for health care is not a form that allows the hospital or health care provider to make decisions for the patient if the patient is incapacitated.

d. A durable power of attorney for health care is not a form that allows an attorney to make medical decisions for a patient.

(Oropella et al., 2016, Chapter 81).

10 **The correct answer is D.**

Rationales:

a. A living will is a guideline created by a patient for a specific set of medical circumstances that lists acceptable and unacceptable types of treatments for those medical circumstances.

b. A durable power of attorney for health care, or health care proxy, is a surrogate named by the patient to make medical decision for the patient if the patient is incapacitated and unable to make decisions for self.

c. A POLST is a guide that helps patients with advanced illness and their families discuss care options in the event of exacerbations and end-of-life scenarios.

d. Shared decision making is when clinicians engage with the patient, family, and health care team to assist in decision making while keeping the patient's goals and interests in the forefront.

(Oropella et al., 2016, Chapter 81).

11 **The correct answer is D.**

Rationales:

All of the above are included in the focus of palliative care.

(Oropella et al., 2016, Chapter 81).

Clinical Pearl

When communicating end of life discussions, providers should consider asking "what would the patient want us to do for him/her?" as opposed to asking the family what they would want. This alleviates the burden from the family, shifting the decisions to those made by the patient. This changes the dynamic of the family from decision-makers to communicators of the patient's wishes.

12 **The correct answer is D.**

Rationales:

a. Opioid analgesics and acetaminophen are examples of drugs that alter the pain perception in the CNS.

b. Nonsteroidal anti-inflammatory drugs (NSAIDs) are examples of drugs that inhibit the production of pain mediators.

c. Local anesthetic agents used for neuraxial blocks are examples of pain medications that interrupt neural impulses.

d. "All of the above" is the correct answer.

(Pandharipande & McGrane, 2019).

13 **The correct answer is A.**

Rationales:

a. The goal of providing adequate pain relief for patients suffering from acute pain is not to keep them quiet and to stop their complaining.

b. One goal of providing adequate pain relief for patients suffering from acute pain is to provide optimum patient comfort.

c. One goal of providing adequate pain relief for patients suffering from acute pain is to help control anxiety and agitation.

d. One goal of providing adequate pain relief for patients suffering from acute pain is to prevent the development of chronic pain syndromes.

(Pandharipande & McGrane, 2019).

14 **The correct answer is C.**

Rationales:

a. It is necessary for the nurse practitioner to be aware of national standards when prescribing opioids.

b. The nurse practitioner knows that it is necessary to adequately evaluate patients at regular intervals if prescribing them opioid medications.

c. This answer is incorrect because it is necessary to consistently document patient compliance and the use of pain assessment tools if prescribing opioids.

d. It is necessary for the nurse practitioner to engage interventions that have safeguards in place for both the patient and the nurse practitioner when prescribing opioids.

(Hudspeth, 2011).

15 **The correct answer is A.**

Rationales:

a. This charting is complete, as it documents his current medication list, plan for follow-up, a standardized method of evaluation, and review of database.

b. This charting is incomplete as it is missing his current medication list and plan for follow-up.

c. This charting is incomplete because there is no standardized method of evaluation of the pain medication listed.

d. This charting is incomplete because there is no documentation of review of database for other prescriptions or visits to other providers for pain issues.

(Hudspeth, 2011).

References

Hudspeth, R. S. (2011). Avoiding regulatory complaints when treating chronic pain patients with opioids. *Journal of the American Academy of Nurse Practitioners, 23*, 515–520.

Oropella, J. M., Pastores, S. M., & Kvetan, V. (2016). *Critical care.* New York, NY: McGraw Hill Education.

Pandharipande, P., & McGrane, S. (2019). Pain control in the critically ill adult patient. In J. A. Melin (Ed.), *UpToDate.* Retrieved September 3, 2019, from https://www.uptodate.com/contents/pain-control-in-the-critically-ill-adult-patient

CHAPTER 15

Nutrition

Rachel A. Schroy, DNP

Disease Questions

Nutrition Requirements

1 Standard tube feedings are made up of carbohydrates (glucose), lipids, and proteins. Which of the three nutritional fuels provides the highest energy yields?

a. Carbohydrates (glucose)

b. Lipids

c. Proteins

d. All are equal

2 A 28-year-old male is mechanically intubated with septic shock secondary to pneumonia. His current continuous intravenous medications are norepinephrine at 12 µg/min, vasopressin at 0.04 units/min, propofol at 20 µg/kg/min, and fentanyl at 25 µg/hr. Which medication does the adult-gerontology acute care nurse practitioners (AGACNP) have to take into consideration when

determining the amount of nonprotein calories needed for nutritional support in this patient?

a. Norepinephrine

b. Vasopressin

c. Propofol

d. Fentanyl

3 Deficiency in this vitamin can cause the following complications: cardiomyopathy, Wernicke encephalopathy, peripheral neuropathy, and lactic acidosis.

a. Thiamine

b. Vitamin E

c. Vitamin C

d. Niacin

4 For critically ill patients who are not severely malnourished or obese, what is the recommended daily caloric need?

a. 15 kcal/kg/d

b. 10 kcal/kg/d

c. 35 kcal/kg/d

d. 25 kcal/kg/d

5 When determining the daily energy and protein requirements for a patient to initiate enteral tube feeding, at what minimum BMI does the AGACNP need to use ideal body weight instead of actual body weight in the setting of obesity?

a. For body mass index (BMI) >30

b. For BMI > 40

c. For BMI > 50

d. For BMI > 60

6 Due to the hypercatabolic state of critically ill patients, which of the following nutritional requirements increases?

a. Carbohydrates

b. Lipids

c. Protein

d. All of the above

7 What is the recommended time frame after admission to intensive care unit (ICU) that enteral tube feeding should be initiated in patients who have no contraindications and who cannot take an oral diet themselves?

a. Within 5–7 days

b. Within the first 6–12 hours

c. Within the first 24–48 hours

d. Within the first 72 hours

8 Absolute contraindications to enteral tube feeding include all of the following EXCEPT:

a. Low-dose vasopressor requirements

b. High-dose vasopressor requirements

c. Complete bowel obstruction

d. Bowel ischemia

9 A 21-year-old female was admitted less than 24 hours ago presenting with acute hypoxic respiratory failure requiring intubation due to suspected aspiration pneumonia. She is severely malnourished secondary to chronic anorexia nervosa and bulimia. Tube feeds were started on this patient yesterday evening at a rate of 55 mL/hr. This morning's laboratory findings are potassium 2.2 mEq/L, phosphorous 1.7 mg/dL, and magnesium 1.1 mg/dL. The AGACNP is concerned she may be developing which of the following?

a. Hypokalemia

b. Refeeding syndrome

c. Gastroparesis

d. Hypomagnesemia

10 The AGACNP has started tube feeds on a mechanically ventilated patient. All of the following are recommended practices to decrease the risk for ventilator-associated pneumonia (VAP) EXCEPT:

a. Elevating the head of bed to 30°–45°

b. Routine oral care with chlorhexidine

c. Monitoring tube feed residual volumes and holding them for residual volumes of 150+ mL

d. Having a subglottic secretion drainage port on the endotracheal tube

11 When planning to start total parenteral nutrition (TPN) on a patient, where should the tip of the intravenous catheter lie?

a. In the median cubital vein

b. In the superior vena cava

c. Near the axillary vein but distal to the shoulder

d. In the cephalic vein

12 When should parenteral nutrition (PN) start for a critically ill patient who was well nourished prior to admission to ICU but who is not a candidate for enteral nutrition?

a. Within 24–48 hours of admission to ICU

b. Within the first 24 hours of admission to ICU

c. Within the first 72 hours of admission to ICU

d. After the first 7 days of admission to ICU

13 The AGACNP is prescribing TPN for a 50-kg male with a BMI of 30%. Because he is critically ill, the goal daily caloric requirement is 25 kcal/kg/daily and daily protein requirement is 1.5 g/kg/d. Each gram of protein provides 4 kcal. What is his total daily protein caloric need?

a. 1,250 kcal

b. 75 kcal

c. 300 kcal

d. None of the above

14 The AGACNP is prescribing TPN for a 50-kg male with a BMI of 30%. He is critically ill, and the plan is to provide 25 kcal/kg/d. His carbohydrate caloric requirements will be 50% of his total daily caloric requirements. The AGACNP has determined that his daily protein caloric needs are 300 kcal. After his carbohydrate and protein daily caloric needs are determined, the remainder of his total caloric needs is from lipids. Knowing that 1 g of lipid is equal to 10 kcal, how many grams of lipids will he need daily?

a. 32.5 g daily

b. 390 g daily

c. 625 g daily

d. 50 g daily

15 The AGACNP is prescribing TPN for a 50-kg male with a BMI of 30%. He is critically ill, and the plan is to provide 25 kcal/kg/d. The AGACNP has determined that he will need daily 75 g of protein, 169 g of carbohydrates, and 32.5 g of lipids. The AGACNP now wants to determine his daily total volume for the TPN using standard concentrations per liter of fluid: 100 g of protein, 700 g of carbohydrate, and 300 g of lipid. There is also an extra 100 mL of additives. What is the daily total volume of TPN in mL? (Round to the nearest whole number.)

a. 1,000 mL

b. 2,500 mL

c. 1,355 mL

d. 1,199 mL

16 One complication of PN is translocation. What is the pathophysiology of how bacterial translocation occurs when PN is the only form of nutrition?

a. The high dextrose infused concentrations promote intravascular bacterial growth, which then becomes a systemic infection.

b. The lack of nutritional bulk in the gastrointestinal (GI) system causes bowel atrophy and loss of bowel mucosa, which results in increased risk for infections secondary to enteric pathogens.

c. The oxidizable lipids in the PN concentrations may promote systemic inflammation.

d. The lack of lipid stimulation in the small bowel prevents gallbladder contraction resulting in increased bile stasis and sludge accumulation, which can lead to infection.

Disease Answers/Rationales

1 **The correct answer is B.**

Rationales:

a. Glucose provides the lowest energy yield of the three nutritional fuels. It yields 3.7 kcal/g of energy.

b. Lipids provide the highest energy yield of the three nutritional fuels. It yields 9.1 kcal/g of energy.

c. Protein is not the highest energy–yielding nutrient of the three nutritional fuels. It yields 4 kcal/g of energy.

d. All three nutritional fuels provide different amounts of energy as discussed above.

(Marino, 2014, p. 848).

2 **The correct answer is C.**

Rationales:

a. Norepinephrine does not supply nutritional calories.

b. Vasopressin does not supply nutritional calories.

c. Propofol is made with 10% lipid emulsion and supplies 1.1 kcal/mL, which would need to be considered when determining a patient's daily nonprotein caloric needs.

d. Fentanyl does not supply nutritional calories.

(Marino, 2014, p. 850).

3 **The correct answer is A.**

Rationales:

a. Thiamine deficiency can present as wet beriberi (cardiomyopathy and peripheral edema) or dry beriberi (Wernicke encephalopathy, peripheral neuropathy). Thiamine deficiency causes a disruption in normal glucose metabolism that results in lactic acidosis production, so thiamine deficiency is something to consider in patients with unexplained lactic acidosis.

b. Vitamin E deficiency is not associated with the mentioned complications. Vitamin E helps prevent cellular injury from lipid peroxidation.

c. Vitamin C deficiency, also known as scurvy, is not associated with the above-mentioned complications. Scurvy presents with fatigue, signs of bleeding (ecchymoses, petechiae), and inflamed and bleeding gums.

d. Niacin deficiency is not associated with the above-mentioned complications. Niacin deficiency would show symptoms of weakness, anorexia, weight loss, glossitis, and mouth soreness.

(Jameson et al., 2018; Marino, 2014, pp. 851–853; Papadakis, McPhee, & Rabow, 2020; Teagarden, Leland, Rowan, & Lutfi, 2017).

4 **The correct answer is D.**

Rationales:

a. This is not a recommended daily caloric need for any patient population. Even in settings of obesity when hypocaloric nutrition is recommended, this range is too severe.

b. This is not a recommended daily caloric need for any patient population. Even in settings of obesity when hypocaloric nutrition is recommended, this range is too severe.

c. This is not a recommended daily caloric need for any patient population and could lead to overfeeding and complications associated with overfeeding.

d. The standard recommendation to determine a critically ill patient's daily caloric need is 25 kcal/kg/d. The gold standard to assess a patient's daily caloric requirement is to use indirect calorimetry (IC) to determine energy requirements. Unfortunately, IC is not practical due to the expense of the machine, time needed to run the test, and lack of trained personnel.

(Marino, 2014, p. 848; McClave et al., 2016, pp. 159–211; Oropello, Pastores, & Kvetan, 2017).

5 **The correct answer is C.**

Rationales:

a. For BMI of 30–50, it is recommended to use actual body weight with goal daily caloric intake being 11–14 kcal/kg.

b. For BMI of 30–50, it is recommended to use actual body weight with goal daily caloric intake being 11–14 kcal/kg.

c. For BMI > 50, it is recommended to use ideal body weight with goal daily caloric intake being 22–25 kcal/kg.

d. It is recommended to use ideal body weight with goal daily caloric intake being 22–25 kcal/kg when the MBI is >50.

(McClave et al., 2016, pp. 159–211).

6 **The correct answer is C.**

Rationales:

a. Increased daily carbohydrates alone do not help counteract the effects of being in a hypercatabolic state seen in critical ill patients.

b. Increased daily lipids alone do not help counteract the effects of being in a hypercatabolic state seen in critical ill patients.

c. Protein is the most important nutritional fuel to protect against the hypercatabolic effects of a critically ill state and maintain lean muscle. Recommended daily protein requirements for critically ill patients is 1.5 g/kg compared to 0.8 g/kg for healthy individuals.

d. Increased daily nonprotein calories alone are not enough to counteract the effects of the hypercatabolic state of critical illness, which is the common concentration of enteral nutritional formulas. Therefore, protein supplements may need to be added to meet the recommended goal of 1.2 g/kg/daily of protein.

(Marino, 2014, Chapter 48; McClave et al., 2016, pp. 159–211).

Clinical Pearl

Nutritional support to the acutely ill is imperative. Protein–calorie malnutrition is often underdiagnosed, and failure to treat can lead to failure to heal and extended lengths of stay.

7 **The correct answer is C.**

Rationales:

a. Critically ill patients are in a hypercatabolic state, so delaying starting enteral nutrition results in decreased muscle mass for the patient. Also, early enteral nutrition decreases mortality and infectious complications.

b. There is no increased benefit to start enteral nutrition earlier than 24 hours compared to starting a little later.

c. Society of Critical Care Medicine (SCCM) and American Society for Parenteral and Enteral Nutrition (ASPEN) recommend starting enteral nutrition within 24–48 hours after ICU admission to reap the benefits of the protective actions it provides against infection.

d. Critically ill patients are in a hypercatabolic state, so delaying starting enteral nutrition results in decreased muscle mass for the patient. Also, early enteral nutrition decreases mortality and infectious complications.

(Marino, 2014, pp. 859–860; McClave et al., 2016, pp. 159–211).

8 **The correct answer is A.**

Rationales:

a. Low-dose and decreasing vasopressor requirements are not a contraindication for initiating enteral nutrition. Enteral nutrition should be started in this setting with close monitoring for any sign of intolerance, in which case tube feeds should be discontinued.

b. Shock state requiring high-dose vasopressor support is a contraindication for initiating enteral nutrition.

c. Bowel obstruction is a contraindication for initiating enteral nutrition.

d. Bowel ischemia is a contraindication for initiating enteral nutrition.

(Marino, 2014, p. 860; Oropello et al., 2017).

9 **The correct answer is B.**

Rationales:

a. Hypokalemia is present, but there is a bigger issue going on given her multiple electrolyte abnormalities in the setting of being severely malnourished and recently started on enteral nutrition.

b. Refeeding syndrome occurs in about 50% of the severely malnourished patients after nutrition is reintroduced. In severe cases of refeeding syndrome, patients can experience neurological complications and cardiac failure. For patients at risk for developing refeeding syndrome, nutrition should be slowly increased to goal with close monitoring of electrolytes and aggressive electrolyte repletion.

c. The electrolyte abnormalities are not common occurrences in gastroparesis.

d. Hypomagnesemia is present, but there is a bigger issue going on given her multiple electrolyte abnormalities in the setting of being severely malnourished and recently started on enteral nutrition.

(Oropello et al., 2017).

10 **The correct answer is C.**

Rationales:

a. The Centers for Disease Control and Prevention (CDC) recommend elevating the head of the bed to 30°–45° for intubated patients receiving eternal nutrition. This recommendation is based on level III quality of evidence but because it is simple, low risk, and possibly beneficial to the patient, it is a recommended practice.

b. The CDC recommends oral care with chlorhexidine based on grade II quality of evidence.

c. Monitoring residual gastric volumes has no impact on VAP rates or length of time intubated. Monitoring gastric volumes is actually a common cause of inadequate nutrition in the ICU, and it has been found that monitoring patients for vomiting or signs of regurgitation is just as effective.

d. Using endotracheal tubes that have a subglottic secretion drainage port is a practice recommendation for VAP prevention based on level II quality of evidence.

(Klompas et al., 2014, pp. 915–936; Marino, 2014, p. 868).

11 **The correct answer is B.**

Rationales:

a. TPN infusion must occur through a central venous catheter due to the hypertonic formulations. The median cubital vein is a superficial vein.

b. Placement of a catheter tip in or near the superior vena cava is considered a central line and is appropriate to use for TPN infusion.

c. TPN infusion must occur through a central venous catheter due to the hypertonic formulations. Catheter placement with the tip terminating distally from the shoulder is not a central venous catheter.

d. TPN infusion must occur through a central venous catheter due to the hypertonic formulations. A catheter terminating in the cephalic vein is not considered a central venous catheter.

(Oropello et al., 2017).

12 **The correct answer is D.**

Rationales:

a. In well-nourished critically ill patients, PN doesn't provide much benefit over risk in the first week of admission to ICU. One exception would be a patient who is chronically on PN prior to admission to ICU; such patients should continue their regular PN.

b. In well-nourished critically ill patients, PN doesn't provide much benefit over risk in the first week of admission to ICU. Studies have shown increased infection morbidities and increased mortality with the use of early PN compared to delaying PN therapy for the first week.

c. In well-nourished critically ill patients, PN doesn't provide much benefit over risk in the first week of admission to ICU. Studies have shown increased infection morbidities and increased mortality with the use of early PN compared to delaying PN therapy for the first week.

d. As discussed above, early PN offers little benefit compared to risks for well-nourished critically ill patients prior to ICU admission. Delaying the initiation of PN beyond 7 days, though, would put the patient at increased risk for deterioration of nutritional status.

(McClave et al., 2016, pp. 159–211; Oropello et al., 2017).

13 **The correct answer is C.**

Rationales:

a. His total daily protein caloric needs would be determined as $60 \times 1.5 = 75$ g; $75 \times 4 = 300$ kcal.

b. His total daily protein caloric needs would be determined as $60 \times 1.5 = 75$ g; $75 \times 4 = 300$ kcal.

c. This is correct. His total daily protein caloric needs would be determined as $60 \times 1.5 = 75$ g; $75 \times 4 = 300$ kcal.

d. The correct answer is provided, option C.

14 **The correct answer is A.**

Rationales:

a. This answer is correct. To determine his daily lipid requirements: $50 \times 25 = 1,250$ kcal/d; $1,250/2 = 625$ kcal of carbohydrates a day; 625 (the noncarbohydrate half of calories) $- 300 = 325$ kcal/d of lipids; $325/10 = 32.5$ g of lipids/day.

b. To determine his daily lipid requirements: $50 \times 25 = 1,250$ kcal/d; $1,250/2 = 625$ kcal of carbohydrates a day; 625 (the noncarbohydrate half of calories) $- 300 = 325$ kcal/d of lipids; $325/10 = 32.5$ g of lipids/day.

c. To determine his daily lipid requirements: $50 \times 25 = 1,250$ kcal/d; $1,250/2 = 625$ kcal of carbohydrates a day; 625 (the noncarbohydrate half of calories) $- 300 = 325$ kcal/d of lipids; $325/10 = 32.5$ g of lipids/day.

d. To determine his daily lipid requirements: $50 \times 25 = 1,250$ kcal/d; $1,250/2 = 625$ kcal of carbohydrates a day; 625 (the noncarbohydrate half of calories) $- 300 = 325$ kcal/d of lipids; $325/10 = 32.5$ g of lipids/day.

Clinical Pearl

Complications of parenteral nutrition include catheter-related issues as well as metabolic consequences if not managed properly. Potential catheter-related complications include thrombosis and infection. Metabolic consequences may include hyperglycemia, electrolyte derangements secondary to refeeding, transaminitis, trace mineral deficiencies, and acalculous cholecystitis.

15 **The correct answer is D.**

Rationales:

a. Protein: 75 g/$0.1 = 750$ mL; carbohydrate: 169 g/$0.7 = 241$ mL; lipid: 32.5 g/$0.3 = 108$ mL. $750 + 241 + 108 + 100 = 1,199$ mL/daily

b. Protein: 75 g/$0.1 = 750$ mL; carbohydrate: 169 g/$0.7 = 241$ mL; lipid: 32.5 g/$0.3 = 108$ mL. $750 + 241 + 108 + 100 = 1,199$ mL/daily

c. This answer is correct. Protein: 75 g/$0.1 = 750$ mL; carbohydrate: 169 g/$0.7 = 241$ mL; lipid: 32.5 g/$0.3 = 108$ mL. $750 + 241 + 108 + 100 = 1,199$ mL/daily

d. Protein: 75 g/$0.1 = 750$ mL; carbohydrate: 169 g/$0.7 = 241$ mL; lipid: 32.5 g/$0.3 = 108$ mL. $750 + 241 + 108 + 100 = 1,199$ mL/daily

16 **The correct answer is B.**

Rationales:

a. Catheter-related bloodstream infections occur when bacteria are seeded due to poor insertion sterility practices or poor catheter care after insertion. Whence bacteria are seeded, PN's high glucose concentrations can promote bacterial growth.

b. Translocation occurs when there is a lack of nutritional bulk in the bowel leading to changes that cause loss of bowel mucosa. The mucosa of the bowel is a protective barrier which, when healthy, protects against invasive enteric pathogens.

c. The statement in this answer describes how PN can promote inflammation. The type of lipids used in PN may promote more oxidant-induced injury in the settings of severe sepsis.

d. The cholestasis caused by PN-only nutrition can lead to acalculous cholecystitis with the pathophysiology described in answer D. Answer D is not a description of how translocation occurs with PN.

(Marino, 2014, Chapters 48 and 49).

References

Jameson, J. L., Fauci, A. S., Kasper, D. L., Hauser, S. L., Longo, D. L., & Loscalzo, J. (Eds.). (2018). *Harrison's principles of internal medicine* (20th ed.). New York, NY: McGraw-Hill Education.

Klompas, M., Branson, R., Eichenwald, E. C., Greene, L. R., Howell, M. D., Lee, G.,… Berenholtz, S. M. (2014). Strategies to prevent ventilator-associated pneumonia in acute care hospitals: 2014 update. *Infection Control & Hospital Epidemiology, 35*(8), 915–936. doi:10.1017/s0899823x00193894

Marino, P. L. (2014). *Marinos the ICU book* (4th ed.). Philadelphia, PA: Wolters Kluwer Health/Lippincott Williams & Wilkins.

McClave, S. A., Taylor, B. E., Martindale, R. G., Warren, M. M., Johnson, D. R., & Braunschweig, C. (2016). Guidelines for the provision and assessment of nutrition support therapy in the adult critically ill patient. *Journal of Parenteral and Enteral Nutrition, 40*(2), 159–211. doi: 10.1177/0148607115621863

Oropello, J. M., Pastores, S. M., & Kvetan, V. (2017). *Critical care.* New York, NY: McGraw Hill Medical.

Papadakis, M. A., McPhee, S. J., & Rabow, M. W. (Eds.). (2020). *Current medical diagnosis and treatment 2020* (59th ed.). New York, NY: McGraw-Hill Education.

Teagarden, M. A., Leland, D. B., Rowan, C. M., & Lutfi, R. (2017, October 8). Thiamine deficiency leading to refractory lactic acidosis in a pediatric patient. *Case Reports in Critical Care, 2017,* 5121032. https://doi.org/10.1155/2017/5121032

CHAPTER 16

Prevention and Screening

Traci Stahl, MSN, FNP-BC, AGACNP-BC

Disease Questions

1 The adult-gerontology acute care nurse practitioner (AGACNP) is called to discharge a 76-year-old man admitted for acute type I myocardial infarction who underwent cardiac catheterization and placement of stent to the left anterior descending artery (LAD). Primary health prevention measures would include which of the following?

a. Follow up with gastroenterology for colonoscopy.

b. Increase rosuvastatin to 40 mg by mouth daily.

c. Obtain annual influenza vaccination.

d. Attend cardiac rehab for 6 weeks.

2 The leading cause of cancer-related death in women is:

a. Breast cancer

b. Colorectal cancer

c. Lung cancer

d. Melanoma

3 The US Preventative Services Task Force (USPSTF) recommends annual low-dose CT (LDCT) scan for high-risk adults. All of the following patients should receive LDCT scan EXCEPT:

a. A 55-year-old female who currently smokes 2 packs per day (ppd)

b. A 72-year-old male who quit smoking 5 years ago

c. A 50-year-old male with Stage 3 small cell lung cancer (SCLC)

d. A 65-year-old male who quit smoking at age 52

4 A 38-year-old male with history of obesity with body mass index (BMI) 33, 5-pack-year smoker, and hypertension. Discharge instructions should include:

a. Follow-up with primary care physician (PCP) for low-density CT lung

b. Referral to intensive multicomponent behavior intervention

c. Follow-up with cardiology

d. Referral to weight loss surgery

5 Which of the following is a recommended method of annual colorectal screening for a 59-year-old male with no family history of colorectal cancer?

a. Digital rectal examination (DRE)

b. Colonoscopy

c. Cologuard

d. In-office fecal occult blood testing

6 A 38-year-old nonsmoking female is being discharged after an elective vein stripping procedure. Her vital signs at discharge are as follows: temperature 97°F, pulse 84, respiratory rate 20, and BP 130/80. Discharge teaching should include which of the following recommendations?

a. Encourage use of seat belt.

b. Follow up with PCP for annual mammogram testing.

c. Follow up with PCP for pneumonia vaccine.

d. Follow up with PCP for routine blood pressure monitoring.

7 B.D. is a 68-year-old male being discharged to home after an ischemic stroke event. An example of a treatment plan for tertiary intervention is:

a. Clopidogrel 75 mg daily

b. Simvastatin 80 mg daily

c. Repeat CT scan of the brain in 3 months

d. Referral to physical therapy

8 All of the following increase the risk of stroke in postmenopausal women EXCEPT:

a. Hypertension

b. Hypercholesterolemia

c. Diabetes

d. Oral contraceptives

9 A 38-year-old Vietnamese woman reports that her mother died at the age of 43 from liver cancer. The nurse practitioner (NP) knows the patient is at risk for:

a. Hepatitis B

b. Malaria

c. Tularemia

d. Tyrosinemia

10 A 49-year-old African American female is being discharged to home s/p repair of femur fracture after a fall in her home. The NP should advise follow-up with her PCP for which of the following?

a. Pneumonia vaccine

b. Bone mineral density screening

c. Tdap booster

d. Colorectal cancer screening

11 Who is at greatest risk for cervical cancer?

a. A 32-year-old female with diagnosis of human papilloma virus (HPV) at age 25

b. An 18-year-old female with more than three sexual partners

c. A 30-year-old woman with current diagnosis of breast cancer

d. A 40-year-old African American female

12 Which of the following patients should NOT receive the measles/mumps/rubella (MMR) vaccination?

a. A 45-year-old male with AIDS and normal T-cell count

b. A 5-year-old female with mother who is 36 weeks pregnant

c. A 26-year-old female who is at 12 weeks' gestation

d. A 35-year-old female who is currently breast-feeding

13 A 42-year-old male with no past medical history (PMH) presents to the emergency room with the following symptoms: pupillary constriction, weight loss, epistaxis, and confusion. He is most likely showing signs of which type of drug use?

a. Heroin

b. Methamphetamine

c. Anabolic steroid

d. Cocaine

14 The NP is discharging a patient after a left total knee replacement surgery. The patient informs the NP that her son is an intravenous drug abuser and she is "afraid I am going to find him dead in my house one day". The NP will provide the patient with which of the following?

a. Lorazepam 0.5 mg no. 15 by mouth every 8 hours for anxiety

b. Referral to psychiatry

c. Naloxone HCL 0.4 mg/mL injection; dispense 1 syringe

d. Ambien 10 mg no. 15 by mouth as needed for sleep

15 Which of these tests effectively screens for cervical cancer?

a. ECG

b. Blood test

c. Pap test

d. Colposcopy

Disease Answers/Rationales

1 **The correct answer is C.**

Rationales:

a. A is an example of secondary prevention. Secondary prevention measures are those interventions that lead to early diagnosis and thus prompt treatment of disease and illness. Colonoscopy helps with the early detection of colon cancer.

b. B is an example of tertiary prevention. Tertiary prevention measures help to improve quality of life and decrease complications in those people already affected by a disease process. This patient has already been diagnosed with coronary artery disease after cardiac catheterization was conducted and revealed disease of LAD requiring stent procedure.

c. C is correct because primary health prevention measures are measures that prevent the onset of illness before the disease process begins. Vaccinations are included in these measures.

d. D is also a form of tertiary prevention. Cardiac rehab will benefit this patient who is already diagnosed with coronary artery disease.

(Ali & Katz, 2015, pp. S230–S240).

2 **The correct answer is C.**

Rationales:

A total of 45% of all cancer deaths in women is attributed to breast cancer. The most common cancers are lung, breast, and colorectal. The most common cause of cancer-related death in women is lung cancer.

(Smith et al., 2019).

3 **The correct answer is C.**

Rationales:

a. This is incorrect because high-risk patients include current smokers.

b. This is incorrect because discontinuation of screening is recommended once a patient has not smoked for 15 years or longer. This patient has not quit smoking for more than 15 years.

c. This is correct because discontinuation of screening is recommended for individuals with limited life expectancy.

d. This is incorrect because this patient has not quit smoking for more than 15 years.

(Smith et al., 2019).

4 **The correct answer is B.**

Rationales:

a. This is incorrect because LDCT is recommended for current smokers between the ages of 55 and 74. This patient is 38 years of age.

b. This is correct because USPSTF recommends clinicians offer or refer adults with BMI > 30, to intensive multicomponent behavioral interventions. This patient has a BMI of 33.

c. This is incorrect because the PCP can safely manage hypertension. Cardiology is not required.

d. This is incorrect because dietary modifications and pharmacotherapy are first-line treatment.

(Yang & Colditz, 2015, pp. 1412–1413).

5 **The correct answer is B.**

Rationales:

a. This is incorrect because DRE is used to examine the prostate and can be useful in detecting abnormal structure of the prostate prompting further testing for prostate cancer.

b. This is correct because colonoscopy is a visual-based examination that will show the presence of polyps. It also can be done less frequently than other modes of testing.

c. This is incorrect because Cologuard is a stool-based test that is not as effective in catching polyps as a visual-based test.

d. This is incorrect because the fecal occult blood test can be performed in the office and is helpful at detecting SIGNS of colorectal cancer. Actual polyp detection is not possible. This type of testing must also be performed more frequently.

(Kwaan & Jones-Webb, 2018, pp. S95–S100).

6 **The correct answer is A.**

Rationales:

(Based upon the leading causes of death by age group)

a. The leading cause of death for people up to age 39 is motor vehicle accident (MVA).

b. This is incorrect because mammograms are recommended to be started at the age of 40.

c. This is incorrect because the pneumonia vaccination is recommended starting at age 60.

d. This is incorrect because blood pressure is within guidelines.

(National Center for Health Statistics, August 2019).

7 **The correct answer is D.**

Rationales:

a. This is incorrect because administration of antiplatelet agents after an ischemic stroke is an example of secondary intervention as it is used to help prevent another stroke.

b. This is incorrect because the use of statin agents is an example of secondary prevention. It is used to help prevent the occurrence of another stroke.

c. This is incorrect because repeating another CT scan of the brain is not indicated.

d. This is correct because the goal of physical therapy is to help improve quality of life. This is a goal of tertiary prevention measures.

(Ali & Katz, 2015, pp. S230–S240).

8 **The correct answer is D.**

Rationales:

A, B, and C are all risk factors associated with menopause.

D is the correct answer because oral contraception is typically not prescribed in postmenopausal women.

(Lisabeth et al., 2009, pp. 1044–1049).

9 **The correct answer is A.**

Rationales:

a. A is the correct answer because recent community-based screening studies have shown a high prevalence of hepatitis B infection in Asian populations.

b. B is incorrect because children under the age of 5 are the most vulnerable group affected by malaria.

c. C is incorrect because tularemia is caused by bacteria carried by animals. Veterinarians, zookeepers, and park rangers are most at risk.

d. D is incorrect because tyrosinemia is a rare autosomal recessive genetic metabolic disorder that causes liver disease in children.

(Liver cancer risk factors, August 2019).

10 **The correct answer is B.**

Rationales:

a. A is incorrect because the patient is less than 65 years of age and no risk factors are identified.

b. B is the correct answer because bone fracture in a woman less than age 65 years of age is a risk factor for osteoporosis.

c. C is incorrect because although it is important to have the Tdap booster every 10 years, in this question, the focus is directed at the bone fracture in a young woman, which is not typical.

d. D is incorrect because colorectal cancer screening is recommended for African American men and women starting at age 50.

(Weinstein & Ullery, 2000, pp. 547–549).

11 **The correct answer is A.**

Rationales:

a. A is the correct answer because an infection with HPV is a risk factor for cervical cancer.

b. B is incorrect because having more than one sexual partner increases the risk of sexually transmitted diseases (STDs).

c. C is incorrect because breast cancer does not increase the risk of cervical cancer.

d. D is incorrect because African American woman are at higher risk for colorectal cancer.

(Curry et al., 2018, pp. 689–690).

Clinical Pearl

Prevention is always better than cure.

12 **The correct answer is C.**

Rationales:

a. A is incorrect because people with AIDS but who have no sign of immunosuppression are still candidates for the MMR vaccine.

b. B is incorrect because children with other household members of pregnant women should be vaccinated.

c. C is the correct answer because the MMR is a LIVE virus and should not be given to pregnant women.

d. D is incorrect because there is no contraindication for breast-feeding women.

(Centers for Disease Control and Prevention, 2017, pp. 207–227).

13 **The correct answer is A.**

Rationales:

a. A is the correct answer because signs of heroin use include pupillary constriction, weight loss, epistaxis, and scratching.

b. B is incorrect because signs of methamphetamine use include pupillary dilation, hyperactivity, weight loss, and rapid eye movements (REM)

c. C is incorrect because signs of anabolic steroid use include hyperactivity, paranoia, and weight gain.

d. D is incorrect because signs of cocaine use are pupillary dilation, weight loss, and epistaxis.

(U.S. Department of Health and Human Services, 2006).

14 **The correct answer is C.**

Rationales:

a. A is incorrect because the patient is more concerned about the safety of her son.

b. B is incorrect because the patient is not showing physical signs of anxiety nor is she requesting consultation.

c. C is the correct answer because it is permissible to prescribe naloxone to a person who has a family member who is an addict at risk for overdose.

d. D is incorrect because the patient is not reporting sleep difficulty.

(Department of Health, July 2019).

15 **The correct answer is C.**

Rationales:

a. A is incorrect because the ECG is a cardiovascular screening tool.

b. B is incorrect because there is no blood test specific to detect cervical cancer.

c. C is the correct answer as annual Pap is the appropriate screening tool for cervical cancer.

d. D is incorrect because colposcopy is a diagnostic test used for cervical cancer detection. It is NOT a screening test.

(Curry et al., 2018, pp. 689–690).

References

Ali, A., & Katz, D. (2015). Disease prevention and health promotion. *American Journal of Preventive Medicine, 29,* S230–S240.

Centers for Disease Control and Prevention. (2017). *Measles and the Vaccine to Prevent It* (pp. 207–227). Retrieved from www.cdc.org

Curry, S., Alex, K., Owens, D., et al. (2018). Screening for cervical cancer: US Preventative Services Task Force Recommendation Statement. *Obstetrical and Gynecological Survey, 73*(12), 689–690.

Department of Health. (July 2019). Retrieved from https://www.health.pa.gov/topics/disease/Opioids/Pages/Naloxone.aspx

Kwaan, M., & Jones-Webb, R. (2018). Colorectal cancer screening in black men: Recommendations for best practices. *American Journal of Preventive Medicine, 55,* S95–S100.

Lisabeth, L., Beiser, A., et al. (2009). Age at natural menopause and risk of ischemic stroke. *Stroke, 40*(4), 1044–1049.

Liver cancer risk factors. (August 2019). Retrieved from https://www.cancer.org/cancer/liver-cancer/causes-risks-prevention/risk-factors.html

National Center for Health Statistics. (August 2019). Retrieved from https://www.cdc.gov/injury/images/lc-charts/leading_causes_of_death_by_age_group_2017_1100w850h.jpgon

Smith, R., Andrews, K., Brooks, D., et al. (2019). Cancer screening in the Unites States, 2019: A review of current American Cancer Society guidelines and current issues in cancer screening. *CA: A Cancer Journal for Clinicians, 69*(3), 184–210. Retrieved from https://doi.org/10.3322/caac.21557.

U.S. Department of Health and Human Services. (2006). *Detoxification and substance abuse treatment.* Retrieved from https://www.ncbi.nlm.nih.gov/books/NBK64115/pdf/Bookshelf_NBK64115.pdf. (Accessed July 2019)

Weinstein, L., & Ullery, B. (2000). Identification for at-risk patients for osteoporosis screening. *American Journal of Obstetrics and Gynecology, 183*(3), 547–549.

Yang, L., & Colditz, G. (2015). Prevalence of overweight and obesity in the United States: 2007–2012. *JAMA Internal Medicine, 175*(8), 1412–1413.

Index